FOURTH EDITION

Primer
of
Epidemiology

Gary D. Friedman
M.D., S.M. in Hyg., F.A.C.P.

Director
Division of Research
Kaiser Permanente Medical Care Program

Lecturer
Department of Epidemiology and Biostatistics
University of California School of Medicine
San Francisco

Lecturer
Department of Biomedical and Environmental Health Sciences
University of California School of Public Health
Berkeley

McGraw-Hill, Inc.
Health Professions Division

New York St. Louis San Francisco Auckland Bogotá Caracas
Lisbon London Madrid Mexico City Milan Montreal New Delhi
Paris San Juan Singapore Sydney Tokyo Toronto

PRIMER OF EPIDEMIOLOGY

234567890 DOCDOC 987654

ISBN 0-07-022454-4

This book was set in Times Roman
by Huron Valley Graphics.
The editors were J. Dereck Jeffers and Susan Finn;
the production supervisor was Gyl A. Favours;
the cover designer was Nicoletta Barolini.
R.R. Donnelley and Sons was printer and binder.

The book is printed on acid-free paper

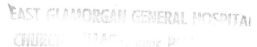

Library of Congress Cataloging-in-Publication Data

Friedman, Gary D.
    Primer of epidemiology / Gary D. Friedman. — 4th ed.
        p. cm.
    Includes bibliographical references and index.
    ISBN 0-07-022454-4 :
    1. Epidemiology. I. Title.
    [DNLM: 1. Epidemiology. WA 105 F911p 1994]
    RA651.F68 1994
    614.4—dc20
    DNLM/DLC
    for Library of Congress   93-47357

Contents

Preface

Epidemiology is not a rapidly changing discipline. However, seven years have passed since the third edition was prepared and my review of that edition revealed a number of subjects that needed to be introduced or elaborated in light of today's epidemiological and medical literature. A brief history of this book will provide some perspective.

The first edition, which appeared in 1974, was written to be a brief, simple, clear introduction to epidemiology for health care professionals. At that time there were few texts available and the discipline was generally poorly understood but becoming increasingly important in our understanding of disease etiology. The second edition, published in 1980, contained an elaboration and updating of some methodological concepts and factual information, but most important, problems to be solved were added to each chapter to enhance the book's educational value. In 1987, the third edition appeared, again with updating of methodology, concepts, vocabulary, and scientific developments. The major addition was a chapter to introduce the reader to multivariate analysis, which had become standard and, to many, incomprehensible fare in the literature.

In addition to the usual updating of studies and references in this fourth edition, some important concepts and methods were introduced for the first time. These included: the proportional mortality rate and its use in occupational studies, the coefficient of variation, the kappa coefficient and intraclass correlation coefficient, open versus closed cohorts, Kaplan-Meier survival analysis, quality-adjusted life years (QALYs), some principles concerning confounding variables, Poisson regression, receiver operating characteristic (ROC) curves, and others. Because of the growing importance and changing view of case-control studies, the chapter concerning them was considerably revised, including the addition of a fairly detailed description of a modern population-based case-control study of cancer, which employed random digit dialing to find controls. Although somewhat counter to my belief in the importance of brevity, I continue to feel that a fairly extensive description of a few illustrative studies helps the reader to better understand epidemiological investigations and what they yield. Most other texts describe their illustrative studies in just a paragraph.

Finally, to enhance the value of the book further, I added a Quick Review chapter that briefly lists the important concepts, principles, and methods in all of the other chapters. This should be helpful to students and others who want a quick "brush-up" or need to refresh their memories for examinations.

I would like to acknowledge again those persons who provided help and advice in preparing all editions after the first. Second edition: Dr. Loring G. Dales and Dr. Robert A. Hiatt, May Kuwatani and Ruth Friedman; Third edition: Professor Nicholas P. Jewell and Professor Byron W. Brown, Bruce Fireman and Ruth Friedman. For assistance with the present edition I would like to thank Dr. Charles P. Quesenberry, Jr., and Ruth Friedman.

Gary D. Friedman

Preface to the First Edition

It has seemed to me that many health-care professionals do not have an adequate understanding or appreciation of what epidemiology is all about or how it relates to their own work. Furthermore, one frequently finds a failure in communication between the clinician and the epidemiologist despite their common concern over human health and disease. I believe it is fair to say that most students of medicine and other health sciences regard epidemiology as a boring and irrelevant subject which they study only because they are required to. Another common view of epidemiology among health-care professionals is that it is highly esoteric or mathematical and too complex for them to understand.

With those problems in mind I have attempted to write a concise textbook for physicians, medical students, and other health-care professionals that would explain epidemiologic concepts clearly and simply. I have also tried to bridge the gap in communication between the clinician and epidemiologist in a variety of ways, such as providing a number of clinical examples throughout the book, explaining to the clinician why the epidemiologic emphasis on the study of groups rather than individuals is necessary, and trying to show the relevance of epidemiology to the major concerns of the clinician such as diagnosis and choice of therapy. Also, I have described several interesting epidemiologic studies to illustrate various methods of investigation. Rather than showing just tables of data to illustrate the results of these studies, I have tried to describe them in sufficient detail so the reader will come away with a real feeling for what it is like to carry out an epidemiologic study. I have attempted, also, to provide some much sought-after practical advice on how to conduct a simple epidemiologic or clinical study and on critical reading of the medical literature. Finally, there is some discussion of epidemiology in relation to the study of problems currently of great social and political importance—the changing health care system and environmental hazards.

Some epidemiologists may be disappointed at the lack of discussion of some of the epidemiologic classics such as Snow's studies of cholera or Goldberger's studies of pellagra. Despite the importance and beauty of these studies, I believe that most students are much more interested in examples that relate to current health and social problems.

Few, if any, of the ideas and concepts in this book are original. I am deeply indebted to those who trained me in epidemiology and related subjects and to the many colleagues and friends with whom I have worked over the past decade for all I have learned from them. A number of the examples, references, and other materials that appear here were suggested to me by colleagues, to whom I am most grateful. It would be impossible for me to name all who, in one way or another, helped me to write this book, but I hope they are aware of my appreciation.

I would like to single out for special thanks Dr. Loring G. Dales, Dr. Mark J. Yanover, and my wife, Ruth, who read the entire manuscript carefully during its preparation and made many valuable suggestions. I am grateful to Mrs. Agnes M. Lewis for carefully typing the manuscript and drawing some of the figures, and to Dr. Morris F. Collen for his advice and encouragement.

Gary D. Friedman

$\underline{\text{P}\text{rimer}}$
$\underline{\text{of}}$
$\text{E}\underline{\text{pidemiology}}$

Chapter 1

Introduction to Epidemiology

EPIDEMIOLOGY: DEFINITION, PURPOSE, AND RELATION TO PATIENT CARE

Epidemiology is the study of disease occurrence in human populations. The primary units of concern are *groups* of persons, not separate individuals. Thinking in epidemiologic terms often seems foreign to clinicians and other health care professionals, who are trained to think of the problems of each particular patient.

Whether one focuses on individuals or groups should depend on what one is trying to accomplish. In caring for a patient, the need to individualize the diagnosis and treatment for that unique person is obvious. However, groups must be studied in order to answer certain important questions. These questions often relate to the etiology and prevention of disease and to the allocation of effort and resources in health care facilities and communities.

Some examples of questions that require the epidemiologic study of human populations are:

When can we expect the next influenza epidemic?
Why are we seeing so much coronary heart disease these days?
How can cancer of the uterine cervix best be prevented?

How often should healthy patients be given medical checkups and what examinations and tests should these checkups include?

Clinical studies of the natural course of disease or the effects of treatments also focus on groups and are often called *clinical epidemiology*. Traditionally, epidemiologists have been concerned with disease patterns in natural populations such as communities or nations. Clinical studies are concerned with groups of patients. The methods of investigation are similar, so that knowledge of epidemiology is useful to the clinical investigator.

In addition to being related to clinical research, epidemiology is intimately involved in clinical practice. Clinicians regularly use epidemiologic knowledge in the diagnosis and treatment of disease. Accordingly, after the elements of epidemiology are presented in subsequent chapters, the relationship of epidemiology to clinical research and to medical care will be described.

How Epidemiology Contributes to Understanding Disease Etiology

Each scientific discipline in medicine is uniquely able to answer certain questions. If our goal is to understand how a particular disease occurs, each discipline can attack the problem at its own level and contribute to our understanding.

It is sometimes implied that the purpose of epidemiology is to provide clues to etiology which can later assist the laboratory scientist in arriving at the real answer. This is a distorted view. There are certain questions that can be answered only outside the laboratory. For example, a new vaccine may be developed and prepared by biologists and biochemists, but only epidemiologists can determine whether the vaccine is successful in preventing disease. Similarly, laboratory scientists can identify carcinogenic compounds in tobacco smoke and can produce lung cancer in experimental animals by forcing them to inhale cigarette smoke. However, the argument that cigarette smoking causes human lung cancer would remain unconvincing if epidemiologists had not also demonstrated that lung cancer occurs more often in cigarette smokers than in nonsmokers.

The routes of transmission—and thus, the potential methods

of prevention—of acquired immune deficiency syndrome (AIDS) were clearly indicated by epidemiologic findings before the AIDS virus was identified (Friedland and Klein, 1987). Careful observations of the history and characteristics of persons with AIDS, compared to what was known or presumed about those not afflicted, showed that transfer of infected blood by transfusion for medical reasons, intravenous drug use, sexual contact, or other means, and intrauterine or other perinatal mother-to-infant routes were the primary ways that the disease was transmitted. Epidemiologic evidence also provided assurance that close nonsexual personal contact and insect bites were not involved in the spread of AIDS.

Causation of Disease   A moment's thought about any disease reveals that more than one factor contributes to its occurrence. For example, tuberculosis is caused not merely by the tubercle bacillus. Not everyone exposed to the tubercle bacillus becomes ill with tuberculosis. Other factors that clearly contribute to the occurrence of this disease—poverty, overcrowding, malnutrition, and alcoholism—have been identified. Amelioration of these other factors can do much to prevent this disease.

Epidemiologists have organized the complex multifactorial process that leads to disease in various ways. One useful way to view the causation of some diseases, particularly certain infectious diseases, is in tripartite terms: the agent, the host, and the environment. For acute rheumatic fever, the agent is the beta-hemolytic streptococcus. However, not all persons infected with this organism develop the disease. Thus, considerations of host susceptibility are important. Constitutional factors appear to play a role not only in whether the disease develops but also in the localization of cardiac damage. Important environmental factors include social conditions such as poverty and crowding as well as nonhuman aspects of the environment such as season, climate, and altitude.

Another epidemiologic view of disease etiology is as a *web of causation*. This concept of disease causation considers all the predisposing factors to a disease and their complex relations with each other and with the disease. One current view of the multiple factors leading to myocardial infarction well illustrates a causal web (Fig. 1-1). (Despite the apparent complexity of this diagram, it is

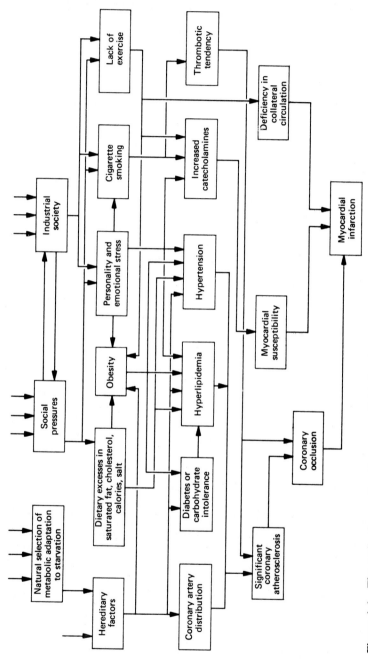

Figure 1-1 The web of causation for myocardial infarction: a current view.

undoubtedly an oversimplification and will certainly be modified by further study.) Note that many interrelated factors ultimately lead to myocardial infarction. Each of the factors mentioned is also influenced by a variety of other factors not shown, leading to as complex a causal web as one chooses to construct. Nevertheless, based on the information presented, it can be seen that a variety of actions could reduce the occurrence of myocardial infarction. These actions include dietary modifications, treatment of hypertension, and changing public attitudes toward smoking and exercise.

It is tempting to search for a primary cause or the most important or direct of the many causal factors. The benefits of this search are perhaps more philosophical or psychological than practical. For disease prevention, it may be most practical to attack a causal web at a spot that seems relatively remote from the disease. To prevent malaria, we do not merely try to destroy the malaria parasite; rather, we drain swamps to control the mosquito population, since this is a practical and effective approach. Similarly, economic development and general improvements in living conditions seem to have done more to reduce mortality from tuberculosis than any chemotherapeutic agent directed specifically at the tubercle bacillus.

Definition and Classification of Diseases

No discussion of disease causation would be complete without some comment about the relatively arbitrary and varying ways in which diseases are defined.

What physicians are faced with are ill persons! However, it has been convenient and valuable to divide ill persons into categories and to give each category a name. We call each category a disease. Ill people do not always fit well into our categories, as any physician who tries to practice medicine using only the textbooks will discover.

We name diseases to reflect something about our perception or understanding of what the disease entails. Some disease names are merely descriptive of some aspect such as appearance (e.g., erythema multiforme) or subjective sensation (e.g., headache). Some names probe a bit deeper but are still descriptive of pathologic anatomy, often defined by gross or microscopic appearance (e.g., fracture of the femur or adenocarcinoma of the colon). On the other hand, the disease name may focus on some real or supposed causative factor; for example, pneumococcal pneumonia implies a pulmonary infection by the pneumococcus.

As knowledge about disease causation increases, descriptive disease names are often changed to terms implying a causal factor. Many ill persons formerly identified by a variety of descriptive terms are thus reclassified under a single causal heading. Similarly, a single descriptive heading may have encompassed a variety of causally defined diseases. One of the former names for tuberculosis was *phthisis,* meaning "wasting away." However, "wasting" dominates the clinical picture in only a portion of tubercular patients, and tuberculosis is only one of the causes of wasting.

Because causal names for diseases immediately imply a means for prevention or therapy, the change of a descriptive name to a causal name can drastically alter the manner in which a particular health problem is handled. Just think, for example, of how the attitudes of society would change if lung cancer, chronic bronchitis, thromboangiitis obliterans, and other predominantly smoking-caused diseases were grouped together and renamed "cigarette disease"? However, causal names can also narrow our view. When the focus on one causal factor such as an infectious agent is reflected in the disease name, we often tend to regard the infectious or other agent as the only cause and often forget that other factors also are operating.

In summary, disease names are important tools for thought and communication. However, they must be viewed in proper perspective. They tend to mask differences among patients, and they have a way of influencing and narrowing our thinking. Disease names may even become "the thing itself," whereas the emphasis should be on the ill person. Furthermore, disease names are transitory. The naming and classifying of ill persons has changed markedly throughout history and will continue to change.

PROBLEMS

1-1 Indicate whether each of the following questions is best answered by:

(A) An epidemiologic study of a population

(B) A clinical study of a group of patients

(C) Some other type of study

a What is the most effective drug for preventing joint deformity in rheumatoid arthritis?

b Which has a stronger affinity for myoglobin: oxygen or carbon monoxide?

c If we establish in our community a program of periodic vaginal examinations with Papanicolaou smears, will we reduce the death rate from cancer of the uterine cervix?

d If dogs are made to exercise regularly, will they have a better chance of surviving an induced myocardial infarction?

e Does a supervised and carefully graded exercise program prevent sudden death in persons recovering from myocardial infarction?

f Does regular exercise during leisure time help prevent myocardial infarction in persons with sedentary occupations?

1-2 Some medical scientists believe that excessive dietary intake of saturated fat and cholesterol is the chief cause of coronary heart disease. Assume for a moment that they are correct and consider dietary fat and cholesterol to be the *agent* in the agent-environment-host approach to disease causation. From the two top rows of the web of causation shown in Fig. 1-1, identify the environmental factors and the host factors. Now note the various elements of the web of causation that would be affected by a program of regular exercise.

1-3 State whether each of the following diseases is named after a cause, a manifestation, or both. Name the cause or give the type of manifestation or both.

a Ingrown toenail

b Pneumonia

c Asthma

d Leptospirosis
e Alcoholic cerebellar degeneration

BIBLIOGRAPHY

Friedland GH, Klein RS: Transmission of the human immunodeficiency virus. *N Engl J Med* **317**:1125–1135 (1987).

MacMahon B, Pugh TF: *Epidemiology: Principles and Methods* (Boston: Little, Brown, 1970), chaps. 1, 2, and 4.

Chapter 2

Basic Measurements in Epidemiology

There is one thing I would be glad to ask you. When a mathematician engaged in investigating physical actions and results has arrived at his conclusions, may they not be expressed in common language as fully, clearly, and definitely as in mathematical formulae? If so, would it not be a great boon to such as I to express them so?
Michael Faraday
Letter to James Clerk Maxwell

Epidemiology is a quantitative science. Its measured quantities and descriptive terms are used to characterize *groups* of persons.

Counts

The simplest and most frequently performed quantitative measurement in epidemiology is a count of the number of persons in the group studied who have a particular disease or a particular characteristic. For example, it may be noted that 10 people in a college dormitory developed infectious hepatitis or that 16 stomach cancer patients were foreign-born.

Proportions and Rates

For a count to be descriptive of a group, it must be seen in proportion to it; that is, it must be divided by the total number in

9

the group. The 10 hepatitis cases would have quite a different significance for the dormitory if the dormitory housed 500 students than if it housed only 20. In the first case the proportion would be 10/500, or 0.02, or 2 percent. (Percentage, or number per 100, is one of the most common ways of expressing proportions. Number per 1000 or per 1 million or per any other convenient base may be used.) In the second case the proportion would be 10/20, or 0.50.

The use of denominators to convert counts into proportions seems almost too simple to mention. However, a proportion is one basic way to describe a group. *One of the central concerns of epidemiology is to find and enumerate appropriate denominators in order to describe and to compare groups in a meaningful and useful way.*

Certain kinds of proportions—*rates*—are used frequently in epidemiology. The various types of rates involve or imply a time relationship. The two most commonly used rates, which every physician should understand and remember, are the prevalence rate and the incidence rate.

Prevalence Rate

$$\text{Prevalence rate} = \frac{\text{number of persons with a disease}}{\text{total number in group}}$$

Prevalence describes a group at a certain point in time. It is like a snapshot of an existing situation. For example, *the prevalence of electrocardiographic abnormalities at our screening examination was 5 percent;* or, *the prevalence of diarrhea in the children's camp on July 13 was 33 percent;* or, *the prevalence of significant hyperbilirubinemia in full-term infants on the third postpartum day is 20 percent.* As can be seen by the above examples, the point in time is not necessarily a true geometric point with no length but a relatively short time, such as a day. Nor does the point have to be in calendar time. It can refer to an event which may happen to different persons at different times, such as an examination, or the third postpartum day.

Incidence Rate

Incidence rate

$$= \frac{\text{number of persons developing a disease}}{\text{total number at risk}} \text{ per unit of time}$$

Incidence describes the rate of development of a disease in a group over a period of time; this time period is included in the denominator. In contrast to prevalence, which is like a snapshot of *all* cases, incidence describes the continuing occurrence of *new* cases of a disease. For example, *the incidence of myocardial infarction is about 1 percent per year in men aged 55 to 59 in our community;* or, *at the height of the epidemic the incidence of chickenpox in first-grade children was 10 percent per day.*

Not everyone in a study population may be at risk for developing a disease. For example, persons suffering from a chronic disease for which there is no cure are usually removed from the denominator population at risk.

It is useful to distinguish between "instantaneous" incidence and cumulative incidence, which can be viewed as the probability of developing a disease over a period of time. The instantaneous rate, also called incidence density or the hazard rate, is based on an idealized view of disease development as a continuous process that can be described as a rate of change at any instant of time (much like the "first derivative" for those readers familiar with differential calculus). Cumulative incidence describes what happens to a specific group that is observed over a long period of time; for example, 15 percent may have developed a particular disease in a 10-year period. Both instantaneous and cumulative incidence rates are versions of the same basic concept: new cases per number at risk per unit of time. However, they differ slightly in that the instantaneous rate of 15 cases per 100 persons at risk per 10 years (or 0.015 per year) applied continuously to 1000 people over a 10-year period would yield somewhat fewer than 150 cases—actually 139. This is because as new cases develop in the group of 1000 real people under observation, the population still at risk becomes steadily smaller.

Another way to express incidence is in terms of new cases per person-time. This is particularly useful when one is studying a group whose members are observed for different lengths of time. *Person-time* is simply the sum of the observation periods at risk for all persons in the group being studied. It is usually expressed as person-years, but other units such as person-days or person-months may be used if more appropriate. Person-time incidence is equivalent to instantaneous incidence. Although hard to visualize, it helps to think of person-time as another way of expressing the fact that incidence rates have both persons at risk and time in the denominator (e.g., new cases per 1000 persons per year). Person-time simply merges the two (new cases per 1000 person-years).

In the medical literature the word *incidence* is often used to describe prevalence or simple proportion. For example, the *incidence of gallstones is 20 percent in middle-aged women;* or, *in our autopsy series the incidence of liver cirrhosis was 12 percent.* This imprecise use of incidence should be avoided, since the specific concept of incidence, defined as a *rate* of development, is a useful one.

Other Rates   Some other rates, often used in epidemiology, are described below.

Period prevalence rate
$$= \frac{\text{number of persons with a disease during a period of time}}{\text{total number in group}}$$

Sometimes one wishes to have a measure of all the disease affecting a group during a period of time, such as the year 1990, rather than at a point in time. The period prevalence of a disease in 1990 is the prevalence at the beginning of 1990 plus the annual incidence during 1990.

Mortality, or death, rate
$$= \frac{\begin{array}{c}\text{number of persons dying}\\ \text{(due to a particular cause or due to all causes)}\end{array}}{\text{total number in group}} \text{ per unit of time}$$

A mortality rate is analogous to an incidence rate but refers to the process of dying rather than the process of becoming ill.

Any rate may refer to a subgroup of a population. An example is the age-specific mortality rate.

Age-specific mortality rate

$$= \frac{\text{number of persons dying in a particular age group}}{\text{total number in the same age group}} \text{ per unit of time}$$

Case fatality rate

$$= \frac{\text{number of persons dying due to a particular disease}}{\text{total number with the disease}}$$

Case fatality rate refers to the proportion of persons with a particular disease who die. The time period is usually not specified but may be, if desired, as with incidence.

Proportional mortality rate

$$= \frac{\text{number of deaths due to a particular cause}}{\text{total number of deaths}}$$

A *proportional mortality rate* is simply the proportion of all deaths that are due to a particular cause. It is used when the living population at risk for the observed deaths cannot readily be enumerated, in the hope that a high proportional mortality rate for a particular condition reflects a high true mortality rate for that condition. While this assumption is often correct, a high proportional mortality can also be caused by a deficiency of deaths from other causes.

A variety of other disease rates have been used (Feldman, 1981). In most rates the numerator must include only persons who are derived from the denominator population. The denominator is considered the total population at risk of being or becoming part of the numerator. Thus, these rates can be viewed as a statement of probability that a condition exists (prevalence) or will develop (incidence) in the population at risk.

Some rates depart somewhat from the ideal of having the

numerator derived from the denominator population at risk. This is done for convenience, because of the ready availability of data that approximate the ideal. Consider the maternal mortality rate.

Maternal mortality rate
$$= \frac{\text{number of deaths from puerperal causes during a year}}{\text{number of live births during the same year}}$$

Actually, the true population of mothers at risk for puerperal death includes those who have had stillbirths as well as those who have had live births. The legally required registration and counting of live births makes the live-birth denominator much more accessible.

Handling Changing Denominators   When a denominator population is growing or shrinking during the period of time for which a rate is to be computed, it is customary to use the population size at the *midpoint* of the time interval as an estimate of the average population at risk. To compute an incidence rate for the year 1988, for example, the denominator would be the population at risk as of July 1, 1988.

Usage of the Word "Rate"   Although terms such as "prevalence rate" and "cumulative incidence rate" are still commonly used, many modern authorities (e.g., Walker, 1991) would restrict the usage of the word "rate" to measures involving instantaneous or person-time changes and omit it from measures that can be viewed as proportions, such as prevalence and cumulative incidence. Do not be surprised, therefore, to find the word "rate" missing from these expressions.

Comparison of Rates Using Differences or Ratios: Attributable Risk and Relative Risk

Differences   It is often desired to compare a rate in one group with that in another. One may simply note both rates and observe that one is larger than the other. By subtracting the smaller from the larger, one may obtain the magnitude of the *rate difference*.

The difference between two incidence rates is sometimes called *attributable risk* if the two groups being compared differ in some other aspect that is believed to play a causal role in the disease. For example, in Hammond's (1966) study of smoking and mortality the lung cancer mortality rate in nonsmokers aged 55 to 69 was 19 per 100,000 persons per year as compared to 188 per 100,000 in cigarette smokers. The difference between the two lung cancer mortality rates was 169 per 100,000 per year. This is the lung cancer risk attributable to smoking *if* smoking is the only important difference between the groups in factors affecting the development of lung cancer. Only the *excess* rate in smokers should be attributed to smoking—not the entire smokers' incidence rate—since some nonsmokers develop lung cancer, too.

When viewed as a proportion of the incidence in a group, the attributable risk is known as the *attributable fraction* or the *etiologic fraction* (*attributable risk percent* if expressed as a percent). The *attributable fraction in the exposed* is simply the difference in rates between the exposed and nonexposed divided by the rate in the exposed. In the example above, the attributable fraction in the exposed would be 169 (difference) divided by 188 (rate in the exposed), which equals 0.9, or 90 percent. In other words, 90 percent of lung cancers that developed in this group of smokers were attributable to smoking. The *attributable fraction in the (entire) population* also can be illustrated by the above example. Suppose, for simplicity, that there were equal numbers of smokers and nonsmokers, 100,000 of each. In one year, 169 of the 188 cases of lung cancer in the smokers were due to smoking and 19 cases in the nonsmokers were not due to smoking. Thus, of all 207 cases, 169, or 82 percent, were attributable to smoking. The attributable fraction in the population may be easily computed by taking the difference between the incidence in the population and the incidence in the unexposed and dividing by the incidence in the population (here, 207/200,000 less 19/100,000 divided by 207/200,000, which again equals 82 percent).

Unfortunately, the attributable fraction is often referred to simply as the attributable risk. It is important to distinguish between a difference between rates and the fraction of the total rate accounted for by that difference. The total rate under consideration may be either the rate in the exposed persons or the rate in the entire group.

Ratios Another way to compare two rates is by determining the ratio of one to the other, that is, dividing one by the other. In the smoking and lung cancer example, the ratio of the rate in smokers to the rate in nonsmokers was 188/19, or 9.9. The smokers had a 9.9 times greater risk of dying from lung cancer than did the nonsmokers. The ratio of two rates is sometimes called the *relative risk,* a general term. More specifically, the ratio of two instantaneous incidence rates is usually called the *rate ratio,* and the ratio of two cumulative incidence rates, the *risk ratio.* Other terms include *morbidity ratio* or, when death rates are compared, *mortality ratio.* The latter two terms are usually used when morbidity and mortality are compared to a standard or benchmark. They are also used in the equivalent ratio comparison of cases observed to cases expected given the standard rates.

When any of these ratios is calculated in a way that takes into account differences between the groups to be compared with respect to age or other characteristics (explained in Chap. 11), it is said to be "standardized"—thus we have the terms *standardized rate ratio,* abbreviated *SRR,* and *standardized morbidity (or mortality) ratio,* abbreviated *SMR.* Whether standardized or not, the ratio of two proportional mortality rates is the *proportional mortality ratio,* or *PMR.*

Ratio Comparisons of Several Groups to a Single Standard
When one wishes to compare several different rates, it is often convenient to determine the ratio of all the different rates to a single standard or reference group. In the study of smoking and lung cancer, smokers were divided according to the number of cigarettes currently smoked per day. Nonsmokers were again used as the standard of comparison, and their mortality rate was arbitrarily designated as 1.0. In comparison, the ratios for male smokers aged 55 to 69 were 3.5 for smokers of 1 to 9 cigarettes per day, 8.8 for smokers of 10 to 19 cigarettes per day, 13.8 for smokers of 20 to 39 cigarettes per day, and 17.5 for smokers of 40 or more cigarettes per day.

Quantitative Attributes

In considering counts, proportions, and rates, we have been dealing with qualitative differences between people—presence or absence of disease or possession of one versus another attribute. Other characteristics of groups that must be considered lie on a quantitative scale. These characteristics include such measures as height, weight, blood pressure, antibody titer, and diameter of tuberculin skin-test reaction. Epidemiology requires appropriate measures so that groups can be described and compared with respect to these quantitative attributes.

In discussing such measures, one must mention some concepts that are usually presented in books or courses on biostatistics or statistics (see Colton, 1974, or Freedman et al., 1978). In this introduction to epidemiology it is not necessary to present statistical aspects in great detail, but certain basic measures do deserve mention. Parenthetically, it might be well to remark that one need not be highly talented in mathematics to understand or carry out epidemiologic studies. While some studies in epidemiology do require sophisticated statistical methods, many problems can be handled well by the simple quantitative measures described here.

Distributions   The most complete summary of a quantitative measurement made on a group of persons is the *distribution*. The distribution reveals how many members, or what proportion, of the group were found to have each value or each small range of values out of all the possible values that the quantitative measure can have. In addition, the counts or proportions (or percentages) may be cumulated by adding each successive amount to all those that preceded it. A distribution of serum uric acid values for 1734 nonsmoking white men aged 40 to 49 is shown in Table 2-1. Note that both numbers and percentages are shown for both the distribution and the cumulative distribution.

A distribution may be displayed graphically as a histogram, in which bars represent the numbers or proportions of subjects in each *class interval*. The uric acid distribution in Table 2-1 is shown in Fig. 2-1 as a histogram. Note that in plotting a histogram the

Table 2-1 Distribution and Cumulative Distribution of Serum Uric Acid Concentrations: Nonsmoking Men, Ages 40–49

Serum uric acid, mg/100 mL	Distribution		Cumulative distribution	
	Number	Percent	Number	Percent
1.0–2.9	10	0.6	10	0.6
3.0–3.9	68	3.9	78	4.5
4.0–4.9	315	18.2	393	22.7
5.0–5.9	565	32.6	958	55.3
6.0–6.9	431	24.8	1389	80.1
7.0–7.9	229	13.2	1618	93.3
8.0–8.9	85	4.9	1703	98.2
9.0–11.9	31	1.8	1734	100.0
Total	1734	100.0		

Mean = 5.93 mg/100 mL

Standard deviation = 1.31 mg/100 mL

Range = 1.32 to 11.12, or 9.8 mg/100 mL

Median = 5.84 mg/100 mL

Interquartile range = 5.07 to 6.79, or 1.72 mg/100 mL

Source: Kaiser-Permanente multiphasic examination data, 1964–1968, tabulated by AB Siegelaub, M.S.

Note: To convert uric acid units from mg/100 mL to μmol/L, multiply values by 59.48.

area of each bar communicates the number or proportion of subjects represented. If all bars represent class intervals of the same width, then the area is proportional to the height. If some bars (class intervals) are wider, as are the extreme right and left bars in Fig. 2-1, their height must be scaled down proportionally.

Another way to display a distribution is by plotting a series of points. Each point shows the midpoint of an interval and the number or proportion of subjects falling into that interval. The points may be connected by straight lines, yielding a polygon, or they may be connected so as to form a smooth curve. The uric acid distribution in Table 2-1 is shown as a curve in Fig. 2-2.

Cumulative distributions are usually shown graphically by curves. Figure 2-3 shows the cumulative distribution curve for the same uric acid data.

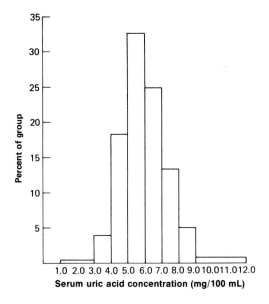

Figure 2-1   Percentage distribution of serum uric acid levels in Table 2-1, displayed as a histogram.

Means   The *mean,* or arithmetic average, is one of the so-called measures of central tendency of the values for the whole group. It is computed by adding all the individual values together and dividing by the number in the group. When one wishes to compare two or more groups, it may be cumbersome to compare their entire distributions. Comparing means is much simpler. In many cases, for comparative purposes, the mean is a reasonably good representation of the group's values, and it can be expressed with just one number.

It should always be remembered though that the mean is only one feature of a distribution and that two differently shaped distributions may have the same mean. It is often important to know more about the distribution than just the mean. In some cases we may be most interested in knowing how many people are at one extreme of the distribution.

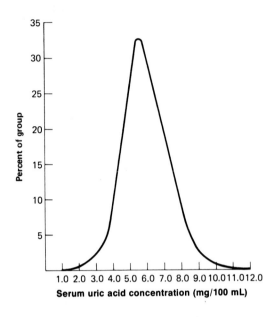

Figure 2-2 Percentage distribution of serum uric acid levels in Table 2-1 displayed as a curve.

Standard Deviations   A good supplement to the mean in describing a group is the *standard deviation,* which is a measure of dispersion or variation. One way to compute it is to (1) square the difference between each value and the mean, (2) add the squared differences, (3) divide that sum by the total number of values minus one, and (4) find the square root of the result of (3). The mean tells where the values for a group are centered. The standard deviation is a summary of how widely dispersed the values are around this center. The standard deviation is also needed in comparing means of different groups to see how likely it is that a difference between two means could have occurred by chance, using statistical significance tests.

Ranges   The *range* of a distribution, the difference between the lowest value and the highest value observed, is, of course, another measure of dispersion. It is often less valuable than the

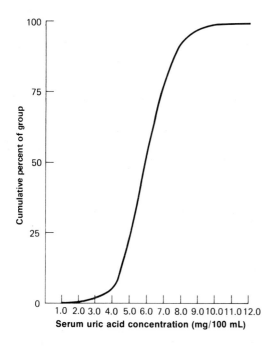

Figure 2-3   Cumulative percentage distribution of serum uric acid levels in Table 2-1, displayed as a curve.

standard deviation, however, since it tells us mainly about only two members of a group and not about how all the others are arranged between them. One extremely high or low value, due to a measurement error, can affect the range greatly.

Quantiles: Values That Divide a Group into Equal Parts
Another way to describe a group on a quantitative scale or to classify each member of a group on such a scale is to divide the group into *quantiles,* or equal subgroups, along the scale. The simplest division is into two parts: the lower half and the upper half. The point on the scale that divides the group in this way is called the *median.* In the uric acid distribution shown in Table 2-1 the median value is 5.84 mg/100 mL. (When the median lies within an interval, e.g., between 5.0 and 6.0, we interpolate to estimate

just where it lies.) One-half of the group has values this high or higher and one-half has values this low or lower. Note that the median value can also be read from the cumulative distribution curve (Fig. 2-3) by observing the uric acid value that corresponds to the 50 percent point on the curve.

Just as one can compare two groups by their means, so one can also compare them by their medians. Although used less often than means, medians have a few virtues that make them appropriate in certain situations. One such situation occurs in a group that has a few members with extreme values. The mean is substantially affected by these extreme values but the median is not. Suppose one wishes to summarize the weights of 22 women attending an obesity clinic. With one exception, the weights are evenly distributed from 180 to 220 lb (that is, 180, 182, 184, etc.). When the exception, a patient who weighs 420 lb, leaves the group, the mean weight of the clinic patients drops by 10 lb but the median drops by only 1 lb. Medians are affected little by extreme values.

Another virtue of the median is its usefulness when some values are missing, but known to be above or below a certain level. Suppose one wishes to compare the age at death of two groups of 50-year-old women exposed to different amounts of ionizing radiation. To use the mean age at death, one must wait until all members of each group die. Conclusions cannot be drawn from the mean age of just some of the deaths, since an early difference between the two groups may be later counterbalanced by a difference in the opposite direction. By the time all the women have died, it is probable that the investigator also will be dead or at least no longer interested in the study. Thus it is important to obtain an earlier answer. The median age at death is one such early measure, since it can be determined as soon as half the women in each group have died.

Groups may be divided into more than two parts. Three equal parts are known as *terciles,* or *tertiles,* four equal parts as *quartiles,* five as *quintiles,* and ten as *deciles.* The finest division commonly used is into 100 parts, or *percentiles.* Percentiles are often useful for ranking individuals in relation to the total group. (Note that the borderlines between any divisions may be read from the cumulative distribution curve.)

Just as groups can be compared with respect to their medians, they can also be compared as to their borderlines between quartiles and so on. Similarly, persons in the upper quartile of a value can be compared with those in each of the other quartiles. Also, one may wish to have a measure of dispersion in a group analogous to the standard deviation. The size of the interval between two percentiles, for example, the 20th and 80th, can be used. One such measure of spread is the *interquartile range,* the interval between the top of the lowest quartile and the bottom of the highest quartile. Note that the interquartile range can easily be read from a cumulative distribution curve as in Fig. 2-3.

Quantiles may prove helpful in determining which of two quantitative variables has a stronger relationship to disease. In a particular population the incidence of coronary heart disease may increase a certain amount with each 20 mmHg increase in systolic blood pressure and a different amount with each 20 mg/100 mL increase in serum cholesterol, but this tells us nothing of the relative importance of the two attributes because the units of measurement for blood pressure and cholesterol are completely different and thus are not at all comparable. A more appropriate contrast would be to note the increase in the incidence of coronary heart disease as one moves up the scale of each measurement by quantile divisions such as deciles or quartiles.

A good example of such a comparison is shown in Fig. 2-4. In the Framingham Heart Study two serum lipid measures, cholesterol and the cholesterol/phospholipid ratio, were compared to determine which was the better predictor of the subsequent development of coronary heart disease. The study population was divided into quartiles of each of the two lipid values. As shown by the morbidity ratios in the figure, the risk of coronary heart disease was clearly related to cholesterol, the incidence being distinctly higher in each successive quartile. In contrast, the increase in risk with each increasing quartile of the cholesterol/phospholipid ratio was slight, showing that the latter measure was clearly an inferior predictor.

This use of quantiles for comparing the strength of relationships must not be done uncritically. The strength can depend greatly on the variability of a measurement in the population

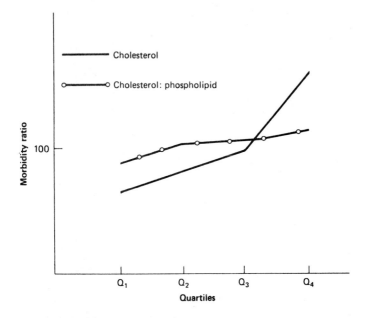

Figure 2-4 Risk of developing coronary heart disease in 10 years in subjects classified into quartiles of cholesterol and cholesterol/ phospholipid ratio. Men, ages 30–59 years at entry. Framingham Heart Study. *(Reproduced in modified form, by permission, from Kannel et al., 1964.)*

studied. If variability is limited (for example, age restricted to one decade rather than ranging throughout adulthood), the strength of a relationship may appear to be weaker than it otherwise would.

Epidemiologic Measurements in Perspective

In summary, epidemiology requires that groups of people be described and compared in a quantitative fashion. However, the particular characteristics of interest may be either qualitative or quantitative in nature.

When qualitative attributes are considered, persons with a particular attribute are counted, and the proportion of the total group studied that they constitute is determined. Since disease is the main concern of epidemiology, proportions of groups with disease or rates of disease are given primary attention. Disease rates are usually considered with respect to time. Disease present at one particular time is measured by a prevalence rate. Disease developing over a period of time is measured by an incidence rate.

Comparing disease rates among different groups is of primary importance. These comparisons are often expressed as differences between rates or as ratios of one rate to another.

Quantitative attributes are also important. It is often necessary to consider the entire distribution of the quantitative measure in a group. However, this distribution may be described in a summary fashion by such measures as the mean and the standard deviation. Breaking the group into equal parts according to ranking on a quantitative scale (quantiles) serves many useful purposes.

Obviously, the measurements described in this chapter do not exhaust the repertory of the epidemiologist. Other measurements have been used, and new ones will be invented for specific purposes. The simple measures described here are established, time-tested, and widely understood.

PROBLEMS

2-1 Suppose that in January 1976, 1000 adult residents of a community accepted an invitation to be examined for hypothyroidism at a local clinic. Eight persons were found to have the disease; it was newly discovered in three, and five were already under treatment. The same group was examined again in January 1978. Six new cases of hypothyroidism were discovered; of these, two had developed symptoms several months before and had been diagnosed and treated by their personal physicians. It was learned that of the eight hypothyroid persons discovered at the 1976 examination, one had discontinued medication and died of myxedema heart disease in 1977.

Otherwise, all persons examined in 1976 came to the second examination.

a   What was the prevalence of hypothyroidism, treated or not, in the examined group in January 1976? In January 1978?

b   What was the annual incidence of hypothyroidism in the group?

c   What was the 2-year-period prevalence of hypothyroidism?

d   What was the case fatality rate of hypothyroidism?

e   Of all cases detected at the two examinations, what proportion was newly discovered?

f   If only 900 of the original 1000 persons were still living in the community and came to the examination in January 1978, would any of your answers to the questions above be changed? If so, how?

2-2   In a certain noisy factory, workers are provided with earplugs and are expected to wear them. An industrial hygienist inspecting the plant found that 100 of the 500 workers in the factory were not wearing their earplugs because they regarded them as uncomfortable and as a nuisance. When all the workers were given a hearing test, it was found that 16 of the earplug wearers and 40 of the nonwearers had developed significant hearing loss. All had had normal hearing at their preemployment examinations 4 years earlier, when the plant opened.

a   What was the risk of hearing loss attributable to not wearing earplugs?

b   What proportion of hearing loss in the nonwearers was attributable to not wearing earplugs?

c   What proportion of the hearing loss in all the workers was attributable to not wearing earplugs?

d   What was the relative risk in nonwearers as compared to wearers?

2-3   The serum uric acid distribution shown in Table 2-1 was derived from nonsmoking men aged 40 to 49. The serum uric acid distribution for the corresponding cigarette smokers is shown in Table 2-2. Calculate the percent distribution and the cumulative distribution in both numbers and percents. Plot

Table 2-2   Distribution of Serum Uric Acid Concentrations: Male Cigarette Smokers, Ages 40 to 49

Serum uric acid, mg/100 mL	Number
1.0–2.9	29
3.0–3.9	214
4.0–4.9	720
5.0–5.9	1107
6.0–6.9	842
7.0–7.9	368
8.0–8.9	133
9.0–11.9	56
Total	3469

the noncumulative distribution as a histogram; plot it in other forms, too, if you wish.

2-4 A hospital contains twelve 20-bed wards. A census reveals the following bed occupancy in the wards.

Ward	No. of patients
1	12
2	15
3	18
4	3
5	6
6	9
7	11
8	16
9	15
10	14
11	14
12	11

What is the mean patient population per ward? The standard deviation? The median? The range? The interquartile range?

BIBLIOGRAPHY

Colton T: *Statistics in Medicine* (Boston: Little, Brown, 1974), chap. 2.

Feldman J: Indices of community health, in D Clark and B MacMahon (eds.), *Preventive and Community Medicine,* 2d ed. (Boston: Little, Brown, 1981), chap. 4.

Freedman D, Pisani R, Purves R: *Statistics* (New York: Norton, 1978).

Hammond EC: Smoking in relation to death rates of one million men and women, in W Haenszel (ed.), *Epidemiological Approaches to the Study of Cancer and Other Chronic Diseases,* National Cancer Institute Monograph 19, U.S. Department of Health, Education, and Welfare, January 1966, pp. 127–204.

Kannel WB, Dawber TR, Friedman GD, Glennon WE, McNamara PM: Risk factors in coronary heart disease: An evaluation of several serum lipids as predictors of coronary heart disease: The Framingham Study. *Ann Intern Med* **61**:888–899 (1964).

Walker AM: *Observation and Inference: An Introduction to the Methods of Epidemiology* (Newton Lower Falls, MA: Epidemiology Resources Inc., 1991), chap. 1.

Chapter 3

Observations Used
in Epidemiology

A wide variety of observations and measurements have been used by epidemiologists in their efforts to *describe* and *explain* the occurrence of disease in human populations. There are so many factors that influence human health and disease that almost any aspect of persons and their environments may be fair game for study. Depending upon what is being explored, epidemiologic studies may require the collaboration of scientists from other medical specialties and a variety of other disciplines. Ophthalmology, psychology, physical anthropology, bacteriology, and meteorology are just a few examples.

While we need not consider all varieties of data that may be used, certain types of observations recur frequently enough to deserve discussion. Health care professionals must have some appreciation of the nature and limitations of these data sources. Not only are they used in scientific study, but they also provide the basis for vital decisions in day-to-day patient care.

Measures of Data Quality: Validity and Reliability

Observations or measurements, whether made by human or machine, involve some degree of error. Errors affect two important aspects of data quality—*validity* and *reliability.*

Validity   Validity, or accuracy, is a measure of how closely the observations correspond to the actual state of affairs. As a clinical illustration, consider a patient with a rapid irregular heartbeat due to atrial fibrillation. Measurement of the patient's heart rate by the radial pulse is considered inaccurate or lacking in validity because some heartbeats produce a pulse too weak to be felt at the wrist. Compared to the true heart rate, the radial pulse rate is *biased* toward lower values, resulting in what is commonly known as a *pulse deficit.*

Reliability   Reliability, or reproducibility, is a measure of how closely a series of observations of exactly the same thing match one another. If the cholesterol concentration of two portions of the same serum specimen is measured in an automated chemical analyzer, ideally the two results should be exactly the same. To the extent that they are not, the analyzer is said to lack reliability.

Effects of Lack of Validity and Reliability

Observations may be highly reliable but invalid. The cholesterol concentration on duplicate specimens may always agree within 5 mg/100 mL. Yet the readings may consistently be about 30 mg/100 mL too high.

This lack of validity does not necessarily rule out the use of the data. In some instances, knowing a person's absolute level of cholesterol may not be as important as knowing how that person ranks in his or her group. If the values for all members of the group are 30 mg/100 mL too high, each person in the group will still be properly ranked in relation to the others. However, if one wishes to compare the mean cholesterol for that entire group with the mean of a group for whom serum cholesterol has been measured accurately, the comparison will be unfair, or biased.

Now consider the effects of unreliability. If a group of observations is unreliable, most of them will also be invalid due to departures from the true values. However, if the unreliability is due to fluctuations that center around the true value, then the average, or mean, of a large series of observations may be quite a valid measure of the true average, or mean. In this case many individuals will be improperly ranked relative to one another if the ranking is based on one measurement for each. However, a comparison of the mean cholesterol of one large group with that of another may be quite fair and unbiased.

Measurement of Reliability

For quantitative variables, especially laboratory measurements, reliability is often measured in terms of the *coefficient of variation*. This is simply the standard deviation of the set of repeated measurements used to estimate reliability divided by their mean, ordinarily expressed as a percentage. Although the standard deviation itself is a measure of variability, it is put into better perspective by relating it to the mean, because the larger the measured values, the more absolute variability is to be expected.

For qualitative variables, a frequently used index of reliability or agreement between observers is known as Cohen's *kappa coefficient* (Cohen, 1960). This measure has the desirable feature of showing how much more agreement there is than would be expected by chance. It can also be used to assess the validity of a measure to be evaluated against a "gold standard" of truth. Consider two physicians performing digital rectal examinations on a group of 50-year-old men to determine whether the prostate gland is enlarged or of normal size. One finds 30 percent of the men to have an enlarged prostate, and the other 40 percent. If two purely random selections of the men were carried out, one identifying 30 percent and the other 40 percent, agreement by chance would be expected in 30 percent × 40 percent, or 12 percent of those selected, plus 70 percent × 60 percent, or 42 percent of those not selected, totaling 54 percent. The interphysician agreement should be compared with 54 percent agreement expected by chance rather than with no agreement at all. Let us say that both physicians agreed in labeling 24 percent of the men as having prostatic enlargement and 52 percent of the men as not having it, totaling 76 percent agreement. Cohen's kappa, which equals 0 when there is no better than chance agreement and 1 when there is perfect agreement but has negative values when there is less than chance agreement, equals

$$\frac{\text{Observed agreement} - \text{chance agreement}}{1 - \text{chance agreement}}$$

In this example we have $(0.76 - 0.54)/(1 - 0.54) = 0.22/0.46 = 0.48$, indicating moderately good agreement. Kappa has been extended to situations where more than one rater is to be compared and where the variable is polychotomous rather than dichotomous (see Fleiss, 1981, for references).

Usual Sources of Variation in Measurements

Not all the fluctuations in measurements or observations are attributable to lack of validity or reliability. The attributes themselves usually vary in a variety of ways.

Consider the distribution of blood pressures found in a community survey in which each subject has two measurements made. The major components of variation in the distribution are as follows:

Differences among subgroups—for example, blacks have higher blood pressures, on the average, than whites; older persons have higher blood pressures than younger ones.

Differences among individuals within a subgroup—for example, among black men aged 50, some individuals have higher blood pressures than others.

Differences within each individual—due to a variety of influences, each individual's blood pressure varies from one moment to the next. Some of these intraindividual differences may follow a regular pattern, for example, diurnal variation.

Measurement errors—even if all blood pressures measured were exactly the same, they would appear to vary because of the failings of the observer, be it human or a mechanical device.

Sampling Variation

Another source of error or variation in data, known as *sampling variation,* is due to chance. It can be overcome by studying groups that are sufficiently large.

When we study the occurrence of a disease in a group of men aged 50 to 59 in a community, we would like to think that our findings are applicable to all men of that age decade in that community. The findings would undoubtedly be true of all 50- to 59-year-old men in the community if we studied all of them, but we usually have to take a sample. If the sample is selected in such a way that all men have an equal chance of being chosen, then we have what is called a *random sample.*

Experience and the laws of probability tell us that the larger the sample that is studied, the more likely are the findings to be representative of the total population. Conversely, the smaller the sample, the more likely we are to be misled. If repeated samples are drawn from a population, the findings in each sample will differ from one another—thus the term *sampling variation.* The larger the sample size, the less the variation and the less chance of error.

This fact may be readily seen in the classic example of a large bag full of an equal mixture of black and white marbles. If an observer tries to determine what proportion of the marbles are white by pulling out only two marbles, there is a 25 percent probability of picking out two white marbles and concluding erroneously that all the marbles are white. If this observer pulls out four marbles instead, the chances of getting all white marbles is much less, only 1 in 16, or about 6 percent. One may apply the laws of probability to compute the likelihood of this false conclusion with any size sample; the result corresponds with our intuitive feeling that the more marbles one looks at, the less the chance of concluding that those in the bag are all white.

Thus, the larger the sample or group studied, the smaller the probability that chance error may occur. Statistical significance tests (such as *t* or chi-square tests and a variety of others described in statistics texts) are used to measure the probability of chance errors, given the size and characteristics of the study population and the question that is being asked. The result of a test of statistical significance is a probability level, or *p* value, as frequently seen in medical journal articles. The expression $p < 0.05$ means that there is less than a 5 percent probability that the observed result could have occurred by chance error.

Another way to measure and describe sampling variation is with *confidence limits,* or *confidence intervals.* Confidence limits, or the confidence interval around a measurement or value (such as a mean or a relative risk), indicate the range of values that probably contains the true value in the underlying population. This will be discussed further in Chap. 11.

Clinical Observations

Clinical observations are the primary basis for decisions as to the presence or absence of a particular disease. The most basic clinical observations constitute the clinical history and physical examination. These are usually obtained by physicians, nurses, and other specially trained physicians' assistants.

The means for obtaining a history and physical examination need not be described here, but some comment about their limitations is in order. Many physicians have had memorable experiences in the unreliability of the medical history interview when they were medical students. Consider this all-too-familiar example. In preparation for rounds with the professor of cardiology the student devotes 10 minutes to careful questioning of the patient concerning nocturnal dyspnea and is convinced that the patient indeed becomes short of breath at night and must sit up in bed in order to breathe more easily. After presenting the history during rounds the next day, the embarrassed student hears the patient tell the professor that he or she has never been short of breath at night.

The physical examination is no more reliable. If the patient is examined by half a dozen physicians, there will often be one or two who will hear (or not hear) a faint diastolic murmur not heard (or heard) by the others. The same degree of disagreement may be expected concerning the palpability of an elusive spleen. Differences in observer skill cannot be denied. Yet the murmur-hearers and spleen-feelers hold the psychological advantage, and objectivity probably suffers as a result.

The measurement of blood pressure with a sphygmomanometer has provided a convenient tool for the study of observer error in clinical medicine. It is a very sobering experience to be among a group viewing a movie prepared by Wilcox (1961) which shows a series of 14 views of a descending column of mercury in a sphygmomanometer accompanied by Korotkov's sounds amplified from a stethoscope. The group is asked to record the systolic and diastolic pressure for each measurement displayed. Even though all observers are seeing the same column of mercury and hearing the same sounds, the differences in the recorded results are striking. The greatest surprise comes when the viewers, learning that some of the early and late scenes are exactly the same, find discrepancies in their own readings for duplicate measurements.

When the results of a series of blood pressure measurements are tabulated, one human source of error that usually comes to light is *digit preference*. Physicians may tend to record values rounded off to a last digit of 5 or 0, or a preference for even over odd numbers becomes apparent (Fig. 3-1). Also noted has been a tendency to slant borderline values downward to avoid making unpleasant diagnoses.

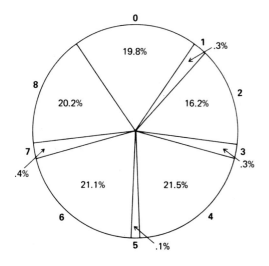

Figure 3-1   Percentage distribution of terminal digits on both systolic and diastolic blood pressure readings by an examining physician in the Los Angeles Heart Study. *(Reproduced, by permission, from Chapman, Clark, and Coulson, 1966.)*

Observations of Medical Specialists

Physicians in certain medical specialties make particular observations that are supposed to provide highly objective evidence as to the presence or absence of disease. Radiologists have the x-ray, cardiologists have the electrocardiogram, and pathologists have their stained microscopic sections. Implicit in giving a pathologist the last word in a clinicopathologic conference is perhaps the feeling that a pathologist's observations, in addition to shedding light on difficult problems, are more reliable and valid than those of a bedside clinician.

A few of these specialists have made important contributions to our knowledge of the extent of observer variation in medicine. They have had the interest and courage to participate in studies to compare observations of the same visual object by different members of the same specialty or to compare duplicate observations by the same individual. The lack of reliability, even in these so-called objective measurements, has been striking (Koran, 1975).

Perhaps the classic series of studies in this area was carried out by Yerushalmy (1969) and his associates in the field of radiology. In one such study 14,541 entering college students received 70-mm chest photofluorograms. Each film was interpreted twice by two physicians and once by six others. Follow-up study of students with films read as "positive" by more than one reader was accomplished by 14- by 17-in chest film interpreted by a group of radiologists. The final interpretation regarding the presence of pulmonary tuberculosis was "roentgenologically positive" for 177 students, "roentgenologically urgent" for 61, and "clinically active" for 13. Each of these students, of course, had initial films that had been read by eight different readers. The percentages of original readings that were falsely read as negative were as follows:

	False Negatives, %
Roentgenologically positive	26.9
Roentgenologically urgent	25.4
Clinically active	25.0

Thus about one-quarter of all these nontrivial cases were missed the first time by competent x-ray readers.

Another series of 1256 14- by 17-in films were interpreted by a group of five competent radiologists and tuberculosis specialists. The number of films read as positive for tuberculosis by each reader was 56, 59, 62, 70, and 109, respectively. The radiologist who identified 109 did not include all those identified by the reader who identified only 56. Similarly, each reader read a different number as being positive when he read the films a second time. In each case some of the films first read as positive were read as negative by the same reader on another occasion.

The presence or absence of significant disease was not the only subject of inter- and intraobserver disagreement. Commonly accepted descriptive terms for pulmonary lesions such as *active, inactive, fibrotic, soft, hard,* and *cavity* showed great differences among readers. After 2 years of work in trying to develop a reliable classification scheme to describe pulmonary lesions, the group of radiologists concluded that they had failed. "It was disappointing to find that many conferences and much practice, together and apart, failed to increase reliability and agreement to a useful degree."

Interpretation of serial radiographs, the basis for many clinical decisions about tuberculosis patients, was also found to be grossly inconsistent. In making a judgment as to whether two x-ray films taken at different times showed progression, regression, or stability of disease, two readers disagreed with each other in about one-third of cases and a single reader disagreed with himself in about one-fifth of cases.

Clinical Diagnoses

Diagnoses are inferences or conclusions based on clinical and laboratory observations. Not only may these observations be incorrect, but the reasoning leading to the conclusions may also be in error. Yet even if the observations are complete and accurate and the reasoning is sound, differently trained physicians use different criteria for making the same diagnosis. Also leading to observer variation is the fact that one physician may have access to more laboratory tests or other specialized data. Furthermore, different terms may be used to refer to the same clinical condition, and a single term (for example, "arteriosclerotic heart disease") may have different meanings to different physicians.

Thus, clinical diagnoses by themselves are indeed undependable indicators of disease for scientific study. Whenever possible, specific criteria should be established for making diagnoses. These criteria should be adhered to carefully and described clearly so that the work may be evaluated or repeated by others.

Medical Chart Review

Both epidemiologic studies and patient care frequently rely upon the review and abstraction of information from medical records. Just as is found for other types of observations, the reading of charts involves substantial amounts of error. Even if the information is relatively complete and the various handwritings are legible, two chart readers will often extract differing information. Usually, however, matters are much worse, with missing information and cryptic or illegible physicians' notes.

Evaluating Quality of Care

Increasing attention is being paid to the quality of care that physicians and other health care professionals provide. Judgments about the quality of physicians' care have traditionally been made by other physicians on the basis of medical chart review. Such judgments, however, may vary considerably from one physician to the next. (See Koran, 1975, for a review of the reliability of these and other clinical observations and judgments.) Furthermore, they often correlate poorly with the outcome of care. There is now a growing preference to evaluate quality of care by focusing on the outcomes achieved rather than by reviewing medical records to see what was, or was not, done.

Disease Reporting

Physicians are legally required to report certain diseases to the local public health authorities at the time of diagnosis. The primary purpose of this is to detect the onset of epidemics of certain serious diseases and to provide information so that appropriate community-wide control measures can be undertaken. In addition to their usefulness in disease control, these data may be used to measure disease incidence in the community.

Despite official requirements, many diseases are underreported. For example, it has been estimated that only about one-fourth of all the reportable cases of sexually transmitted diseases are actually reported, despite the continuing concern in many communities about their high prevalence. Desire to avoid social stigma for patients, the pressures of other work, and laxity are among the reasons that have been given for underreporting.

This problem is not restricted to certain infectious diseases. In the 1950s and 1960s the American Medical Association and the U.S. Food and Drug Administration carried out special programs to encourage physicians to report instances of suspected adverse drug reactions. The purposes of these programs were to obtain some measure of the frequency of occurrence of various drug reactions and to provide a means of receiving early warnings of as-yet-unsuspected side effects of drugs. The response of physicians was quite disappointing. By and large, busy physicians do not wish to take the time to fill out the reporting forms. In a study of various approaches to detecting adverse drug reactions in a hospital, a system that required physicians to fill out a drug reaction card at the time of discharge was judged "completely unsatisfactory," since intensive daily surveillance of just one service yielded 4 times as many reactions as were reported by the cards from the entire hospital (Cluff et al., 1964).

Some legally mandated or other organized recording of specific diseases, such as for cancer registries, does not depend on physicians. Specially trained personnel visit hospitals and other medical facilities to abstract information about patients with these conditions. Case identification, characterization, and follow-up by well-run registries contributes importantly to the epidemiologic study of cancer and other diseases.

Death Certificates and Mortality Statistics

Mortality data for nations, states, and communities, as obtained from death certificates, have played an important role in epidemiologic research for more than a century. Many major problems and inaccuracies are associated with death certificates. (See Feinstein, 1968, for detailed discussion.) Nevertheless, they constitute a widely implemented collection of data about fatal illnesses that can be used to study disease occurrence on a local, national, or international scale.

Death certificate diagnoses are usually clinical diagnoses and are thus subject to all the vagaries described above. In addition, several diseases may have contributed to the patient's death, but under current procedures, only one underlying cause is to be selected. Before 1949 in the United States, coding rules automatically led to the choice of one underlying cause out of several possibilities. For example, if both diabetes mellitus and heart disease were listed on the death certificate, diabetes was coded as the underlying cause even if the doctor felt that heart disease was more to blame. Starting in 1949, the physician was asked to indicate the underlying cause. While this may have been an improvement, it resulted in some sudden changes in apparent mortality rates (e.g., a drop in diabetes mortality, as would be expected); it also forced physicians to oversimplify many complex situations where multiple causes might have been involved. For this reason, many authorities have urged the adoption of a multiple-cause coding system for death certificates. If mortality statistics are to become more meaningful, it would be helpful if physicians were trained in uniform and proper procedures for filling out death certificates.

Other changes in diagnostic classifications as reported in the *International Classification of Diseases,* now in its tenth revision, have lead to abrupt changes in reported mortality rates for the diseases affected. Studies of time trends in disease mortality must take into account these coding changes as well as the technological advances that lead to increased diagnoses of particular conditions and changes in the fashion of allocating deaths to one disease instead of another. Figure 3-2, from a study by Reid and Evans (1970), which shows time trends in mortality rates for nephritis, hypertension, and both combined among men aged 45 to 54 in England and Wales, illustrates several of these factors. The gaps in the curves reflect changes in disease classification. The sharp rise

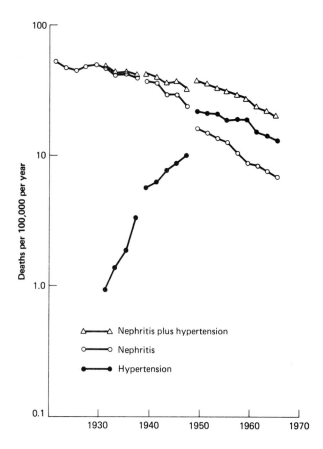

Figure 3-2 Mortality rates from nephritis, hypertension, and both combined, among males aged 45–54 years in England and Wales, from 1931–1966. *(Reproduced, by permission, from Reid and Evans, 1970.)*

in the death rate for hypertension between 1931 and 1950 probably reflects the increased use of the sphygmomanometer and an increased awareness of the importance of hypertension. The reciprocal changes in hypertension and nephritis deaths may represent an increasing tendency to attribute uremia to kidney damage produced by hypertension rather than by inflammation.

Responses to Questionnaires

The clinical history is only one of many kinds of data that may be obtained by questionnaires. Data relating to social status or exposures to environmental hazards can also be obtained in this manner.

It does not seem necessary to belabor the frailties of human observations and their written or oral communications any further, except to encourage again a reasonably skeptical attitude toward the results of questionnaire studies and to show some examples of problems commonly encountered.

Nonresponse   If given a choice, a substantial proportion of individuals will not answer questions. In 1971 a questionnaire was mailed to 8250 Kaiser Foundation Health Plan members who were participating in a study to evaluate periodic checkups involving multiphasic screening. Because of the incomplete response to one mailing, four subsequent mailings were sent out to nonrespondents. The percentage of the total group responding to each mailing is shown in Table 3-1. The final nonresponse rate of 20.4 percent (100 percent minus 79.6 percent) is not at all unusual for a mailed questionnaire.

Nonresponse can also occur under more controlled or supervised conditions. As part of a multiphasic examination at Kaiser-Permanente, patients were given a self-administered series of ques-

Table 3-1   Response to Five Mailings of a Questionnaire by 8250 Kaiser Health Plan Members*

Mailing	Percentage of total study group responding
First	43.4
Second	15.4
Third	8.6
Fourth	7.0
Fifth	5.2
Total	79.6

*Data tabulated by Barbara A. Campbell, M.A.

tions about their smoking habits. The answers to the questions about smoking were used to classify examinees in a study of the characteristics of smokers and nonsmokers (Friedman et al., 1972). In doing so, it was found that about 12.7 percent of 111,024 persons did not answer at least one of the crucial questions about present or past smoking habits.

Nonresponse would not constitute a serious problem if it merely reduced the number of subjects available for study; however, it may also lead to a biased study sample if the respondents and nonrespondents differ with respect to health or some other characteristic being studied. Unfortunately, this is frequently the case.

Inconsistent or Otherwise Unusable Responses   It is surprising how often persons will answer both "yes" and "no" to the same questionnaire item or provide otherwise inconsistent responses. In the study of smoking just referred to, 2.3 percent of subjects did not indicate that they smoked cigarettes but then gave a positive response to some duration of smoking or quantity of cigarettes smoked. Because of this and other serious inconsistencies, plus the omissions described above, 16.5 percent, or about one-sixth, of the total subjects had to be excluded.

Overreporting of Disease Symptoms   Patients who either deny or exaggerate disease symptoms are well known to physicians. In a study of the reliability of a self-administered questionnaire (Collen et al., 1969) it was found that, on the average, one-fifth of persons who answered "yes" to a symptom question the first time denied the symptom when the questionnaire was administered again at the same examination. Physicians who perform follow-up examinations after patients have answered a symptom questionnaire often find that positive responses to questions about serious symptoms either cannot be substantiated or appear nonsignificant upon careful history taking. As an example of the likely overreporting of symptoms on a self-administered questionnaire, 15.9 percent of 1950 young women aged 15 to 19, taking Kaiser-Permanente multiphasic examinations, answered "yes" to the following question, describing symptoms almost pathognomonic of angina pectoris: "In the past year have you had repeated pain (or pressure or tight feeling) in your chest when you walked fast or uphill and that left after a few minutes rest?"

Presenting Oneself in a Favorable Light   The universal trait of wanting to present oneself in a favorable light can introduce considerable bias into epidemiologic studies. Persons tend to deny sexually transmitted disease and drug abuse and to underestimate their alcohol consumption.

Household Surveys

Information about medical conditions and other pertinent social and personal characteristics is frequently obtained by household interview survey. Assessments of health and social problems by survey may be the basis of determining priorities for community or national policy. Thus, the limitations of this study method should be well understood.

Problems associated with survey data and the techniques of obtaining representative samples of individuals for questioning have been a major concern of social scientists. In the health field, the *National Health Survey* (NHS) has been authorized by the United States Congress to carry out surveys by the household interview method since 1957. In the course of this work, NHS scientists have carried out important methodologic studies to determine the accuracy of interview-acquired information.

In one such study (Madow, 1967), the chronic conditions reported by patients were compared to the chronic conditions recorded by physicians in their medical records during a 1-year period. Overall, 45.3 percent, or almost half, of the chronic conditions recorded by the physicians were not reported by the patients despite the fact that patients were given a fairly comprehensive checklist of conditions to jog their memories.

Thus, interview data about illness are apt to be incomplete. As might be expected, conditions for which the patient made more frequent doctor visits were more apt to be reported, as were those for which a doctor was seen more recently. Furthermore, conditions were more likely to be reported in an interview if they affected the person's way of life by causing, for example, pain, worry, or limitations in work, diet, or beverage consumption.

Laboratory Data

Mechanical, electrical, and chemical measurements are also subject to error. Well-run clinical laboratories maintain continuing quality control programs to monitor the validity and reliability of their measurements. When significant errors occur, monitoring permits institution of prompt corrective action.

Yet, even with the most careful quality control, significant errors occur, due to both known and unknown factors. Many of these factors cannot be controlled within the laboratory. For example, exposure of a blood specimen to light can cause a breakdown of bilirubin and significantly lower the serum bilirubin concentration before the specimen reaches the laboratory. Similarly, ingestion of a variety of drugs can affect the measurement of important blood constituents. A well-known example is the effect of iodide-containing drugs on the protein-bound iodine test of thyroid function.

STUDYING RELATIONSHIPS IN IMPERFECT DATA: THE VALUE OF INVESTIGATING LARGE GROUPS

This section is, to the author, one of the most important in this book. It will attempt to bridge a serious gap in understanding and communication between the scientifically minded clinician and the epidemiologist.

As will be developed more fully in the next chapter, one of the primary concerns of the epidemiologist, like that of other scientists, is the study of *relationships*. The epidemiologist focuses on relationships between diseases and other human or environmental attributes by studying population groups.

The clinician, on the other hand, focuses on the individual patient and strives to obtain complete and accurate information in order to provide the best possible diagnosis and treatment. Based on an appropriate concern for the patient's welfare, he or she can tolerate few avoidable errors in this information. Accustomed to high standards in the pursuit of information and the expenditure, if necessary, of many hundreds of dollars per patient in laboratory tests and specialized diagnostic procedures, the clinician becomes intolerant of the use of relatively low-quality data such as questionnaires or death certificates in epidemiologic studies.

A case in point is the difficulty in convincing some neurologists of the validity of epidemiologic studies of stroke that do not include an evaluation of all study subjects by a neurologist. Neurologists spend years learning the subtleties of the neurologic examination and the fine points of differentiating strokes from a variety of other neurologic conditions (many of which are quite rare). To many physicians with such a background it is inconceivable that one would undertake a scientific study of stroke based, say, on identification of cases simply by asking, "Have you ever had a stroke?"

Yet in a study of a large population, the human and financial resources to provide a neurologist's examination for all subjects are not available now, nor will they be in the foreseeable future. So let us compromise and have any ill persons in whom the attending physician suspects a stroke evaluated by a neurologist. This approach is more workable and can be employed in special intensive population studies such as the Framingham Study (described in Chap. 8). Yet even there, practical difficulties arise: a person who has a stroke that is rapidly fatal or that occurs out of town will probably not be seen by a neurologist.

Epidemiologists are not in favor of bad data. We want the best we can get. But experience has shown that important relationships can be discerned, even in data of relatively poor quality, because studying large groups provides power to overcome error. With some validity to the data and large enough numbers of study subjects to minimize sampling error, one may still derive valuable information from poor-quality data.

Consider the following numerical example. Suppose that we want to determine whether stroke is related to hypertension and we can only use a questionnaire that asks "Have you ever had a stroke?" and "Have you ever had high blood pressure?" The questionnaire is administered to 10,000 persons aged 65 to 74. Let us postulate that the true state of affairs for this population happens to be that 200 persons have had a stroke and 2000 have had high blood pressure. Of the stroke cases, 150 had high blood pressure. The "true" population breakdown is shown in Table 3-2.

A slight digression here may be of value to the reader who is unfamiliar with the presentation of data in a *two-by-two,* or *four-fold,* table, frequently used in epidemiology and exemplified by Table 3-2. These tables show the relationship of one "yes or no," or dichotomous, variable to another. The presence or absence of one disease or characteristic is indicated at the left and the presence or absence of the other is shown at the top.

Table 3-2 shows how the population is divided into the four possible subgroups according to each of the two characteristics. The number 150 in the upper left corner indicates that there are 150 persons with a history of both stroke and hypertension. The number 1850, to the right of the 150, represents 1850 persons with a history of hypertension but no history of stroke. The sum of 150 and 1850, or 2000, is shown at the far upper right and represents all persons with a history of hypertension. The 8000 persons without a history of hypertension are shown in the second row. Of the 8000, the 50 on the left have a history of stroke. The 7950 next to them do not have a history of stroke. The total of 50 plus 7950, or 8000, is shown to the right. Totals of the columns are shown below and represent the 200 persons

Table 3-2   "True" Breakdown of a Population of 10,000 Persons, Ages 65 to 74, According to the Presence or Absence of a History of Hypertension and a History of Stroke
(Fictitious Data)

| | | Stroke history (true) | | |
		Present	Absent	Total
Hypertension history (true)	**Present**	150	1,850	**2,000**
	Absent	50	7,950	**8,000**
	Total	**200**	**9,800**	**10,000**

with a history of stroke and the 9800 without. The grand total of the population, or 10,000, is shown at the lower right-hand corner.

Returning now to the argument at hand, the prevalence of a history of stroke in those with a history of high blood pressure is 150/2000, or 7.5 percent. The prevalence of a stroke history in those without a hypertension history is 50/8000, or 0.625 percent. Thus, if one could only know the true situation, one would find that hypertensives were 12 times (7.5/0.625) more likely to have a history of stroke than were nonhypertensives.

Now let us estimate that our questionnaire elicits positive responses to the stroke question from only 160, or four-fifths, of the stroke cases and, in addition, that 196, or 2 percent, of the 9800 nonstroke cases answered "yes" to the stroke question by mistake. Let us also assume that only one-half of hypertensives were aware of, and reported, their elevated blood pressure and that 5 percent of nonhypertensives erroneously reported that they were hypertensive.

As a result of these errors, some of the persons from each "true" category will be moved to each of the four "reported" categories. For example, consider the 150 persons with "true" strokes and "true" hypertension. Only half report their hypertension. Of the 75 reporting either hypertension or nonhypertension, one-fifth do not report their stroke. So the 150 "true" stroke cases with hypertension will be distributed into the four "reported" categories as shown in Table 3-3.

Table 3-3   Parceling Out the 150 Persons with a "True" History of Both Stroke and Hypertension into Four Categories According to What They Will Report on the Questionnaire
(Fictitious Data)

		Stroke history (reported)	
		Present	**Absent**
Hypertension history (reported)	**Present**	60	15
	Absent	60	15

One may go through this exercise with each of the other three "true" categories and divide each into the four "reported" categories. If one then adds up all the persons in each of the "reported" categories, the (rounded) result is as shown in Table 3-4.

Now the observed prevalence of a history of stroke in prior hypertensives is 88/1400, or 6.3 percent. This is about twice the 3.1 percent prevalence (268/8600) in prior normotensives. *Despite the poor quality of the data, the relationship between hypertension and stroke, while not as strong as in reality, may still be perceived.* Thus, the study of relationships in groups of people can, to some degree, overcome certain kinds of error.

This is not an argument for using poor data when better are obtainable. One must always be aware of the limitations of the data used and how inaccuracies and biases may affect one's findings. In the example it was assumed that the failure to report hypertension was equally true of persons with and without stroke. If stroke affected memory so as to further diminish the reporting of hypertension in the stroke case group, then the study might have missed the stroke-hypertension relationship completely or might even have led to the opposite conclusion. Thus, data can be, and often are, so bad as to be unrevealing or even misleading, despite large numbers.

The example given illustrates a frequent characteristic of epidemiologic studies. When relationships are observed in data with an appreciable number of misclassified subjects (for example, persons

Table 3-4   Findings in the Total Population Based upon What They Report on the Questionnaire
(Fictitious Data)

		Stroke history (reported)		
		Present	**Absent**	**Total**
Hypertension history (reported)	**Present**	88	1,312	**1,400**
	Absent	268	8,332	**8,600**
	Total	**356**	**9,644**	**10,000**

with a disease classified as nondiseased), the results are usually conservative. That is, the relation in real life is greater than that which is revealed by the data. This is always true when the misclassification is *nondifferential,* which means that when two characteristics are studied in relation to each other, misclassification in one does not vary according to the other. In this example we observed that the nondifferential misclassification of patients regarding their blood pressure or stroke status reduced an actual twelvefold increase of stroke in hypertensives to an observed twofold increase. If, however, there are severe misclassification problems affecting over half the subjects or *differential* misclassification affecting one subgroup of subjects much more than another (for example, persons with stroke much more than persons without), then the resulting data can exaggerate, or reverse, as well as understate a relationship, and the findings may be totally misleading (see Fleiss, 1981; Rothman, 1986).

Unless such gross distortions are present, the study of large groups allows one to detect important relationships, using poor data that are intolerable in conscientious patient care. This, then, is the explanation to the clinician of the seeming tolerance of epidemiology for inadequate data.

PROBLEMS

3-1   Two automated blood cell counters are tested twice using a prepared suspension of leukocytes containing 8000 cells per cubic millimeter. The cell counts by device A are 8400 per cubic millimeter the first time and 8350 per cubic millimeter the second. Device B's counts are 8200 and 7850.

  a   Which device gives leukocyte counts with greater validity?

  b   Which device gives leukocyte counts with greater reliability?

  Which device would you use for:

  c   Evaluating the effectiveness of treatment for a particular patient's infection by monitoring the trend in the patient's daily leukocyte count?

  d   Screening a group of workers exposed to a bone marrow–depressing chemical to detect those with leukocyte counts less than 4000 per cubic millimeter for further clinical evaluation?

e Determining the mean leukocyte count in a study group consisting of 100 sets of identical twins?

f Determining which twin in each set has the higher leukocyte count?

3-2 In the cardiology department of a medical school, students are tested twice by having them listen to heart sound recordings of the same 20 patients presented in different order 1 week apart. Ten of the patients have diastolic murmurs and the other ten have systolic murmurs. To facilitate the grading process, 100 students are judged by how closely their decisions about the timing of the murmurs approach the true 50-50 split between systolic and diastolic. Only three students report equal division into systolic and diastolic murmurs at both sessions. Do you agree that these three students show excellent validity and reliability in their assessment of the timing of murmurs? Explain your answer.

3-3 In an article about a new analgesic drug, the authors report that the drug relieves pain better than does a placebo and that "the difference is statistically significant ($p<0.01$)." What does $p<0.01$ mean?

3-4 In a study of precursors of stroke carried out by Friedman et al. (1968), elderly patients with and without stroke were compared with respect to the frequency of previous cardiovascular conditions. Medical charts in a large clinic were reviewed by two abstractors. The presence of physicians' diagnoses such as angina pectoris and congestive heart failure (before any stroke had occurred) were noted and recorded on special forms for later tabulation and analysis. What major sources of error could this procedure have introduced into the study? Try to think of at least three or four.

3-5 At the present time, would the underlying cause of death be recorded accurately on a larger proportion of death certificates of 45-year-olds or of 75-year-olds? Explain your answer.

3-6 In an epidemiologic study of about 84,000 persons (Klatsky et al., 1977), alcohol consumption was assessed by questionnaire. Compared with nondrinkers and persons consuming two or fewer drinks per day, those drinking three or more drinks per day had higher blood pressures, on the average, and a greater prevalence of clinically significant hypertension.

   a What bias would you expect in the measurement of alcohol consumption by questionnaire?

   b A critic of the study suggested that this bias would invalidate the finding that consumption of three or more drinks per day was associated with higher blood pressure. Do you agree? State the reason for your answer.

3-7 A psychologist has developed a test for school children that is supposed to identify who will commit violent crimes during adolescence and young adulthood. In one school 10 percent of the 200 children tested show a positive result, indicating criminal potential. Half of these children do indeed go on to commit violent crimes, whereas only 5 percent of those who test negative do so. Calculate Cohen's kappa to measure how well the test result agrees with the outcome.

BIBLIOGRAPHY

Chapman JM, Clark VA, Coulson AH: Problems of measurement in blood pressure surveys: Inter-observer differences in blood pressure determinations. *Am J Epidemiol* **84**:483–494 (1966).

Cluff LE, Thornton GF, Seidl LG: Studies on the epidemiology of adverse drug reactions: I. Methods of surveillance. *J Am Med Assoc* **188**: 976–983 (1964).

Cohen J. A coefficient of agreement for nominal scales. *Educ Psychol Meas* **20**:37–46 (1960).

Collen MF, Cutler JL, Siegelaub AB, Cella RL: Reliability of a self-administered questionnaire. *Arch Intern Med* **123**:664–681 (1969).

Feinstein AR: Clinical epidemiology: II. The identification rates of disease. *Ann Intern Med* **69**:1037–1061 (1968).

Fleiss JL: *Statistical Methods for Rates and Proportions, 2d ed.* (New York: Wiley, 1981).

Friedman GD, Loveland DB, Ehrlich SP, Jr: Relationship of stroke to other cardiovascular disease. *Circulation* **38**:533–541 (1968).

Friedman GD, Seltzer CC, Siegelaub AB, Feldman R, Collen MF: Smoking among white, black and yellow men and women: Kaiser-Permanente multiphasic health examination data, 1964–1968. *Am J Epidemiol* **96**:23–35 (1972).

Klatsky AL, Friedman GD, Siegelaub AB, Gérard MJ: Alcohol consumption and blood pressure: Kaiser-Permanente multiphasic health examination data. *N Engl J Med* **296**:1194–1200 (1977).

Koran LM: The reliability of clinical methods, data and judgments. *N Engl J Med* **293**:642–646, 695–701 (1975).

Madow WG: *Interview Data on Chronic Conditions Compared with Information Derived from Medical Records*. National Center for Health Statistics Report, ser. 2, no. 23, U.S. Department of Health, Education, and Welfare (1967).

Reid DD, Evans JG: New drugs and changing mortality from noninfectious disease in England and Wales. *Br Med Bull* **26**:191–196 (1970).

Rothman KJ: *Modern Epidemiology* (Boston: Little, Brown, 1986).

Wilcox J: Observer factors in the measurement of blood pressure. *Nurs Res* **10**:4–20 (1961).

Yerushalmy J: The statistical assessment of the variability in observer perception and description of roentgenographic pulmonary shadows. *Radiol Clin North Am* **7**:381–392 (1969).

Chapter 4

Basic Methods of Study

In the two preceding chapters the reader has been introduced to the data employed in epidemiology and the basic measurements that are used to describe groups of persons. It is now appropriate to consider the major types of epidemiologic investigation. Each type of study uses these tools in a particular way and has a unique logical framework. In addition, each type of study is especially appropriate for the unique circumstances surrounding any particular investigation—the aims of the investigation, the populations available for study, and the human and financial resources that can be brought to bear on the problem.

Relationships

Much of the effort of medical scientists in understanding the etiology of disease and in developing appropriate therapies involves a study of the relationship of one type of event or characteristic or *variable* to another. Consider the following questions as examples:

Does exposure to cold, wet weather predispose to the common cold?

What is the influence of the serum potassium concentration on the contractility of the heart?

Is obesity related to the occurrence of gallstones?

What is the effect of vitamin C deprivation on wound healing?

Which part of the hemoglobin molecule carries the oxygen?

Does BCG vaccination provide protection against pulmonary tuberculosis?

In Table 4-1 these questions are listed together with the relationship that should be studied to help answer each. In a two-variable relationship one is usually considered the *independent* variable which affects the other, or *dependent,* variable.

The relationships that are studied need not be only between one variable and a second. Often, the investigator must be concerned with the interrelationships of three or more variables. For example, to better understand the relationship of potassium to the force of cardiac contraction, calcium concentration must also be taken into account. Whether or not obesity is related to gallstone

Table 4-1   Examples of Relationships Studied in Order to Answer Certain Questions

Question	Suggests study of the relationship between variables	
	Independent variable	**Dependent variable**
Does exposure to cold, wet weather predispose to the common cold?	Daily weather conditions	Incidence of common cold
What is the influence of the serum potassium concentration on the contractility of the heart?	Serum potassium concentration	Stroke output of the heart
Is obesity related to the occurrence of gallstones?	Skinfold thickness	Prevalence of gallstones
What is the effect of vitamin C deprivation on wound healing?	Vitamin C content of the diet	Tensile strength of healing wounds
Which part of the hemoglobin molecule carries the oxygen?	Portion of hemoglobin molecule	Affinity for oxygen
Does BCG vaccination provide protection against pulmonary tuberculosis?	Presence or absence of vaccination	Incidence of tuberculosis

occurrence may depend on racial characteristics and the type of diet eaten, both of which must be considered and assessed as additional independent variables.

Observational versus Experimental Studies

There are two basic approaches to investigating the relationship between variables. In *observational* studies, nature is allowed to take its course, and changes or differences in one characteristic are studied in relation to changes or differences in the other, if any. In *experimental* studies, the investigator actively intervenes and makes one variable change and then sees what happens to the other. In doing so, he or she tries, as much as possible, to prevent other important variables from affecting the outcome. By controlling the experimental situation in this way, the investigator may conclude that the intervention or manipulation of the independent variable actually affected, or caused the change in, the dependent variable.

Epidemiology includes both observational and experimental studies. An example of an epidemiologic experiment was the large-scale field trial of poliomyelitis vaccine in which two large groups of children, comparable in all important respects (e.g., age, health, socioeconomic status, and likelihood of exposure to poliomyelitis virus), received vaccine and placebo, respectively, with follow-up to measure the subsequent incidence of poliomyelitis (described in Chap. 9).

Because of the difficulties of performing well-controlled experiments on human populations and the availability of an abundance of observational data, epidemiologists have tended to concentrate on observational studies. In doing so, they have tried to "control" the important extraneous variables by their data-analysis methods. Also, they are always on the lookout for "natural experiments"— spontaneous occurrences that approximate experiments by virtue of a change in one independent variable apparently unaccompanied by changes in other important variables. An example might be the sudden graded exposure to ionizing radiation received in 1945 by the population of Hiroshima, which has permitted the study of the relationship of different doses of radiation exposure to the subsequent development of a variety of diseases.

Such dreadful natural experiments are rare (thank goodness) and the observational epidemiologist has to rely on other techniques and criteria for determining the possible effects of additional variables.

Observational studies fall into two main categories, descriptive and analytic. These studies, in turn, may be subdivided into cross-sectional, or prevalence, studies, case-control studies, and cohort, or incidence, studies, depending on the groups of persons investigated and the time relationships involved. (Case-control studies are probably best included only in the analytic category.) These will be described subsequently. Attention also will be paid to defining the relationship between prospective and retrospective studies and to clarifying the confusion that revolves around this distinction.

Descriptive versus Analytic Studies

There are two fundamental objectives of observational epidemiologic studies. One is to *describe* the occurrence of disease or disease-related phenomena in populations. The other is to *explain* the observed pattern of occurrence of disease. Seeking the latter objective involves the identification of causal, or etiologic, factors.

Descriptive studies usually involve the determination of the incidence, prevalence, and mortality rates for diseases in large population groups according to basic group characteristics such as age, sex, race, and geographic area. In this way, the general distribution of disease in the population is described.

Studies attempting to explain disease occurrence are often referred to as *analytic* studies. The starting point for an analytic study is often a descriptive finding that raises certain questions or suggests certain hypotheses that require further investigation. In analytic studies the investigator tries to answer a specific question or group of questions.

The distinction between descriptive and analytic studies is not clear-cut. A large-scale descriptive study may (perhaps unexpectedly) provide abundant and impressive data that give a clear answer to a specific question. In an analytic study, designed to answer specific questions, data collected incidentally may be of great descriptive interest and raise further questions for investigation.

Despite this fuzziness, it is often useful to categorize epidemiologic studies in this manner. Descriptive studies usually involve a more diffuse, superficial, or general view of a disease problem. Analytic studies narrow down on a specific question and may require a more rigorous study design and data analysis.

Cross-Sectional, or Prevalence, Studies

Cross-sectional, or *prevalence,* studies examine the relationship between diseases and other characteristics or variables of interest as they exist in a defined population at one particular time. The presence or absence of disease and the presence or absence of the other variables (or, if they are quantitative, their level) are determined in each member of the study population or in a representative sample at one particular time. The relationship between a variable and the disease can be examined in two ways, either (1) in terms of the prevalence of disease in different population subgroups defined according to the presence or absence (or level) of the variables or, conversely, (2) in terms of the presence or absence (or level) of the variables in the diseased versus the nondiseased.

Cohort, or Incidence, Studies

Instead of measuring the relationships of attributes to existing disease, as do prevalence studies, *cohort,* or *incidence,* studies look more directly at attributes or factors related to the *development* of disease. A study population free of the disease under investigation is identified at a particular time. The attributes of interest are measured initially in this group of persons, known as a *cohort.* Then, these persons are followed up over a period of time for the development of the disease being studied. The relationship of an attribute to the disease is examined by dividing the population into subgroups according to the presence or absence (or level) of the attribute initially and comparing the subsequent incidence of disease in each subgroup.

Case-Control Studies

In *case-control* studies, after the initial identification of cases, that is, location of persons with the disease of interest, a suitable control group or comparison group of persons without the disease is identified. The relationship of an attribute to the disease is examined by comparing the diseased and nondiseased with regard to how frequently the attribute is present or, if quantitative, what the levels of the attribute are in the two groups. Case-control studies are similar to cross-sectional studies if they assess the relationship of existing disease to other variables or attributes. Case-control studies can be made similar to cohort studies of disease development by making sure that only newly diagnosed, or "incident," cases are included.

An Illustrative Example

Cross-sectional, case-control, and cohort studies are discussed in detail in Chaps. 6, 7, and 8, respectively. At this point an example may help to clarify the distinction among these study plans. Suppose we wish to learn whether obesity predisposes to degenerative arthritis of the knees. In a cross-sectional study we would x-ray the knees of a defined population, perhaps all the adults in a community, and determine degree of obesity by measuring height and weight or skinfold thickness. We would then compare the prevalence of osteoarthritis in population subgroups showing various degrees of obesity. Or, we may want to contrast the mean skinfold thickness or other obesity measure in those with osteoarthritis and those without.

In a case-control study of this question, we might collect a group of persons with osteoarthritis of the knees admitted to a local hospital during the past year. For a control group, we might select for each osteoarthritis case a person of the same sex and similar age admitted to the same hospital during the same week for minor elective surgery such as herniorrhaphy or hemorrhoidectomy. We would then compare the recorded heights and weights of the case group with those of the control group to see if, indeed, the osteoarthritis cases were more obese.

To approach this problem by a cohort study, we would go back to a defined adult population and x-ray their knees to exclude persons with existing osteoarthritis. We would then measure skinfold thickness or height and weight to divide the population without osteoarthritis into the obese and nonobese or, preferably, some finer gradations of fatness. We would call them back 10 years later for repeat knee x-rays, which would demonstrate new cases of osteoarthritis. Then we would compare the incidence of osteoarthritis in the various fatness groups.

Remembering our original question, "Does obesity *predispose* to osteoarthritis?" the cohort study approach seems to provide the most direct answer, since we looked for obesity *before* the osteoarthritis developed. The cross-sectional and case-control studies provided only indirect evidence, since they looked at obesity and disease at the same time. However, the time sequence often can be taken into account in cross-sectional and case-control studies by inquiring about the medical history of the persons being studied. For example, in the osteoarthritis study we also could have asked the patients about their weight 10 years ago, or at age 25, or before their knees started to hurt. Although this information may not be as accurate as that derived from weighing the subjects initially in a cohort study, it does make the time sequence evident in cross-sectional and case-control studies.

Prospective and Retrospective Studies

The question of time sequence leads naturally to consideration of the much discussed *prospective* and *retrospective* studies. It is almost a matter of faith that investigations are unsatisfactory if they are retrospective. One often hears such comments as, "Of course, this study was retrospective, so we cannot be confident of the findings."

Before discussing the merits of prospective versus retrospective studies, it is important to clarify their meaning. Actually, much confusion has resulted because the terms are used in two different ways, leading to such semantic horrors as "retrospective-prospective" studies.

One of the meanings of prospective versus retrospective has to do with the time period during which the data are recorded in relation to the time at which the study effort begins. In this sense, retrospective studies use observations that have been recorded in the past. In contrast, prospective studies involve the collection of observations after the investigation is started.

The other meaning of prospective versus retrospective studies is related not to the time sequence of the observations and the beginning of the study but, rather, to the time sequence of observations of study variables and the occurrence of disease. In this sense, prospective studies are analogous to cohort studies, and retrospective studies are analogous to case-control studies. Prospective, or cohort, studies measure characteristics and wait for disease to develop, while retrospective, or case-control, studies attempt to measure past characteristics in persons already diseased.

It is strongly suggested that this second set of definitions be discarded, since better terms are available, as noted. The advantages and disadvantages of cross-sectional, case-control, and cohort studies will be discussed in Chaps. 6, 7, and 8. The following discussion of prospective versus retrospective studies will consider only the first pair of definitions, relating to when the data were collected.

In prospective studies the investigator can plan and control the methods for making and recording observations, keeping in mind their purpose. In retrospective studies the already-recorded data may have been collected for an entirely unrelated purpose. Therefore these data may well be incomplete and recorded in a manner not appropriate for the desired study.

Consequently, there often are severe problems involved in retrospective studies. Consider a study of changes in the outcome of treatment of congestive heart failure in a particular hospital over a period of several years. In carrying out a retrospective study, the investigator would be plagued by the fact that the criteria for the diagnosis of congestive heart failure vary over the years and vary from doctor to doctor. The recent advent of bedside measurement of central venous pressure, pulmonary wedge pressure, and cardiac output has improved the ability to diagnose the condition. Cases diagnosed many years ago may differ in character and severity from those diagnosed last year. Therefore, observed changes in outcome may be related more to differences in initial severity than to the effects of treatment. If one of the criteria for improvement were weight loss, the investigator might be frustrated to find that admission and discharge weights were not recorded for many patients over the years, ruling them out of this aspect of the study.

If this study were carried out prospectively, the investigator could initially establish criteria for the diagnosis of congestive heart failure and set up objective measures of severity and improvement. In addition, he or she could establish procedures to ensure that all the needed measurements were made uniformly on all patients. Thus, the superiority of a prospective study of this question is obvious.

Not all retrospective data need be of poor quality. If we again consider retrospective studies using hospital charts, a variety of data come to mind that would probably have been recorded accurately and consistently. Examples are time of admission, number of days spent in the hospital, sex of the patient, whether the patient died, and whether any blood transfusions were received.

PROBLEMS

4-1 Select two appropriate labels for each of the following studies. One label should be either *retrospective* or *prospective;* the other should be *cross-sectional, case-control,* or *cohort.* Use the definitions of retrospective and prospective recommended in this chapter.

    a A telephone survey to be conducted next summer to determine whether peptic ulcer is then more frequent in unemployed or in employed adults

    b A study of mortality rates experienced to date by veterans of World War II, comparing men who had served in the Army with those who had served in the Navy

c A study comparing manic-depressive with schizophrenic adult patients in a mental hospital to determine which group more often showed behavior problems prior to illness as recorded in their school records

d A follow-up study to determine whether seventh-grade girls whose parents give permission for them to attend sex education lectures will have a lower rate of teenage pregnancy in the next 5 years than girls whose parents refuse

4-2 Suppose that, in the example described in Prob. 4-1*d,* after parental permission is obtained, girls are assigned by a toss of the coin to either a sex education movie or a series of lectures. The girls are followed up to determine which educational technique results in a lower pregnancy rate. What type of study would this be?

4-3 Indicate for each of the studies described in Probs. 4-1 and 4-2 what the independent and dependent variables are.

4-4 The study described in Prob. 4-1*a* was planned after it was noted in a tabulation of cause-specific mortality rates in cities that the rate of mortality from peptic ulcer was greater in one city where there was a higher unemployment rate than in an adjacent city with a low unemployment rate.

a What type of study was the tabulation of mortality rates in cities, descriptive or analytic?

b Judging from the analytic study described in Prob. 4-1*a,* what hypothesis was derived from the difference between the two cities in their peptic ulcer mortality rates?

BIBLIOGRAPHY

Kelsey JL, Thompson WD, Evans AS: *Methods in Observational Epidemiology* (New York: Oxford University Press, 1986).

Lilienfeld AM, Lilienfeld DE: *Foundations of Epidemiology,* 2d ed. (New York: Oxford University Press, 1980), chaps. 8, 9.

MacMahon B, Pugh TF: *Epidemiology: Principles and Methods* (Boston: Little, Brown, 1970), chap. 3.

Chapter 5

Descriptive Studies

Descriptive epidemiologic studies reveal the patterns of disease occurrence in human populations. They provide general observations concerning the relationship of disease to basic characteristics. These characteristics include such personal items as age, sex, race, occupation, and social class. Also of great importance are geographic location and time of occurrence of disease. Thus, the major characteristics of interest in descriptive epidemiology may be summarized under the categories: person, place, and time.

At first glance, the goal of describing disease occurrence in this way may seem trivial and not worthy of the efforts of medical scientists. However, such studies are of fundamental importance and serve a variety of purposes—chiefly:

1 Alerting the medical community to what types of persons (e.g., young or old, male or female, white-collar workers or blue-collar workers) are most likely to be affected by a disease, where the disease will occur, and when. This information is of great value to physicians in making diagnoses, even though they may not be aware of using it.

2 Assisting in the rational planning of health and medical care facilities (e.g., number of coronary-care-unit beds needed for the cases of myocardial infarction in a particular community).

3 Providing clues to disease etiology and questions or hypotheses for further fruitful study (e.g., low prevalence of tooth

decay in certain areas in the United States suggested further studies concerning the value of fluoride in drinking water).

PERSON

Basic demographic and social characteristics of persons constitute the attributes of greatest concern. Among these characteristics are age, sex, race or ethnic group, marital status, social class or socioeconomic status, religion, and occupation.

Age

Age is one of the most important factors in disease occurrence. Some diseases occur almost exclusively in one particular age group, such as hypertrophic pyloric stenosis in young infants and carcinoma of the prostate in elderly men. Other diseases occur over a much wider age span but tend to be more prevalent at certain ages than at others.

The time of life at which an infectious disease predominates is influenced by such factors as the degree of exposure to the agent at various ages, variations in susceptibility with age, and the duration of the immunity developed after infection. The influence of age-related exposure and duration of immunity is illustrated by the contrast between the single occurrence of chickenpox almost exclusively in young children and the repeated occurrence of gonorrhea, predominantly in adolescents and young adults. Chickenpox is readily transmitted among children playing together or gathering in classrooms, and it produces a lifelong immunity. Gonorrhea is transmitted by sexual contact and results in no immunity.

Many chronic and degenerative diseases such as coronary heart disease and osteoarthritis show a progressive increase in prevalence with increasing age. It is tempting to regard a disease with this age pattern as being due merely to aging itself. It should be remembered, however, that increasing age also marks the passage of time, during which the body is accumulating exposure to harmful environmental influences. For example, the wrinkling and loss of elasticity in skin that we associate with aging can be brought about or accelerated by chronic exposure to sunlight.

Instead of adopting the fatalistic view that a disease is an inevitable consequence of aging, a search for other causative factors should be undertaken. One of the great contributions of epidemiology in the past few decades has been to show that aging is not the primary cause of atherosclerosis and its consequences, as was previously thought, but that a person's habits and manner of living may contribute significantly to this disease process.

To see how age patterns of disease occurrence lead to clues and hypotheses, note the age trend, reported by Lilienfeld (1956), in the incidence of breast cancer among single and married women in New York State (Fig. 5-1). The steady geometric (note the logarithmic scale) increase in incidence with age diminishes sharply in the forties with a lesser continuing increase in the older years. The reduction in the forties of the rate of increase with age suggested the hypothesis that the hormonal changes of the menopause tend to decrease susceptibility to breast cancer. This hypothesis continues to be of great interest to scientists studying the causes of breast cancer.

Current and Cohort Age Tabulations   The tabulation of disease rates in relation to age at one particular time, as in Fig. 5-1, is known as a *current,* or *cross-sectional,* presentation. This shows disease rates as they are occurring simultaneously in different age groups; thus, different people are involved in each age group. The other way to tabulate and analyze age relationships is in terms of *cohorts.* A cohort is a specific group of people identified at one period of time and followed up as they pass through different ages during part or all of their life span.

The results of cross-sectional and cohort age analyses can differ to a surprising degree, and either approach may be more appropriate for a particular problem. In a classic study, Frost (1939) compared cross-sectional and cohort age analyses of tuberculosis death rates in Massachusetts. Figure 5-2 shows the cross-sectional curves for males in the years 1880, 1910, and 1930. First of all, note that at all ages the mortality rates decreased between 1880 and 1930. Also, observe that the shapes of the age curves were chang-

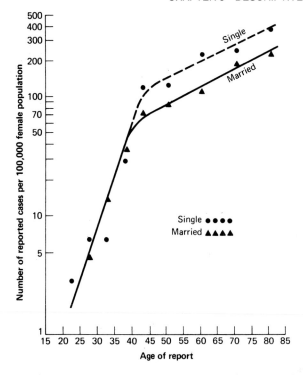

Figure 5-1   Annual age-specific incidence rates of reported cases of female breast cancer, by marital status, New York State exclusive of New York City, 1949. *(Reproduced, by permission, from Lilienfeld, 1956.)*

ing. The 1930 curve was of particular concern to public health workers in the 1930s because it showed tuberculosis mortality rates rising with age in adult life, reaching a maximum between ages 50 and 60. This new age pattern of susceptibility to death from tuberculosis was thought possibly to be due to the failure of many individuals to become infected and acquire immunity during youth.

The matter was clarified, however, by a cohort analysis, shown in Fig. 5-3. Each curve represents the cohort of persons born in the 10-year period leading up to and including the year shown above the curve (e.g., the 1870 cohort included individuals born from 1861 to 1870). In this cohort analysis it is apparent that

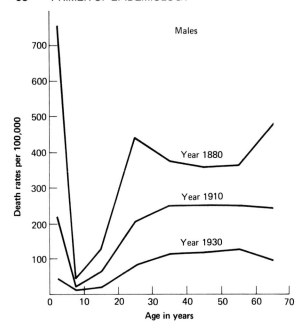

Figure 5-2 Massachusetts death rates from tuberculosis—all forms—
by age, 1880, 1910, 1930. *(Reproduced, by permission, from Frost,
1939.)*

each group experienced its maximum adult risk of tuberculosis
death during the age decade of the twenties with subsequent decline in risk with age. Thus, for any particular group of adults,
there was no increase in susceptibility with age, after all. Rather,
persons in their fifties in 1930 had higher death rates than did
younger persons because they belonged to the 1880 cohort, which
experienced a greater exposure to tuberculosis than any of the
succeeding cohorts.

Note that the frequently quoted calculations of average life
expectancy are determined essentially on a cross-sectional rather
than a cohort basis, using what are known as *life tables* (Hill and
Hill, 1991). The presently observed annual mortality rates for each

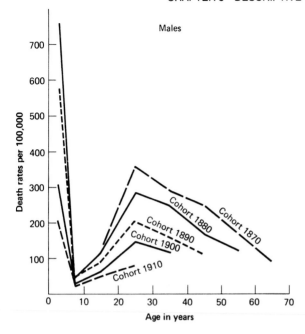

Figure 5-3 Massachusetts death rates from tuberculosis—all forms—by age, in successive 10-year cohorts. *(Reproduced, by permission, from Frost, 1939.)*

year of age are applied successively to a hypothetical population beginning either at birth or at some other starting point. It is assumed that as this hypothetical population ages, year by year, it will experience the same mortality rates for each year of life as are now observed in the current population at each age. Actually, the cohort of persons born now may be exposed to different risks of death as they go through various age periods of life than are experienced by persons who are *now* in those age periods.

Sex

Some diseases occur more frequently in males, others more frequently in females. If sex-linked inheritance can be excluded, a sex difference in disease incidence initially brings to mind the possibility of hormonal or reproductive factors that either predispose or protect. For example, the greater occurrence of coronary heart disease in young men than in young women cannot be explained entirely by sex differences in the so-called coronary risk factors such as blood lipid concentrations, blood pressure, cigarette smoking, diabetes mellitus, and obesity. There may be some important hormonal factor that contributes to the male-female difference—perhaps protection of the female by estrogens before menopause. Similarly, the greater prevalence of gallstones in women than in men is probably attributable, in part, to the effects of repeated pregnancies and, in addition, to hormonal effects on bile composition.

But men and women differ in many other ways, including habits, social relationships, environmental exposures, and other aspects of day-to-day living. The higher prevalence of cirrhosis of the liver and chronic bronchitis in men is at least partly related to the fact that, on the average, men have drunk more alcohol and smoked more cigarettes than have women.

Sex differences in disease occurrence are important descriptive findings and often suggest avenues for further research. No disease can be considered to have a well-understood etiology if it manifests a male or female predominance that is not explained.

Race

Racial differences in disease prevalence have often been noted. In the case of some diseases (e.g., black-white differences in sickle cell anemia and skin cancer), the differences are genetically determined. With other diseases, the explanation may not be so simple, especially when racial differences are accompanied by differences in socioeconomic status.

A case in point is the higher prevalence of hypertension and its complications in blacks than in whites in the United States. Suggested explanations have included (1) increased genetic susceptibility in blacks, possibly reflected in racial differences in kidney function, (2) increased emotional stress in blacks due to racial discrimination, (3) lower average socioeconomic levels in blacks (since in either whites or blacks the prevalence of hypertension is higher in lower socioeconomic groups), (4) less access for blacks to good medical care, (5) a higher prevalence of obesity in blacks, and (6) selection of blacks who were genetically better equipped to conserve salt and to survive the frequent diarrheal diseases aboard slave ships and the other stresses of slavery related to salt metabolism (Howard and Holman, 1970; Gillum, 1979; Wilson and Grim, 1991; Curtin, 1992). It may eventually be shown that some or all of these mechanisms are involved.

Marital Status

Marital status is another important descriptive variable. Married persons have lower mortality rates than single persons, including both overall mortality and mortality from most specific diseases. Whether the married state provides health benefits or whether characteristics favoring long life also predispose to marriage has not been determined.

Of great interest in studies of cancer etiology has been the contrast between cancer of the breast and cancer of the uterine cervix in their relation to marital status. Breast cancer is more apt to develop in single women or women who marry late in life, while cervical cancer is associated with early marriage. Further studies stemming, in part, from these observations suggest that cervical cancer is associated with coital activity at an early age and that having a first pregnancy at an early age may help protect a woman from breast cancer.

The data regarding the relationship of breast cancer incidence to age (see Fig. 5-1) also revealed a higher incidence in single women than in married women in their forties and later age decades. Lilienfeld (1956) suggested the hypothesis that early artificial, or surgical, menopause, occurring more often in married than in single women, might be protective against breast cancer. This hypothesis received some confirmation in an analytic case-control study in which it was found (1) that women with breast cancer less often gave a history of artificial menopause than did control subjects and (2) that married women more often gave a history of artificial menopause than did single women.

Socioeconomic Status

Socioeconomic status, or social class, is a somewhat nebulous concept, but it can be measured fairly conveniently by the occupation or income of the family head, by his or her educational level, or by residence, in terms of the value and amenities of the home or dwelling unit. The British have used occupation to define five social classes: (I) professional, (II) intermediate, (III) skilled, (IV) partly skilled, and (V) unskilled. Using this classification system, the Registrar General for England and Wales has provided descriptive data relating social class to a variety of conditions.

As mentioned above regarding hypertension, many diseases show a distinct social class gradient, with higher rates in the lower socioeconomic classes. Included are rheumatic heart disease, chronic bronchitis, tuberculosis, stomach ulcer, stomach cancer, and nutritional-deficiency diseases.

At the same time, however, low socioeconomic status also appears to confer protection against some diseases. In the series of annual poliomyelitis epidemics that began in 1947, the higher social classes were the most severely affected. It is believed that poor sanitary conditions in economically disadvantaged groups had led to widespread subclinical infection in the first few years of life, resulting in immunity. When "higher" living standards prevent this early infection, poliomyelitis acquired later in childhood is more likely to cause disabling paralysis.

A marked socioeconomic gradient in infant mortality has long been noted. Table 5-1 shows social class and rates of infant mortality (at age under 1 year) per 1000 live births in England and Wales during two time periods, 1930 to 1932 and 1949 to 1953. Note that even though there was a marked improvement by the later time period, social class V still had over twice the infant mortality rate observed in social class I. Infant mortality rates often have been used as an index both of living standards and of

Table 5-1   Infant Mortality Rates in England and Wales as Related to Social Class during Two Time Periods, 1930–1932 and 1949–1953

Social class	Infant mortality rates*	
	1930–1932	1949–1953
I	32.7	18.7
II	45.0	21.6
III	57.6	28.6
IV	66.8	33.8
V	77.1	40.8
All classes	61.6	29.5

*Deaths of infants under 1 year old per 1000 live births. Registrar General's data, Taylor and Knowelden (1964).

availability of medical services in comparing nations or areas within a nation.

PLACE

Where disease occurs is a matter of great importance. Comparison of disease rates in different places may provide obvious clues to etiology or serve as a stimulus to further fruitful investigation. The places of concern may be as large as a continent or as small as part of a room. As illustrative examples, descriptive findings will be presented from international comparisons, comparisons of regions within the United States and Canada, and comparisons of areas in a city.

International Comparisons

Because of the problems regarding the validity of mortality statistics, described in Chap. 3, it is difficult to take seriously small differences among nations in mortality rates for specific diseases. However, it is also difficult to explain away very large differences as due to artifact—that is, where the death rate for a disease in one country is 2 or 3 times as large as the death rate in another. Large differences are particularly impressive when both countries are known to have reasonably good vital statistics systems.

The Unusual Disease Occurrence in Japan Ranking the disease-specific mortality rates of various nations has revealed Japan to be among the highest nations for some diseases and among the lowest for others. Table 5-2 shows some age-adjusted or age-specific mortality rates for stomach cancer, colon cancer, breast cancer, cerebrovascular disease (primarily strokes), and coronary heart disease. Note that among the nations studied, Japan is the highest-ranking country for stomach cancer and cerebrovascular disease and the lowest ranking for breast cancer, colon cancer, and coronary heart disease.

Because of Japan's unusual position among nations regarding these diseases, consideration of the mode of life in Japan has suggested a number of hypotheses for further study. The relatively frequent practice and long duration of breast feeding of infants in Japan helped to raise the question of whether lactation may diminish the risk of developing breast cancer. (Apparently it does not; see MacMahon et al., 1970.) The traditional Japanese diet has come under considerable scrutiny in hopes of finding predisposing factors for stomach cancer and protective factors for colon and breast cancer. Also, the low fat intake in Japan has been thought responsible for the low average serum cholesterol levels observed there and the low incidence of coronary heart disease. Although some portion of the high cerebrovascular death rate may be due to a known tendency of Japanese to attribute any sudden death to a cerebral hemorrhage, the high salt intake of Japanese has come under suspicion as a possible predisposing factor for hypertension and stroke.

Many traditional practices in Japan are changing, and it will be of considerable interest to learn whether disease rates will change in ways that are consistent with the above hypotheses. There are early indications that some of the predicted changes in disease incidence are taking place (Wynder and Hirayama, 1977). Also, the migration of Japanese to places where they adopt new eating and living habits has permitted comparative studies aimed at identifying environmental factors that predispose to disease. Gordon

Rank	Stomach cancer, males, 1964–1965	Colon cancer (except rectum), males, 1964–1965	Breast cancer, females, 1964–1965	Cerebrovascular disease, males, ages 65–74, 1964	Coronary heart disease, males, ages 45–54, 1964
1	Japan (69)	Scotland (16)	Netherlands (26)	Japan (1,680)	Finland (442)
2	Chile (58)	Denmark (14)	England & Wales (24)	Scotland (901)	Scotland (358)
3	Austria (42)	U.S.A.—white (14)	Denmark (24)	Finland (751)	U.S.A. (354)
4	Finland (40)	Canada (13)	Scotland (24)	West Germany (750)	Australia (324)
5	West Germany (37)	New Zealand (13)	Canada (23)	Italy (708)	Northern Ireland (324)
6	Italy (34)	Northern Ireland (13)	New Zealand (23)	Hungary (706)	Canada (311)
7	Portugal (33)	Ireland (13)	South Africa (23)	Austria (663)	New Zealand (293)
8	Netherlands (28)	Australia (12)	Northern Ireland (22)	Northern Ireland (656)	England & Wales (245)
9	Belgium (27)	Belgium (12)	U.S.A.—white (22)	Israel (614)	Israel (214)
10	Switzerland (26)	England & Wales (12)	Switzerland (22)	England & Wales (612)	West Germany (183)
11	Norway (26)	France (12)	Ireland (22)	Australia (611)	Denmark (181)
12	Scotland (25)	Switzerland (11)	Belgium (21)	Czechoslovakia (560)	Norway (164)
13	South Africa (25)	U.S.A.—nonwhite (11)	Israel (21)	Switzerland (530)	Netherlands (162)
14	Ireland (24)	Netherlands (11)	U.S.A.—nonwhite (20)	France (528)	Austria (159)
15	England & Wales (23)	South Africa (11)	Australia (19)	U.S.A. (495)	Belgium (159)
16	Sweden (22)	Austria (10)	Sweden (19)	Norway (492)	Czechoslovakia (151)
17	Northern Ireland (22)	West Germany (10)	West Germany (18)	Denmark (478)	Hungary (147)
18	Denmark (22)	Sweden (10)	Austria (17)	New Zealand (475)	Switzerland (134)
19	France (21)	Norway (8)	Norway (17)	Netherlands (416)	Italy (133)
20	Israel (18)	Italy (8)	France (16)	Canada (414)	Venezuela (131)
21	U.S.A.—nonwhite (18)	Portugal (8)	Italy (16)	Sweden (394)	Sweden (125)
22	Canada (18)	Israel (7)	Finland (14)	Belgium (334)	France (74)
23	New Zealand (17)	Finland (5)	Portugal (13)	Venezuela (281)	Japan (51)
24	Australia (15)	Chile (4)	Chile (9)		
25	U.S.A.—white (9)	Japan (3)	Japan (4)		

*Death rates per 100,000 shown in parentheses (rounded from the original).

Sources: Stomach, colon, and breast cancer: Segi et al. (1969); cerebrovascular and coronary heart disease: World Health Organization (1967).

(1957) compared mortality rates for Japanese in Japan, Hawaii, and the United States mainland and found contrasting trends for cerebrovascular disease and for coronary heart disease. Cerebrovascular disease mortality rates in both sexes decreased, and coronary mortality rates in men increased from Japan to Hawaii to the United States mainland. This suggested that as Japanese were adopting "the American way of life," their susceptibility to the two diseases in question was moving in the direction of that found in other Americans. (The assumption that migrants are genetically similar to those who remain in their native land should always be viewed with caution.) In order to explore in detail the reasons for the above geographic trends in cerebrovascular and coronary disease, parallel data collection methods were established in three epidemiologic studies of Japanese, located in Hiroshima, Japan; Honolulu, Hawaii; and in the San Francisco Bay area (Syme et al., 1975). These studies confirmed the geographic trends (Worth et al., 1975) and showed that biochemical risk factors for coronary heart disease (serum cholesterol, glucose, uric acid, and triglycerides) are lower in Japanese men in Japan than in Hawaii and California (Nichaman et al., 1975). However, differences in prevalence of coronary heart disease are not fully explained by the conventional coronary risk factors and may be due, in part, to cultural factors (Marmot and Syme, 1976).

Comparisons of Regions within Countries

The availability of mortality statistics for states and smaller geographic subdivisions in the United States and other nations has permitted the discovery of interesting place-to-place variations in disease occurrence. Differences in mortality rates between urban and rural areas are a common finding. The higher mortality from lung cancer in cities than in farming areas is consistent with an etiologic role of either cigarette smoking or air pollution, since both are more common in cities.

The North-to-South Gradient of Multiple Sclerosis Geographic variation within nations may take the form of a distinct north-to-south gradient, which suggests that climate or other factors related to latitude may be involved. An example is the find-ing in the United States and Canada of generally higher mortality rates for multiple sclerosis the farther north one looks (Fig. 5-4). Confirmation of the north-to-south trend also comes from other nations and from prevalence rates found in several cities (Fig. 5-5). While hypotheses abound, to date no one has convincingly explained this geographic distribution of multiple sclerosis (Alter, 1968; Raymond, 1986).

Areas within a City

When studying disease occurrence within a city, it is often desirable to plot the occurrence of disease in each census tract, since informa-tion about other characteristics of persons in each tract is available.

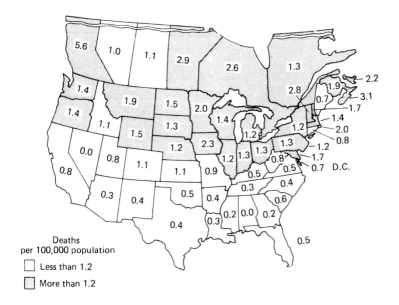

Figure 5-4   Multiple sclerosis mortality rates per 100,000 population in the U.S. states and in Canadian provinces. *(Reproduced, by permission, from Alter, 1968, adapted from Limburg, 1950.)*

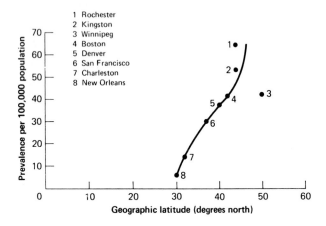

Figure 5-5 Multiple sclerosis prevalence rates in cities of the United States and Canada. *(Reproduced, by permission, from Alter, 1968.)*

Rheumatic Fever in Baltimore   Figure 5-6, from Gordis et al. (1969), shows the distribution in Baltimore census tracts of the homes of hospitalized rheumatic fever cases from 1960 to 1964. Most of the cases occurred in two clusters on either side of the central business district—in the low-income area south of North Avenue, which is shown by a heavy line. Naturally, we cannot form a judgment based only on the "numerator" cases but must relate these to the "denominator" populations in each tract to develop rates.

Thus, annual incidence rates for rheumatic fever were calculated for groups of census tracts in this area. They ranged as high as 40.2 per 100,000, whereas the incidence rate for the entire city was only 15.6 per 100,000.

Studying the high and low incidence areas further revealed that nonwhite children suffered a higher incidence of rheumatic fever than did white children. Only among whites was higher socioeconomic status related to lower incidence of rheumatic fever. When housing characteristics were examined, the degree of crowding was the variable that was most closely related to rheumatic fever occurrence. The authors emphasized the importance of socioeconomic

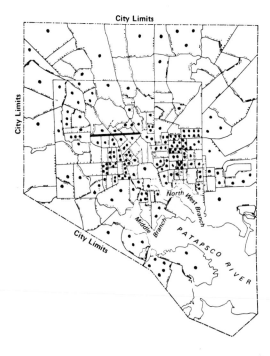

Figure 5-6   Residence distribution of hospitalized rheumatic fever patients, Baltimore 1960–1964. Heavy line shows North Avenue. Each dot represents one patient. *(Reproduced, by permission, from Gordis et al., 1969.)*

conditions in the occurrence of this disease and showed that the higher incidence in nonwhites might have been due to the crowded living conditions in which most Baltimore nonwhites lived.

TIME

The pattern of disease occurrence in time is often an extremely informative descriptive characteristic. A great variety of time trends may be found in the literature; these involve simple increases or decreases of disease incidence or more complex combinations of these changes in time. To provide an introduction to this interesting subject, a few examples of short-term, periodic, and long-term time trends will be described.

Short-Term Increases and Decreases in Disease Incidence

Short-term changes are those increases or decreases in disease incidence that are measured in hours, days, weeks, or months. These are most often observed in the study of epidemics of infectious disease, as will be illustrated below. However, important short-term trends also have been noted in the occurrence of symptoms of, or even deaths due to, chronic noninfectious disease in relation to both natural phenomena, such as heat waves, and stresses created by humans, such as marked increases in air pollution.

Epidemics   An *epidemic,* or *outbreak,* is the occurrence of a disease in members of a defined population clearly in excess of the number of cases usually or normally found in *that* population. In investigating epidemics, a careful tabulation of the distribution of disease-onset times of the affected members of the population, in terms of either counts of cases or incidence ("attack") rates, may be very helpful in determining the initiating causes and mechanism of spread.

For a thorough discussion of the propagation of epidemics, the reader is referred to Last (1986). A few basic principles and technical terms should be mentioned, however, before we consider some examples of time patterns. Epidemics affect only susceptible members of the population, of which there may be many or few. Others in the population are immune due to antibodies related to previous infection, immunization, or passive transfer from mother to infant. Still others may be resistant due to other inherent factors. After a person is exposed to the disease-causing agent, there is an *incubation period* until the disease first appears. Susceptible persons may also develop *inapparent infections,* in which no symptoms or signs become evident. The infectious agent may leave the host during the *communicable period,* which varies in timing and duration from one disease to the next.

Infections are transmitted from one person to another in a variety of ways: by direct personal contact, by touching contaminated objects, or by droplets spraying from one person to another close by, as during talking or sneezing. Evaporation of such droplets may yield *droplet nuclei,* which, like certain disease-carrying dusts, may remain airborne for longer periods and travel longer distances. Other modes of transmission include *vehicles,* such as certain foods or water, and *vectors,* such as arthropods which carry the infectious agent.

Infections are usually introduced into a population directly or indirectly by one or more persons. If all members of the population are immune, an epidemic obviously cannot begin. If a large proportion of the population members are immune, the likelihood of person-to-person spread may be so small that the disease will not be propagated, and *herd immunity* is said to exist. By preventing an epidemic from taking hold in a population, herd immunity extends considerable protection to nonimmune individuals. However, there is nothing magical about the protection afforded by herd immunity. Epidemics can occur among subgroups of susceptibles in a population with a high proportion of immune individuals if the susceptibles are in close contact with one another. Indeed, pockets of such susceptibles do exist in modern urban communities (see Fox et al., 1971).

If the population contains a sufficient proportion of susceptibles and the infection spreads rapidly enough, the disease will show a trend of increasing incidence through time to a maximum, followed by a fairly steady diminution until the disease disappears completely or almost completely. The decrease is due largely to the fact that the population begins to run out of susceptible individuals, as those who were previously susceptible acquire the infection and become immune. As susceptibles become increasingly scarce, the infectious agent, no matter how well and how rapidly transmitted, finds less and less fertile soil in which to grow, so to speak. The rise through time from a negligible incidence rate to a maximum followed by a fall to low levels again appears graphically as a simple *epidemic curve,* usually but not always involving short-term trends of days, weeks, or months.

Figure 5-7 shows an epidemic of measles (rubeola) that occurred among children in Dallas, Texas, from late 1970 almost to the middle of 1971 (Luby et al., 1971). By May 1971 there were 1071 reported cases. The histogram displaying the epidemic's time sequence is of special interest because it shows an abrupt drop after the apparent peak of the epidemic was reached at the end of March. During the 2-week period in which the abrupt fall in case counts began, a special immunization campaign for children was carried out. Although alternative explanations should be considered, it appears that the campaign was helpful in controlling the epidemic by sharply reducing the number of susceptible individuals in the population.

The observed time pattern of an epidemic may provide a strong indication of the mode of initiation and spread. Figures 5-8 and 5-9 show two different outbreaks of the same disease, infectious hepatitis. Figure 5-8 depicts the number of cases by *week* of onset in an epidemic occurring in Barren County, Kentucky, and lasting from June 1970 through April 1971. Figure 5-9 is drawn on a different time scale and shows the number of cases by *day* of onset in an epidemic that occurred in Orange County, California, between August 21, 1971, and September 13, 1971. The essential distinction between the two epidemics is their duration, particularly in relation to the known incubation period of this disease, which ranges from 15 to 50 days and is commonly about 25 days.

Although the communicable period for this disease has not been clearly defined, the clustering of the Orange County cases within such a narrow time interval—the great bulk appearing within 9 days and all within 24 days—suggested that the outbreak resulted from a *point source,* that is, a single common exposure to the virus. With an incubation period measured in weeks, person-to-person spread among the group of cases could not have been a significant factor in an epidemic that ended so soon after it started.

In contrast, the bulk of the Barren County cases occurred over an interval of 4 months and the total epidemic lasted for 10 months, so there was ample time for direct person-to-person spread. This mode of transmission, however, would not be the only possible mechanism consistent with a hepatitis epidemic of this duration. Prolonged exposure of a population to a contaminated food or wa-

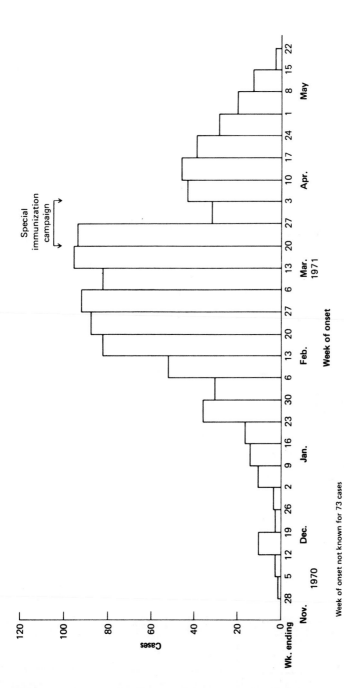

Figure 5-7 Measles cases, by week of onset. Dallas, Texas, December 1, 1970–May 22, 1971. *(Reproduced, by permission, from Luby et al., 1971.)*

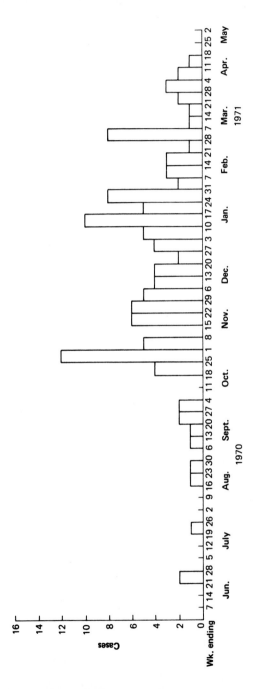

Figure 5-8 Infectious hepatitis cases, by week of onset, Barren County, Kentucky, June 1970–April 1971. (*Reproduced, by permission, from Carman et al., 1971.*)

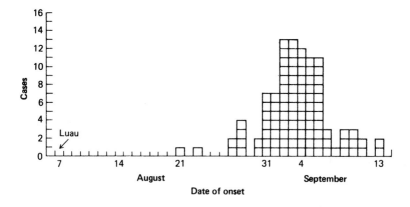

Figure 5-9 Cases of infectious hepatitis in individuals attending luau, by day of onset. Orange County, California, 1971. (Date of onset for one case undetermined.) *(Reproduced, by permission, from Philp et al., 1972.)*

ter supply could also result in a long-lasting epidemic. However, no such mechanism could be incriminated in Barren County.

Further investigation of each epidemic was quite revealing. In Barren County, most of the 118 cases occurred in children attending two elementary schools. The first observed case in June occurred in a boy whose parents frequently baby-sat for other children in the area. Among the children exposed to his parents was a 7-year-old boy, who was the first hepatitis case at one of the schools. The 7-year-old's illness began on September 26. All but one of the cases involving children in that school and their families could be traced directly or indirectly to contact with the 7-year-old. Similarly, at the other school the first illness occurred in a 9-year-old girl on September 21. It was not determined how she became infected, but she spread the disease to a total of 34 persons via 5 children with whom she had contact (Carman et al., 1971).

In Orange County almost all the 99 cases were members of a private sailing club. The only time all the cases were together during the prior year was at a club luau at a remote island off the California coast on August 7. One clue to the vehicle of infection was found in the age distribution of incidence. The attack rate was 6 percent in persons under age 15 and 62 percent in persons age 15 and over.

Detailed analysis of suspect foods revealed that only one item—mai-tai punch—was *not* consumed by *all* persons who remained free of the disease. Sizable proportions of persons *not* eating each of the other foods did become ill, which tended to exonerate these other food items, since if eating something leads to illness, not eating it should be preventive. The description of the food-handling situation at the luau by Philp and his associates (1972) clearly shows how the mai-tai could have served as the vehicle for the fecal-oral transmission of the hepatitis virus.

> All food and beverages were brought to the island by boat. Commercial bottled water for drinking was imported. Little attention, however, was paid to food-handling practices. The only water for handwashing was a single water tap located 85 yards beyond the luau site and 35 yards beyond the two privies available to the group. Handwashing was a rare event. Foods were cooked in an earthen pit for 6 hours to the point of disintegration. Unwashed papaya, pineapple, and oranges were peeled and cut for a fruit mix. Mai-tai punch was prepared from the cut fruits, unwashed fresh strawberries, instant tea, canned pineapple juice, canned lemon-lime drink, bottled water, club soda, and rum. All were mixed in a new plastic garbage can. The punch was served from a 3-tiered fountain made with fiberglass bowls suspended over the garbage can reservoir. Punch was pumped from the can to the top of the fountain, where it flowed over the fiberglass tiers back down into the garbage can. Persons who drank punch filled their cups under one of the streams as it cascaded from one bowl to the next. Many reported punch running over their hands and back into the punch reservoir. Due to the presence of pieces of fruit, particularly strawberries, the pump which forced the punch to the top of the fountain plugged frequently and was unplugged by one or more persons reaching into the bottom of the garbage can and pulling fruit pieces

out of the pump. Persons who unclogged the pump also reported sand at the bottom of the can.

Recurrent, or Periodic, Time Trends

The incidence of certain diseases shows regular, recurring increases and decreases. This regular pattern may exhibit cycles that last several years. Many cycles occur annually and represent seasonal variation in disease occurrence. Seasonal variation is a well-known characteristic for many infectious diseases and is usually based on characteristics of the infectious agent itself, the life pattern of its vector or other animal hosts, or changes in the likelihood of person-to-person spread. For example, waterborne gastrointestinal infections often exhibit a peak occurrence in the later summer months when recreational swimming and other factors facilitate their transmission. Similarly, upper respiratory infections frequently show a seasonal rise in or near winter, aided by the concentration of people indoors where virus-containing airborne droplets are readily transmitted.

Short-term periodic variations also have been observed. For example, death rates from automobile crashes show weekly cycles, with the highest rates occurring on weekends, particularly on Friday and Saturday nights, and the lowest rates on Tuesdays and Wednesdays. This is also true for deaths per person-mile of travel, indicating that the weekly cycles are not simply a reflection of the amount of driving that is done. The rise on weekends probably is due largely to increased alcohol consumption.

Long-Term, or Secular, Time Trends

Some diseases exhibit a progressive increase or decrease in occurrence that is manifested over years or decades. These long-term time trends are often referred to as *secular* trends.

Figure 5-10 shows the mortality rates in United States males of several leading types of cancer from 1930 to 1989. A marked secular increase in mortality from lung cancer has occurred, rep-

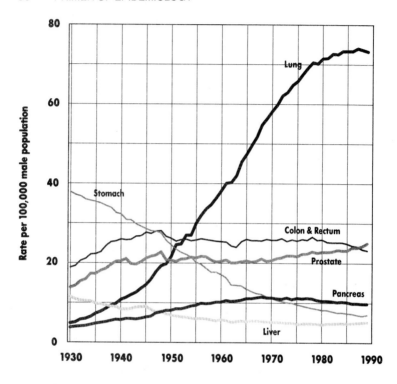

Figure 5-10   Age-adjusted male cancer death rates for selected sites, United States, 1930–1989. *(Reproduced, by permission, from American Cancer Society, 1993. Copyright by the American Cancer Society, Inc.)*

resenting about a 15-fold increase in 1989 as compared to 1930. This increase is believed to be due largely to an increase in cigarette smoking. Figure 5-10 also shows a marked downward trend in stomach cancer mortality. This gratifying change may be at least partly explained by improvements in food preservation and storage and the resulting changes in diet, as people select more fresh fruits and vegetables and less salted and pickled foods (Forman, 1991). Another important long-term downtrend is the recent fall in the death rate for cardiovascular disease in the United States, which started in the mid-1960s for coronary heart disease and earlier for cerebrovascular disease. Between 1972 and 1990, the age-adjusted mortality rate dropped 47 percent for coronary heart disease and 57 percent for stroke (Source: National Center for Health Statistics). Changes in life-style, improvements in prevention and therapy, and possibly other unidentified factors all contributed to this decline (Goldman and Cook, 1984).

As has been discussed, when a marked increase in incidence occurs in a short period of time, it is quite apparent to the medical community and is referred to as an epidemic, an emotionally loaded term that spurs prompt action. Long-term trends are barely perceptible and might go unnoticed were it not for the study of vital statistics. It would be useful, perhaps, to label as *epidemics* the long-term increases such as that noted for lung cancer. If this term were applied, more action might be taken to investigate the causes and to institute control measures.

PROBLEMS

5-1 As mentioned at the beginning of this chapter, three important uses of descriptive epidemiologic data are in:
   (A) Planning appropriate health care and medical care programs or facilities
   (B) Assisting in diagnosis
   (C) Developing hypotheses concerning disease etiology
   Some descriptive findings are listed below. For each finding, indicate which one of the above uses would be *least* appropriate.
   a The incidence of lung cancer has been increasing in the United States over the past few decades.
   b An epidemic of shigella dysentery has just begun in our community.
   c Hypertension is more prevalent and more severe in blacks than in whites in the United States.

5-2 Among nonwhite (largely black) men in the United States, the mortality rate for cancer of the prostate has been increasing dramatically over the past few decades, and this cancer is now the most common among black men. Figure 5-11 shows death rates for prostatic cancer among nonwhites by year of birth (Ernster et al., 1978). Each line represents a different 5-year age group from 45 to 49 through 80 to 84 years of age.

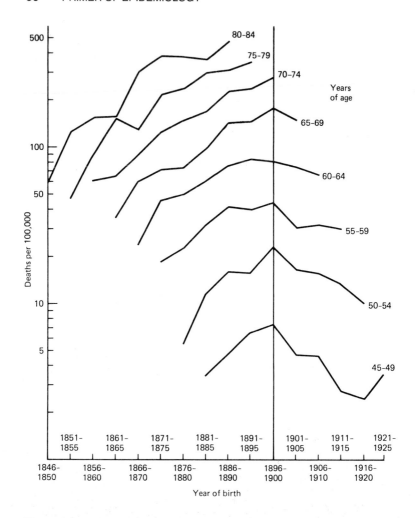

Figure 5-11 Annual age-specific prostatic cancer mortality rates per 100,000 by cohort for U.S. nonwhite males born between 1846 and 1925. *(Reproduced, by permission, from Ernster et al., 1978. Copyright, 1978, by the American Association for the Advancement of Science.)*

a How does the mortality rate for this disease relate to age?

b What term is used to describe the men born in each 5-year time period?

c Describe the relation of prostatic cancer mortality among nonwhites to year of birth.

d Which cohort has generally experienced the highest mortality rates?

e Since death rates have been falling in the younger men in more recent years, why is the overall death rate for prostatic cancer in nonwhites still rising?

f Do you expect the overall prostatic cancer mortality rate in nonwhites to continue to rise? Explain your answer.

g How would you attempt to develop a hypothesis concerning the etiology of cancer of the prostate from these data?

h How does this representation of a cohort analysis differ from that shown in Fig. 5-3?

5-3 The map shown in Fig. 5-12 represents the white male death rates by state economic area for malignant melanoma of the skin. What geographic pattern do you observe? What etiologic factor for skin melanoma does this pattern suggest to you?

5-4 Figure 5-13 shows the distribution of onset times in an epidemic of vomiting and diarrhea that occurred after breakfast on an airliner traveling from Anchorage, Alaska, to Copenhagen, Denmark, on February 2, 1975. (For a complete description see Eisenberg et al., 1975.)

a Which of the following foodborne etiologic agents is most likely responsible for the epidemic?

(1) Chemical toxin: usual incubation period—a few minutes to 2 hours

(2) Staphylococcal enterotoxin: usual incubation period—2 to 4 hours

(3) Salmonella infection: usual incubation period—12 to 24 hours

b Is this most likely a point-source or a continuing-source epidemic? Was it propagated by person-to-person spread? Explain your answers.

c How do you account for the three cases with onset time 8.5 to 9 hours after breakfast?

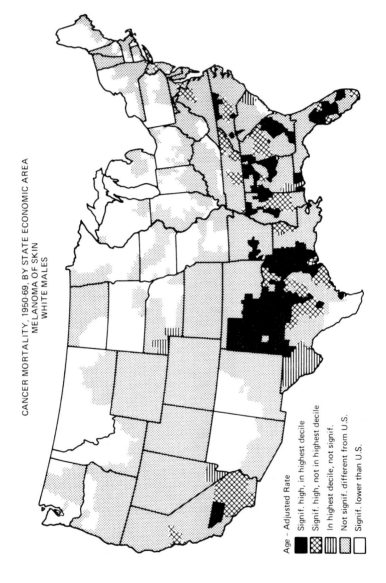

CANCER MORTALITY, 1950-69, BY STATE ECONOMIC AREA
MELANOMA OF SKIN
WHITE MALES

Age - Adjusted Rate

Signif. high, in highest decile
Signif. high, not in highest decile
In highest decile, not signif.
Not signif. different from U.S.
Signif. lower than U.S.

Figure 5-12   Mortality from malignant melanoma of skin by state economic area: white males, 1950–1969. *(Reproduced, by permission, from Mason et al., 1975.)*

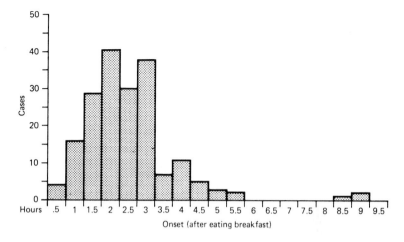

Figure 5-13 Foodborne outbreak on an aircraft, February 1975. *(Reproduced, by permission, from von Magnus et al., 1975.)*

BIBLIOGRAPHY

Alter M: Etiologic considerations based on the epidemiology of multiple sclerosis. *Am J Epidemiol* **88**:318–332 (1968).

American Cancer Society: *Cancer Facts & Figures—1993* (Atlanta: American Cancer Society, 1993).

Carman M, Guerrant WB, Hernandez C: Infectious hepatitis—Kentucky. *Cent Dis Control: Morb Mortal Wkly Rep* **20**:136–137 (1971).

Curtin PD: The slavery hypothesis for hypertension among African Americans: The historical evidence. *Am J Public Health* **82**:1681–1686 (1992).

Eisenberg MS, Gaarslev K, Brown W, Horwitz M, Hill D: Staphylococcal food poisoning aboard a commercial aircraft. *Lancet,* **2**:595–599 (1975).

Ernster VL, Selvin S, Winkelstein W, Jr: Cohort mortality for prostatic cancer among United States nonwhites. *Science* **200**:1165–1166 (June 9, 1978).

Forman D: The etiology of gastric cancer, in IK O'Neill, J Chen, H Bartsch (eds.), *Relevance to Human Cancer of N-Nitroso Compounds, Tobacco Smoke and Mycotoxins* (Lyon: International Agency for Research on Cancer, 1991), pp. 22–32.

Fox JP, Elveback L, Scott W, Gatewood L, Ackerman E: Herd immunity: Basic concept and relevance to public health immunization practices. *Am J Epidemiol* **94**:179–189 (1971).

Frost WH: The age selection of mortality from tuberculosis in successive decades. *Am J Hyg* **30**:91–96 (1939).

Gillum RF: Pathophysiology of hypertension in blacks and whites: A review of the basis of racial blood pressure differences. *Hypertension* **1**:468–475 (1979).

Goldman L, Cook EF: The decline in ischemic heart disease mortality rates: An analysis of the comparative effects of medical interventions and changes in lifestyle. *Ann Int Med* **101**:825–836 (1984).

Gordis L, Lilienfeld A, Rodriguez R: Studies in the epidemiology and preventability of rheumatic fever: I. Demographic factors and the incidence of acute attacks, and II. Socio-economic factors and the incidence of acute attacks. *J Chron Dis* **21**:645–666 (1969).

Gordon T: Mortality experience among the Japanese in the United States. Hawaii and Japan, *Public Health Rep* **72**:543–553 (1957).

Hill AB, Hill ID: *Bradford Hill's Principles of Medical Statistics,* 12th ed. (London: Edward Arnold, 1991), pp. 188–194.

Howard J, Holman BL: The effects of race and occupation on hypertension mortality. *Milbank Mem Fund Q* **48**:263–296 (1970).

Last JM (ed.): *Maxcy-Rosenau: Public Health and Preventive Medicine,* 12th ed. (Norwalk, Conn.: Appleton-Century-Crofts, 1986), pp. 55–68.

Lilienfeld AM: The relationship of cancer of the female breast to artificial menopause and marital status. *Cancer* **9**:927–934 (1956).

Limburg CC: Geographic distribution of multiple sclerosis and its estimated prevalence in the United States. *Proc Assoc Res Nerv Ment Dis* **28**:15–24 (1950).

Luby JP, Dewlett HJ, Dickerson MS: Measles—Dallas, Texas. *Cent Dis Control: Morb Mortal Wkly Rep* **20**:191–192 (1971).

MacMahon B, Lin TM, Lowe CR, Mirra AP, Ravnihar B, Salber EJ, Trichopoulos D, Valaoras VG, Yuasa S: Lactation and cancer of the breast: A summary of an international study. *Bull WHO* **42**:185–194 (1970).

Marmot MG, Syme SL: Acculturation and coronary heart disease in Japanese-Americans. *Am J Epidemiol* **104**:225–247 (1976).

Mason TJ, McKay FW, Hoover R, Blot WJ, Fraumeni JF, Jr: *Atlas of Cancer Mortality for U.S. Counties: 1950–1969,* U.S. Department of Health, Education, and Welfare, DHEW Publication (NIH) 75–780, 1975.

Nichaman MZ, Hamilton HB, Kagan A, Grier T, Sacks ST, Syme SL: Epidemiologic studies of coronary heart disease and stroke in Japanese men living in Japan, Hawaii, and California: Distribution of biochemical risk factors. *Am J Epidemiol* **102**:491–501 (1975).

Philp JR, Hamilton TP, Albert TJ, Stone RS, Pait CF, Roberto RR, Fiumara NJ, Hinman AR, Friedmann C: Hepatitis A outbreak, Orange County, Calif. *Cen. Dis. Control: Hepatitis Surveillance,* Report No. 35, pp. 12–13 (1972). See also *Am J Epidemiol* **97**:50–54 (1973).

Raymond CA: MS prevalence—genes vs. geography. *J Am Med Assoc* **256**:810–815 (1986).

Segi M, Kurihara M, Matsuyama T: *Cancer Mortality for Selected Sites in 24 Countries, no. 5 (1964–1965)*. Department of Public Health, Tohoku University School of Medicine. Sendai, Japan, 1969.

Silverberg E, Lubera J: Cancer statistics. 1986, *Ca-A Cancer J Clinicians* **36**:9–25 (1986).

Syme SL, Marmot MG, Kagan A, Kato H, Rhoads G: Epidemiological studies of coronary heart disease and stroke in Japanese men living in Japan, Hawaii, and California: Introduction. *Am J Epidemiol* **102**: 477–480 (1975).

Taylor I, Knowelden J: *Principles of Epidemiology* (Boston: Little, Brown, 1964), chaps. 6, 7 (infectious epidemics); chap. 12, pp. 318–321 (social class).

von Magnus H, Lautrop H, Gaarslev K, Skovgaard N, Elliott C, Kuhn JR, Tanaka R, Freedman DK, Bennett R, Pullen MM, three EIS officers: Outbreak of staphylococcal food poisoning aboard an aircraft. *Cent Dis Control: Morb Mortal Wkly Rep* **24**:57–59 (1975).

Wilson TW, Grim CE: Biohistory of slavery and blood pressure differences in blacks today: A hypothesis. *Hypertension* **17**(suppl I):I122–I128 (1991).

World Health Organization: Mortality statistics: Cardiovascular diseases, annual statistics, 1955–1964, by sex and age. *Epidemiol Vital Stat Rep* **20**:535–710 (1967).

Worth RM, Kato H, Rhoads GG, Kagan A, Syme SL: Epidemiologic studies of coronary heart disease and stroke in Japanese men living in Japan, Hawaii, and California: Mortality. *Am J Epidemiol* **102**:481–490 (1975).

Wynder EL, Hirayama T: Comparative epidemiology of cancers of the United States and Japan. *Prev Med* **6**:567–594 (1977).

Cross-sectional Studies

In going beyond descriptive observations to delve more deeply into disease etiology, there are, as defined in Chap. 4, three basic types of observational investigations:

1 Cross-sectional, or prevalence, studies
2 Case-control studies
3 Cohort, or incidence, studies

These will be discussed in greater detail here and in the next two chapters. As will be seen, cross-sectional studies are, conceptually, quite straightforward and provide a good basis for subsequent consideration and comparison of the two other study types.

How Cross-sectional Studies Are Carried Out

Initial Steps The question(s) for study must be clearly defined in terms of the relationship between some possible predisposing factor(s) and the disease under investigation. Next, a suitable study population is identified. If this population is small enough to be studied using the human and financial resources available (for example, students in a school, adults in a small town), the entire population can be included. If the target population is too large (for example, children in the United States, men in a large city), a representative sample is selected.

Sampling   Methods for selecting an appropriate sample constitute an important and well-developed field of statistical study and cannot be dealt with comprehensively in this book. The reader should be familiar with a few basic types of samples, since sampling may be necessary in any type of epidemiologic study. For a more complete discussion the reader is referred to Levy and Lemeshow (1980).

The most elementary kind of sample is a *simple random sample,* in which each person has an equal chance of being selected directly out of the entire population. One way to carry out this procedure is to assign each person a number, starting with 1, 2, 3, and so on. Then, numbers are selected at random, usually from a table of random numbers, until the desired sample size is attained.

A *stratified random sample* involves dividing the population into distinct subgroups according to some important characteristic, such as age or socioeconomic status, and selecting a random sample out of each subgroup. If the proportion of the sample drawn from each of the subgroups, or *strata,* is the same as the proportion of the total population contained in each stratum (for example, age group 40 to 59 constitutes 20 percent of the population, and 20 percent of the sample comes from this age stratum), then all strata will be fairly represented with regard to numbers of persons in the sample. This proportionality is often desirable and may simplify data analysis. On occasion, however, the investigator may have to take a larger proportion of the study sample out of one or a few sparsely populated strata in order to make available for study adequate numbers of subjects with certain important characteristics.

A *cluster sample* involves (1) dividing the population into subgroups, or *clusters,* that are not necessarily (and preferably not) homogeneous, as are strata, (2) drawing a random sample of the clusters, and (3) selecting all or a random sample of the persons in each cluster. When each cluster comprises persons in a localized geographic area, cluster sampling is especially useful for national surveys. It is obvious that many more persons can be studied for the same cost if they live in a few United States counties, than if they are scattered all over the country.

Finally, *systematic samples* involve first deciding what fraction of the population is to be studied—for example, one-half or one-tenth—and listing the population in order, perhaps as in a directory or on a series of index cards. Then, starting at the beginning of the list, every second or every tenth person (to continue our example) is selected. To sample in this manner, the investigator must be quite sure that the intervals do not correspond with any recurring pattern in the population. Consider what would happen if the population were made up of a series of married couples with the husband always listed first. Picking every fourth person would result in a sample of men only if one started with the first or third subject or of women only if one started with the second or fourth.

Sampling can be done in multiple stages, such as sampling within strata which are, in turn, within clusters. In this manner, sampling can become quite involved and require expert assistance in planning. Experience has also revealed subtle problems and biases that might not occur to the novice. Sampling by households is a good example. If there is no one home when the interviewer arrives, he or she should come back again rather than go to the house next door, because households with a person at home in the daytime tend to differ from those without. Similarly, the first house seen as one approaches a new block should not be routinely called upon, since persons in corner houses tend to differ from those in the middle of the block.

Data Collection   Once the total study population or sample is defined, the necessary data are collected. Presence of disease may be determined in a variety of ways. For example, in a small town, all or almost all the existing cases of a disease often can be found by contacting all the practicing physicians and reviewing hospital records. Or, the disease can be detected by a special examination of all the residents.

The presence of, or exposure to, the possible causative factors under investigation also should be determined by appropriate tests and measurements. For example, in assessing the possible role of inhaled factors, amount of cigarette smoking can be determined by interview, and air pollution levels in various places of living or work can be determined by appropriate measuring devices.

Data Analysis   The usual way to tabulate the data in a cross-sectional study is to subdivide the population according to the suspected predisposing factors being studied and compare the disease prevalence rates in each subgroup. If the relationship of chronic cough to number of cigarettes smoked is to be studied in a group of middle-aged men, then the group may be divided into appropriate smoking categories, such as: none, less than one-half pack per day, one-half pack or more but less than one pack, one pack or more but less than two packs, and two packs or more. The prevalence rate of chronic cough is then determined for each smoking subgroup and the rates in the subgroups are compared. Of course, before the rates are computed, specific criteria for "chronic cough" must be defined.

Interpretation

In general, the cross-sectional study will show the presence or absence of a relationship between the study variable(s) and existing disease. *Existing* disease, as contrasted with *developing* disease found in a cohort study, implies a need for caution, since existing cases may not be representative of all cases of the disease.

Consider coronary heart disease, for example. One of the important manifestations of coronary heart disease is sudden unexpected death. In a prevalence survey, cases of coronary heart disease showing sudden unexpected death as their first clinical manifestation will be missed because the duration of recognizable disease is so extremely short. It would indeed be remarkable if such an event happened to occur just at the moment the individual was taking the survey examination! From this extreme example it can readily be seen that the shorter the duration of the disease, whether it kills or is cured rapidly, the less chance the victim has of being detected in a one-time prevalence survey. It follows logically, then, that cases of long duration are overrepresented in a cross-sectional study. (This is demonstrated graphically in Prob. 6-2; be sure not to skip it.) The characteristics of these long-duration cases may, on the average, differ in a variety of ways from the characteristics of all cases of the disease being studied.

While we are considering the duration of illness of diseased persons in a prevalence study, it would be worthwhile to digress slightly and point out that there are two basic properties of a disease that are reflected in its prevalence. One is how much disease develops per unit of time, or *incidence;* the other is how long it lasts, or *duration.* In fact, under stable conditions, where the incidence and duration of a disease have remained constant over a period of time, the relationship between prevalence, incidence, and duration can be expressed, when prevalence is less than 10 percent, as a simple mathematical equation: Prevalence equals incidence times mean duration ($P = I\bar{d}$). Thus, if any one of the three measures is unknown, it can be computed from the other two, provided that conditions are stable, as mentioned.

Prevalence cases also can become unrepresentative of all cases when certain types of cases leave the community. Some affected persons may be institutionalized elsewhere or move to another city where there are special facilities for treatment and thus escape local surveillance procedures.

When interpreting the findings of a cross-sectional study, care must be taken to avoid assigning an unsubstantiated time sequence to an association between a trait or other factor and the disease. If it is found, for example, that cancer patients exhibit more anxiety or other emotional problems than the unaffected members of the population, it cannot be assumed that the anxiety preceded the cancer. After all, cancer patients may have good reason to be nervous or disturbed. In contrast, there would be no doubt about the cancer being preceded by such traits as eye color, blood type, or maternal exposure to radiation.

Example 1: Prevalence Studies of Chronic Respiratory Disease in Berlin, New Hampshire

In 1961, Ferris and Anderson (1962) carried out a cross-sectional study of chronic respiratory disease in relation to cigarette smoking and air pollution in Berlin, New Hampshire. This industrial town with almost 18,000 inhabitants is located in a valley near the Canadian border and is almost completely surrounded by mountains. The major industry and chief source of air pollution is a paper and pulp mill.

In this study, the investigators planned to diagnose three disease states—chronic bronchitis, bronchial asthma, and chronic obstructive lung disease—using simple pulmonary function tests and a standardized interview questionnaire about respiratory symptoms. These standardized methods for assessing pulmonary disease, developed and tested in Great Britain and already used in several studies, would permit a comparison of the findings in Berlin, New Hampshire, to those in British and other population groups. At that time there was great interest in the apparent disparity in the relative frequency of chronic bronchitis in Great Britain and the United States, and it was believed that differences in diagnostic criteria and fashions might have been at least partially responsible.

The investigators, in cooperation with the local health department, selected the study sample in two stages. First, using the town's tax roll book, which listed the adults in alphabetical order, they randomly selected 36 pages (clusters). Second, from the 36 pages they systematically selected every second name of those in the 25- to 54-year age stratum and all names of persons aged 55 to 69. Persons aged 70 and over were listed separately in the town records, and a sample of this age stratum was randomly selected.

Before any data were collected, the local physicians and the state health department were contacted and the study was publicized by newspaper and radio. The study subjects were invited by letter to take the study examination at a clinic in the health department. Failure to respond led to a telephoned invitation. If this, in turn, failed, the subject was visited at home and, if the subject agreed, the interview and physiologic testing were carried out there. Through these persistent efforts, over 95 percent of the 1261 selected subjects were examined, with the only nonparticipants being those who were away from home during the survey and a few who refused.

An account of respiratory symptoms was elicited by the standardized interview. Smoking habits, occupational exposures, and previous chest illnesses were also assessed in the interview. Forced expiratory volume, both total (FEV) and during the first second (FEV_1), and peak flow were measured with a recording spirometer.

The presence of disease was defined by strict criteria. For example, the diagnosis of chronic bronchitis required "the report of bringing up phlegm from the chest six times a day on four days a week for three months in a year, for the past three years or more."

Data analysis revealed a greater prevalence of respiratory disease in men than in women. Furthermore, there was a clear relationship of respiratory disease to smoking. For example, in men the age-adjusted prevalence of chronic bronchitis was:

15.0% in those who had never smoked
18.9% in ex-smokers
29.8% in smokers of 1 to 10 cigarettes per day
34.2% in smokers of 11 to 20 cigarettes per day
42.3% in smokers of 21 to 30 cigarettes per day
61.1% in smokers of 31 to 40 cigarettes per day
75.3% in smokers of 41 or more cigarettes per day

The town was divided into areas with low, intermediate, and high degrees of air pollution, according to independent measurements of air quality. Residence of study subjects in these three areas showed only an equivocal relationship to respiratory disease. However, if only male nonsmokers were considered, it appeared that chronic bronchitis was more apt to be found in subjects who lived in residential areas having greater air pollution.

The planned United States—British comparison was later reported by Reid et al. (1964). The findings in Berlin, New Hampshire, were compared with those derived from a random sample of urban and rural adults in Britain examined in a comparable fashion. It was found that the British exceeded the Americans very little in the prevalence of simple chronic bronchitis, characterized by chronic cough and sputum production. However, bronchitis complicated by shortness of breath and repeated acute illnesses was more prevalent in Britain, particularly among urban men.

The prevalence survey in Berlin, New Hampshire, was repeated in 1967 using comparable methods (Ferris et al., 1971). It was noted that the prevalence of respiratory disease symptoms was lower in 1967 and that, on the average, there was some improvement in pulmonary function. Because there also had been a fall in air pollution between 1961 and 1967, the authors concluded that this was the probable explanation for the observed improvement. In their analysis they were careful to consider other possible explanations for the change, such as observer differences and the increasing use of filter-tip cigarettes.

The second survey in 1967 illustrates the usefulness of repeated prevalence studies in assessing time trends in disease or other population characteristics, provided that comparable measurement methods are used. The effort and expense of keeping a population under continuous long-term surveillance often can be avoided by conducting careful cross-sectional studies at fairly wide intervals.

The 1967 sample was resurveyed in 1973 to determine whether the changes in the nature of the local air pollution, such as a decrease in suspended particulates, had had any effect on pulmonary function or on the prevalence of chronic respiratory disease or symptoms. No such effect could be demonstrated (Ferris et al., 1976).

Example 2: Cardiovascular Disease in Evans County, Georgia

In Chaps. 4 and 5, emphasis has been placed on descriptive epidemiologic findings as a source of hypotheses for further analytic studies. Another very important source of ideas and hypotheses has been clinical observations by astute and concerned health care professionals. A physician's observations and interest proved to be a major stimulus for the epidemiologic study of cardiovascular disease in Evans County, Georgia, which began in 1960 as a prevalence study (Cassel, 1971a and b; Hames, 1971; McDonough et al., 1965).

Dr. Curtis Hames, who practiced in the area, was impressed with the difference in frequency with which he found coronary heart disease occurring in whites and blacks. Although coronary heart disease was a common problem in his white patients, he rarely saw it in blacks, despite the fact that many black patients had hypertension and appeared to consume a high animal-fat diet. Furthermore, the male-female difference in susceptibility to coronary heart disease which was so obvious in whites was not apparent in blacks.

To confirm and explain these differences in a systematic fashion, Hames encouraged the interest and participation of epidemiologists and other investigators. Largely due to his excellent rapport with the community, there was nearly complete participation of the selected study subjects.

Evans County is located on flat or slightly rolling terrain about 60 miles inland from the coastal port of Savannah, Georgia; its greatest diameter is 19 miles. The county's economy was, in 1960, primarily agricultural, although its extensive pine forests were a source of lumber, pulpwood, and turpentine. In 1960, the total population was 6952, of which 66.5 percent were white and 33.5 percent were black.

The study sample consisted of a 50 percent random selection of county residents aged 15 to 39 and all residents aged 40 and over. Of the 3377 persons chosen, 92 percent underwent the study examination, which consisted of a medical and dietary history, physical examination, urinalysis, serum cholesterol measurement, electrocardiogram, and chest x-ray. The social class standing of each subject was determined according to the occupation, education, and source of income of the head of the household.

The diagnosis of coronary heart disease required that a subject have either a history of angina pectoris or a history or electrocardiographic evidence of myocardial infarction. Each of these manifestations was defined as definite, probable, possible, or absent according to standard criteria. It is essential for investigators to establish, adhere to, and describe in study reports strict criteria for the diagnosis of disease so that others may know just what kinds of cases were included or excluded. Strict criteria also permit other investigators to reproduce the study findings or at least to understand why their own study results might differ.

The major findings of the Evans County prevalence study included confirmation of the initial clinical observations. Coronary heart disease prevalence was indeed lower in blacks than in whites, the difference occurring only in men. Part of this black-white difference could be explained by social class, since white men of lower socioeconomic status had coronary heart disease prevalence rates approaching the low levels in blacks, almost all of whom were in the lower social bracket. The age-adjusted prevalence rates were:

97 per 1000 in high-social-class whites
40 per 1000 in low-social-class whites
21 per 1000 blacks

The investigators could not explain these racial and social class differences by taking into account differences in other risk factors, including blood pressure, serum cholesterol levels, body weight, cigarette smoking, and dietary intake. However, it was noted that habitual physical activity, as estimated by type of occupation, was inversely related to coronary heart disease prevalence. Men in occupations involving the most physical exertion (for example, manual labor, sharecropping) showed the lowest prevalence of coronary heart disease. Since these occupations were primarily engaged in by blacks and low-social-class whites, it appeared that physical activity might explain their relatively low prevalence of coronary heart disease.

As with the Berlin, New Hampshire, study described above, a second examination procedure was carried out several years later, beginning in 1967. However, this was *not* for the purpose of repeating the cross-sectional study. Rather, the second round of examinations was applied only to the initially examined cohort as part of the follow-up for a cohort study. An initial prevalence survey can be, and often is, used as the first stage of a cohort study, in that it defines and characterizes a *population at risk*—those initially free of the disease being studied. As will be described in Chap. 8, this population at risk can then be followed up for the development of the disease.

The cohort study confirmed the black-white difference in the occurrence of coronary heart disease, but the social class difference in whites was no longer evident. It appeared that this was due to a rapid catching up of the lower-class men to the upper-class men in coronary heart disease risk, during a period when Evans County was changing from an agrarian to an industrial economy. The only subgroup of white men with the same low risk as the blacks were sharecroppers, again suggesting a protective effect of high levels of physical activity.

Exploration of the lower risk of coronary heart disease among blacks has continued to be a major focus of investigation in the

Evans County population. Later findings include black-white differences in lipids and lipoproteins, with blacks having relatively higher levels of HDL-cholesterol (cholesterol in high-density lipoproteins, associated with low risk of coronary heart disease) and whites having relatively higher levels of LDL-cholesterol (cholesterol in low-density lipoproteins, associated with high risk of coronary heart disease). These differences were independent of occupation and social class (Tyroler et al., 1975, 1982). Blacks were also found to have higher levels than whites of fibrinolytic activity in the blood (Szczeklik et al., 1980), which may help to prevent blockage of blood vessels by thrombosis. Nevertheless, black men had a considerably higher risk of developing electrocardiographic left ventricular hypertrophy (Arnett et al., 1992), and this and other electrocardiographic abnormalities conveyed a risk of mortality in black men similar to that found in white men (Strogatz et al., 1987).

Problems

6-1 Specify whether each of the following sampling plans constitutes a simple random sample, a stratified random sample, a cluster sample, or a systematic sample.

    a A sample of students in a high school is chosen as follows: Two students are selected from each classroom by having all in the room draw straws and picking those with the two shortest straws.

    b A target population for a telephone survey is picked by selecting 10 pages from a telephone directory by means of a table of random numbers and calling every person listed on the 10 pages.

    c The number 803 is the first three-digit random number produced by a computer operating under a random number–generating program. A sample of automobile drivers in a state is selected by picking all those whose driver's license number ends with the three digits 803.

    d One die (of a pair of dice) is rolled to decide which one of the six soldiers who volunteered will go on a dangerous mission.

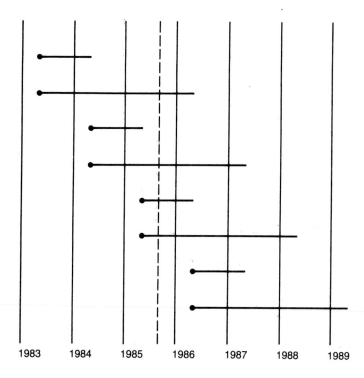

Figure 6-1

6-2 In Fig. 6-1 each horizontal line represents the duration of a case of disease, beginning at the left with a dot. In this simple example one 1-year case and one 3-year case begin in April of every year. Only the cases beginning from 1983 to 1986 are shown. A prevalence, or cross-sectional, study was conducted in September 1985, as represented by the vertical broken line.

   a What was the prevalence of the disease at the time of the study, assuming a population of 100 persons?

   b What was the incidence of the disease in each year from 1983 to 1986, again assuming a population at risk of 100 persons?

   c By the formula $P = I\bar{d}$ compute the mean duration of the disease. How does this compare with the mean duration computed directly by adding up the durations of all eight cases shown and dividing by 8?

d What proportion of all cases shown were 3-year (long-duration) cases? What proportion of cases included in the cross-sectional study were 3-year (long-duration) cases? What principle do these proportions illustrate?

6-3 Improved therapy of childhood leukemia has considerably lengthened the average survival time in recent years. What has this done to the prevalence of the disease? Do you regard prevalence as a good index for comparing two nations with respect to their risk of developing a disease? Explain your answer.

6-4 How can a cross-sectional study serve as the initial phase of a cohort study? Think of two important objectives it can accomplish.

BIBLIOGRAPHY

Arnett DK, Strogatz DS, Ephross SA, Hames CG, Tyroler HA: Greater incidence of electrocardiographic left ventricular hypertrophy in black men than in white men in Evans County, Georgia. *Ethn Dis* **2:**10–17 (1992).

Cassel JC: Summary of major findings of the Evans County cardiovascular studies. *Arch Intern Med* **128:**887–889 (1971a).

————: Review of the 1960 through 1962 cardiovascular disease prevalence study. *Arch Intern Med* **128:**890–895 (1971b).

Ferris BG, Jr, Anderson DO: The prevalence of chronic respiratory disease in a New Hampshire town. *Am Rev Respir Dis* **86:**165–177 (1962).

Ferris BG, Jr, Chen H, Puleo S, Murphy RLH: Chronic nonspecific respiratory disease in Berlin, New Hampshire, 1967 to 1973. A further follow-up study. *Am Rev Respir Dis* **113:**475–485 (1976).

Ferris BG, Jr, Higgins ITT, Higgins MW, Peters JM, van Ganse WF, Goldman MD: Chronic nonspecific respiratory disease, Berlin, New Hampshire, 1961–1967: A cross-sectional study. *Am Rev Respir Dis* **104:**232–244 (1971).

Hames CG: Evans County cardiovascular and cerebrovascular epidemiologic study: Introduction. *Arch Intern Med* **128:**883–886 (1971).

Levy PS, Lemeshow S: *Sampling for Health Professionals* (Belmont, Calif.: Lifetime Learning Publications, 1980).

McDonough JR, Hames CG, Stulb SC, Garrison GE: Coronary heart disease among Negroes and whites in Evans County, Georgia. *J Chron Dis* **18**:443–468 (1965).

Reid DD, Anderson DO, Ferris BG, Jr, Fletcher CM: An Anglo-American comparison of the prevalence of bronchitis. *Br Med J* **2**:1487–1491 (1964).

Strogatz DS, Tyroler HA, Watkins LO, Hames CG: Electrocardiographic abnormalities and mortality among middle-aged black men and white men of Evans County, Georgia. *J Chronic Dis* **40**:140–155 (1987).

Szczeklik A, Dischinger P, Kueppers F, Tyroler HA, Hames CG, Cassel JC, Creagan S: Blood fibrinolytic activity, social class and habitual physical activity: II. A study of black and white men in southern Georgia. *J Chron Dis* **33**:291–299 (1980).

Tyroler HA, Hames CG, Krishan I, Heyden S, Cooper G, Cassel JC: Black-white differences in serum lipids and lipoproteins in Evans County. *Prev Med* **4**:541–549 (1975).

Tyroler HA, Schoenfeld G, Heiss G, Hames CG: Population correlates of HDL apolipoproteins, in G Noseda, C Fragiacomo, R Fumagalli, R Paoletti (eds.), *Lipoproteins and Coronary Atherosclerosis* (Amsterdam: Elsevier, 1982), pp. 95–102.

Chapter 7

Case-Control Studies

Case-control studies are closely related to cross-sectional studies if the cases used are those that exist at one point in time; or they are related to cohort studies if, as is generally preferred, the cases are new or *incident* cases accumulated over a period of time. However, because they generally involve fewer and often more readily accessible subjects, case-control studies are much more often carried out. Among analytic studies, they are usually the first approach used to determine whether a particular personal characteristic or environmental factor is related to disease occurrence.

How Case-Control Studies Are Carried Out

Identification and Collection of Cases Once the study objectives and methods have been clearly defined, the first step in a case-control study is the identification of the cases, or diseased persons, to be studied. (Many rightfully object to the use of the term *case* to refer to a sick human being. Although this dehumanizing term should be avoided in the clinical setting, its use in a research context facilitates clear communication and does not imply any lack of sympathy or concern about the ill.)

As mentioned previously in connection with cross-sectional studies, it is important to set up criteria for the diagnosis and inclusion of cases in the investigation and to describe these criteria carefully when the study is finally reported. It is usually advisable to require objective evidence and documentation of the disease, even if, as a result, some cases will have to be omitted and the size of the case group reduced. Thus, for a study of renal calculi, it may be best to insist that all included cases have stones documented by x-ray evidence or removal by surgery, not diagnosed only by the presence of renal colic. By accepting less well documented cases, the investigator runs the risk of diluting his or her case group with some noncases and lessening the chances of finding differences between the case group and the control group.

This recommendation, of course, applies to disease identification for all types of studies, not just case-control studies. However, as was stressed in the last section of Chap. 3, *misclassification* of a few nondiseased persons as cases and of a few diseased persons as controls, no matter how distressing to the clinician, will probably not prevent the discovery of major case-control differences.

The cases may be identified or *ascertained* by a community-wide search, which is greatly facilitated if a registry of the disease is available. Often cases are ascertained in one or more hospitals, clinics, medical centers, and more recently in health maintenance organizations that provide comprehensive medical care to defined populations of subscribers. The case group will usually be limited to those first diagnosed during a particular time period. For example, one may decide to study all cases of well-documented renal stones initially detected at a particular hospital during the 2-year period, January 1, 1994, to December 31, 1995.

Usually, the inclusion of all patients who meet the diagnostic criteria and the time and place specifications is not possible for a variety of reasons. Some patients will have moved away or died and some will refuse to cooperate; or, some hospital records may be lost so that certain essential information is not available to the investigator. The investigator should report how many cases met the initial criteria for inclusion and how many were finally included. The reasons for omitting cases and the number omitted for each reason should be stated.

When possible, a study should include only incident cases, those which first develop or which are first diagnosed during the period of data collection. This avoids the unrepresentativeness of prevalent cases, discussed with regard to cross-sectional studies in Chap. 6. By using only new cases and selecting controls to be representative of persons at risk for developing the disease, the case-control study aims to identify factors responsible for disease *development,* much like a cohort study. Unfortunately, although more appropriate for study, incident cases are sometimes too few in number to provide reliable findings, especially when the disease is very rare. Also, for some chronic diseases such as hypertension, there may be insurmountable difficulties in specifying a meaningful date of onset, again necessitating the study of prevalent cases. Then, careful consideration should be given to whether a factor associated with prevalent disease increases the duration of disease instead of, or in addition to, causing or predicting its development.

Selection of Control Subjects   Deciding who will constitute the control group or groups is perhaps the most difficult decision to be made in planning a case-control study, and it requires a good deal of skill and judgment. In a cross-sectional, or cohort, study this problem does not arise since the cases may be compared with the entire nonaffected portion of the population. In settling for the simple low-cost case-control study the investigator hopes that almost as much can be learned about the relationship of the disease to other variables by comparing a group of cases and a group of controls. It would be ideal for the controls to be a sample of the population from which the cases are derived, that is, to be representative of the people who would have been in the case group had they developed the disease under study. If this is not feasible, one tries to approach this ideal as closely as possible.

General Principles   One of the most important considerations in selecting controls involves the information to be collected concerning study variables or potential etiologic factors. There should be no major differences between case and control groups with respect to the quality or availability of this information. Availability of information implies both (1) how much information is obtained concerning each case and control, and (2) what proportions of the case and control groups will, or can, supply it. Equal access to important information previously recorded in a similar fashion for both cases and controls—for example, birth weight recorded in the same hospital—may strongly favor the use of a particular control group. If data have to be obtained by interview, then one worries that quality or availability of information may differ due to differences between cases and controls in emotional state, knowledge of the disease studied, educational or socioeconomic status, and location of the interview (for example, at home or in a hospital).

Consideration of the *known* sources of bias in quality and quantity of information about cases and controls and of the fact that there are often biases which are *unknown* usually leads the investigator to seek controls who are generally similar to the cases, except for the essential difference in whether the disease under investigation is present or absent. Yet, this striving for general similarity should not be carried to the point where there is little or no hope of finding case-control differences in the factors under study. For example, by selecting the controls so that they are of similar educational background to the cases, one will minimize case-control differences in the understanding of a printed questionnaire. But this selection procedure will also preclude the study of the relation of educational level to the disease and may seriously impair case-control comparisons of factors related to education, such as socioeconomic status.

When controls are chosen so as to be similar to the cases for a characteristic and when this tends to mask a disease's association with another characteristic of interest, the cases and controls are said to be *overmatched.* This can happen when controls are matched to the cases for a characteristic that is correlated with the possible cause of disease under study but is either not an independent cause of the disease or is part of the pathway through which the possible cause of interest leads to disease (Breslow and Day, 1980). Assume that low socioeconomic status leads to a disease through reduced consumption of fresh fruit. In the above example, matching for educational level is overmatching because low educational level, a correlate of low socioeconomic status, does not in itself lead to the disease. If we matched for fresh fruit consumption, our study of socioeconomic status and the disease would also be overmatched and the relation would be obscured because fruit consumption is "down the causal chain" between socioeconomic status and disease. Overmatching is also said to exist when matching reduces the statistical reliability or increases the cost of a study (Schlesselman, 1982; Rothman, 1986).

In selecting a control group two major questions must be answered:

1 From what source(s) will controls be drawn?
2 What will be the method of selection of controls from the source(s)?

These decisions must take into account the need, mentioned above, for controls that are generally similar, but not too similar, to the cases, plus some very practical considerations—in particular, the control groups that are potentially available and the human and financial resources that can be used for the study.

Selecting a Source of Controls Many sources of controls have been used, including:

1 Patients within the same medical care facility
  a Without regard to their diagnosis
  b Excluding those with certain diseases
  c Including only those with certain diseases believed to be unrelated to the causal factors to be investigated
  d Examined and found to be healthy
2 Persons drawn from outside the facility
  a Sample of general community
  b Sample of members of health maintenance organizations from which cases are derived
  c Friends or acquaintances
  d Fellow employees
  e Neighbors
  f Family members such as spouses or siblings

When one is faced with the practical decision about which source of controls to use, reasons for and against any potential source can usually be mustered, and the reasons the source chosen might have given biased results will be heard from critics after the study is reported. For example, the investigator may decide to select controls for hospitalized renal calculus cases from herniorrhaphy cases in the same hospital, since that hospital serves a particular socioeconomic and ethnic segment of the community, and since, after the acute pain has subsided, the mental status of a kidney stone patient should not be very different from that of a hernia patient (as contrasted with a patient, say, with a stroke or terminal cancer). Yet if an important difference between kidney stone patients and their hernia controls is found, there will usually be the lingering question of whether the difference is related to kidney stones or to hernias. Therefore, it is frequently helpful to have a diagnostically heterogeneous control group or more than one control group, if possible. Similarly, repetition of the study by other investigators in other settings will usually reveal whether some underlying truth about renal calculi has been discovered. MacMahon and Pugh (1970) and Schlesselman (1982) have thoroughly discussed many of these important issues and other factors to be considered in selecting controls.

Selecting Control Subjects from the Source   Selection of the control group from the chosen source usually involves sampling. If resources are limited, the control group will usually be about equal in size to the case group, or, if necessary, smaller than the case group. If resources permit the inclusion of more study subjects but no more cases are available, the control group may be enlarged to decrease sampling variation. For example, the control group may be made 2 or 3 times as large as the case group. Substantial reductions in sampling variation can be achieved by adding more controls—up to about 5 or 6 times as many controls as cases. Beyond five or six per case, additional controls provide little additional reliability.

As already noted, selecting a source places some general limitations on the nature of the control group. In addition, when individual controls are chosen from the source, the investigator will often *match* the controls to the cases with regard to some important characteristics such as age or sex. By matching for a particular characteristic, the investigator tries to eliminate a case-control difference in this characteristic as a possible contributor to a case-control difference in a study variable. While this approach is intuitively appealing, it does not always achieve this objective in case-control studies, and matching must be used with discretion (Rothman, 1986).

Controls are often picked individually, in a *paired* fashion. That is, for each case, one or more controls are picked in some systematic fashion according to preset rules or criteria. In a study of renal calculi, it may be decided to include as controls other urological patients who have no urinary tract stones and no obvious mental impairment due to uremia or other cause and who are matched to the cases with regard to age, sex, race, and date of admission. The selection of an individually matched control for each case might involve selecting the first patient admitted to the urological service after the case who meets the diagnostic and mental status criteria, who is of the same sex and race as the case, and whose age differs by no more than 5 years from that of the case. Some leeway is necessary in matching for quantitative variables such as age and admission date or else no match will be found for most cases. Failure to find matched controls will also occur frequently if matching is attempted on more than a few characteristics.

Another form of matching sometimes used is known as *frequency matching*. Here the investigator does not attempt to match controls to cases individually, but selects controls so as to keep their number with a particular characteristic equal to, or in proportion to, the number of cases with that characteristic. Thus, if the cases consist of 20 persons in their forties, 40 in their fifties, and 70 in their sixties, controls might be selected to have 20, 40, and 70, or perhaps 40, 80, and 140 (twice as many) persons in these respective age decades. Like individual matching, frequency matching helps ensure that the cases can be compared with sufficient numbers of controls in each stratum of the matching variable to provide statistically reliable findings. If there were 70 cases and, say, only 3 controls in their sixties, one could not place much reliance on the contrast in this age group.

A method for identifying general population controls that has become popular is random digit dialing (Waksberg, 1978). Telephone numbers in the community where the cases arose are dialed, often by first selecting at random a "block" of 100 numbers with the same area code and first five digits, and then randomly selecting the last two digits to call one number and then others in the block if the first proves to be nonresidential. When suitable controls are found to reside in the households reached, they are recruited, and if cooperative, they are interviewed or tested in like manner to the cases. This procedure is not as easy as it sounds and entails much cost and effort. Of course, the subjects—controls by necessity and cases for comparability—must have telephones. Unless one is careful, subtle biases can occur with this method of control selection (Greenberg, 1990).

If the disease being studied is known to be uncommon in the group serving as a source for controls, then little, if any, diagnostic effort or documentation is needed to rule out the disease in the selected controls. A simple interview question will often suffice. However, if the disease could occur commonly in controls, a greater effort to rule it out, such as a review of the medical chart, is desirable to minimize misclassification.

Data Collection   Any source of data about the study variables may be used. As has been mentioned, accurate information collected on both cases and controls before the disease developed is ideal. Collecting information after the disease develops may be necessary, but every effort should be made to avoid qualitative and quantitative case-control differences in the data gathered. For example, if possible, the research assistant(s) recording laboratory data for all study subjects should do so without knowing whether particular individuals are cases or controls. Similarly, it may often be desirable to structure data-collecting interviews to avoid discussing disease status altogether or at least until the questions about etiologic variables have been asked.

Data Analysis   Traditionally, the basic case-control comparison is expressed in terms of the proportion of cases versus the proportion of controls who show a particular characteristic. If the characteristic is a quantitative rather than a qualitative "yes or no" attribute, then its distribution in the cases and controls can be compared, as can the important features of distribution, such as the mean, standard deviation, and median.

In considering an attribute as a possible factor in the etiology of a disease it is often more meaningful or natural to express the relationship of the attribute to the disease as it is expressed in a cohort study—that is, as a comparison of the disease rate in those with and without the attribute. Unfortunately, disease incidence rates are not directly obtainable from case-control studies. However, simple methods are available for deriving the easily understood *rate comparisons,* both *relative risk* and *attributable fraction* (defined in Chap. 2), from case-control data.

Case-control studies ordinarily estimate relative risks and rate ratios by the odds ratio, which approximates them closely when the disease is relatively rare. This is true of most chronic diseases, which occur in less than 5 percent of ordinary populations over several years of observation. In recent years it has been recognized that if controls are selected with due respect to the time of disease development in the cases, the classical "rare disease assumption" is not required. Instantaneous rate ratios can be estimated directly if controls are selected to be at risk at the time that each case is diagnosed. Cumulative risk ratios can be estimated directly if controls are sampled from all individuals in the source population that gave rise to the cases, including those who became cases (Rodrigues and Kirkwood, 1990). Nevertheless, odds ratios are most frequently reported and should be understood by all health care professionals.

The odds ratio method for estimating relative risk from case-control studies ignores any prior matching of controls to cases. The odds ratio, or relative odds, is readily determined by the following formula:

$$\text{Odds ratio} = \frac{\text{(no. of cases with characteristic)}}{\text{(no. of cases without characteristic)}}$$

$$\times \frac{\text{(no. of controls without characteristic)}}{\text{(no. of controls with characteristic)}}$$

In Table 7-1 the numbers involved are represented by the letters *a, b, c,* and *d;* thus, in this case the odds ratio is *ad/bc.* A specific example, involving 100 cases and 100 controls, is shown by the

Table 7-1   Results of a Case-Control Study; Matching (If Done) Not Considered*

Attribute	Cases	Controls
Present	a(20)	c(10)
Absent	b(80)	d(90)
Total	(100)	(100)

* Letters a, b, c, d represent numbers of subjects; numbers in parentheses represent specific example described in text.

numbers in parentheses in Table 7-1. The characteristic is present in 20 cases and 10 controls; therefore the odds ratio is $(20 \times 90)/(80 \times 10) = 2.25$. From these case-control data we can say that persons with the characteristic have 2.25 times the chance of developing the disease as those without it.

An even simpler method for estimating relative risk is available if the controls are matched to the cases. In that event, a fourfold table can be set up to describe case-control *pairs,* as shown in Table 7-2. The relative risk is approximated by the ratio b/c, where b is the number of case-control pairs in which *only* the case has the characteristic and c is the number of pairs in which *only* the control has the characteristic. Surprisingly, the information necessary to compute the odds ratio is all contained in the data from these discordant pairs; the other pairs can be ignored. The numbers in parentheses in Table 7-2 constitute a rearrangement of the data in Table 7-1 into one possible set of results for matched pairs.

In this example the relative risk estimate, 18/8, is again 2.25. In real life the results of the two methods do not usually agree so exactly. Generally, the unmatched analysis of matched data gives estimates of relative risk that are biased in the direction of a weaker association (for example, see Prob. 7-2).

The reader interested in further discussion of relative risk estimates from case-control studies should refer to the literature summarized in Rodrigues and Kirkwood (1990) and the classic studies of Mantel and Haenszel (1959), and Cornfield (1951).

Table 7-2   Results of a Case-Control Study Based on Matched Pairs*

Attribute in the case	Attribute in the control	
	Present	Absent
Present	$a(2)$	$b(18)$
Absent	$c(8)$	$d(72)$

*Letters, a, b, c, d represent numbers of pairs; numbers in parentheses represent specific example described in text.

Case-control estimates of attributable fraction are discussed by Schlesselman (1982) and Cole and MacMahon (1971). In brief, the estimated attributable fraction in the exposed is $(r-1)/r$ where r is the relative risk estimate. Correspondingly, the population attributable fraction is $[p(r-1)]/[p(r-1) + 1]$ where p is the proportion of the population exposed. If population exposure data are not available, the proportion of the control group that was exposed may be used for p in the formula.

Interpretation and Some Cautions

If the cases show a higher proportion with an attribute than do the controls (i.e., relative risk greater than 1), or if the distributions or mean levels of an attribute differ, then there is an observed association between the attribute and the disease. Interpreting whether this association implies a cause-and-effect relationship is another matter, involving a number of considerations to be discussed in Chap. 11.

It should also be emphasized that the nature of the cases studied is influenced by their source. For example, cases derived only from a hospital, and not from outpatient clinics as well, may have the most severe form of a disease. Thus, while we have emphasized the problems of control groups, the characteristics of the case group must also be carefully considered in study design and interpretation.

Although matching is an appealingly simple and straightforward method of controlling for extraneous or confounding variables (discussed in Chap. 11), it can introduce unexpected complications and biases into a case-control study. Thus, matching should not be done if it does not contribute in some important way, and if done, a matched-pair or matched-set analysis, like that shown in Table 7-2, should be performed. Problems associated with matching have been thoroughly discussed by Schlesselman (1982) and Rothman (1986).

Example 1: Oral Contraceptives and Thromboembolic Disease

Millions of women now take oral contraceptive tablets to prevent pregnancy. Several questions concerning the safety of these agents have arisen. One major area of concern has been whether oral contraceptives predispose to thromboembolic conditions, particularly thrombophlebitis and its possibly fatal sequela, pulmonary embolism. Following the publication of some clinical case reports in the early 1960s it became apparent that epidemiologic studies were necessary to determine whether women who take oral contraceptives are indeed at greater risk of developing these diseases.

Thrombophlebitis and pulmonary embolism *not* secondary to trauma, surgery, or childbirth develop rather rarely in women during the reproductive years. Thus a cross-sectional or a cohort study of this question seemed impractical, at least as a first approach, since finding an adequate sample of cases would have required the study of many thousands of women. Case-control investigations were therefore undertaken, in both Great Britain and the United States. The United States study by Sartwell and his associates (1969) is an excellent example of the case-control method.

The investigators decided to include as cases women aged 15 to 44 who had been hospitalized with thromboembolic conditions and discharged alive within the previous 3 years. It was necessary to collect the cases from a large number of hospitals to obtain an adequate sample size. All told, there were 48 participating hospitals in five large eastern cities: Baltimore, New York, Philadelphia, Pittsburgh, and Washington, D.C. Cases were excluded from the study if they also had a chronic condition possibly predisposing to thromboembolism, such as diabetes mellitus or hypertension, or a recent precipitating event, such as surgery, pregnancy, trauma, localized infection, or prolonged inactivity. Reasonable medical evidence for thromboembolism was required, and all cases were reviewed independently by two physicians.

The derivation of the final study group of 175 cases was carefully described by the authors and clearly shows the marked attrition that often occurs between *potential* and *actual* numbers of study subjects. In all, 2648 women in the desired age range with thromboembolic conditions within the 3-year period were identified and their hospital records were abstracted. The vast majority of these cases, 2288, were immediately rejected because of having possibly predisposing conditions, and another 99 were rejected for other reasons, such as sterility (which obviates contraceptive use), death, or having moved from the area. Of the 261 women selected as suitable cases, 72 had to be dropped because the interview could not be obtained, and another 14 were excluded because no interview could be obtained from their matched control subjects.

Two matched controls were selected for each case with the expectation that if one could not be interviewed the alternate control would still be available, thus yielding data on one control per case. Matching was based on several criteria:

Hospital	same as case
Sex	all women
Discharge date	same 6-month interval as that of case
Discharge status	all alive
Age	same 5-year span
Marital status	same
Residence	(not stated but presumably the same metropolitan area)
Race	same
Parity	same general class, that is, no pregnancies, one or two pregnancies, three or more pregnancies
Hospital pay status	ward, semiprivate, or private room

Also, controls were excluded in the same manner as the cases, that is, for chronic diseases possibly predisposing to thromboembolism or for sterility. Most control subjects turned out to have acute medical and surgical illnesses, conditions treated by elective surgery, or traumatic injuries.

Cases and controls were interviewed at home. A variety of questions were asked concerning pertinent variables, such as religion, educational level, and smoking habits. To elicit information about contraceptive use, cases and controls were asked to select from a list of 13 methods those which they had used within the 2-year period before they were hospitalized.

Data analysis showed that the overall frequency of employment of *any* birth control method was similar in the 175 cases and controls—114 and 101 users of at least one method, respectively—and many women had used more than one method during the 2-year period. While the case-control differences in proportions using each of the other methods were small and not statistically significant, cases did report using oral contraceptives significantly more often than did controls—67 versus 30 women, or 38 percent versus 17 percent.

Using the matched-pair formula to compute relative risk, the investigators found that users of oral contraceptives were about 4 times as likely as nonusers to develop thromboembolic conditions. Furthermore it could be shown that about one-fourth of the total cases would be attributable to oral contraceptive usage if a cause-and-effect relationship were involved. It was, of course, carefully pointed out that the cases studied were a highly selected group, that is, free of predisposing conditions, unlike most thromboembolism cases.

Further analysis showed that the case-control differences in oral contraceptive use were present in the major subgroups of the study subjects, when the total group was subdivided by such variables as age and marital status. The case-control differences were found for several different thromboembolic conditions including deep thrombophlebitis of the lower extremity, pulmonary embolism, and intracranial vascular conditions.

This and other studies established the increased risk of thromboembolic disease associated with the use of oral contraceptives as originally formulated. Newer birth control pills contain lower and presumably safer doses of hormones. Case-control investigations of the safety of these newer preparations are still being carried out.

Example 2: Pedestrians Fatally Injured by Motor Vehicles

In their concern with learning about the diseases that present complex diagnostic or pathophysiologic problems, medical personnel are apt to forget that injuries and death due to gross physical trauma are major health problems in affluent industrialized societies as well as in "less-developed" areas. In particular, accidents are the leading cause of death in children and young adults in the United States. Automobile accidents lead all other types as a cause of death.

The word *accident* implies that physical injuries produced by automobiles and other energy sources are haphazard and uncontrollable. Among those arguing against this fatalistic concept, Haddon advocated the use of carefully designed and implemented epidemiologic studies as a means of identifying factors responsible for traumatic injuries, so that appropriate preventive measures can be instituted. His research group's interesting study of the characteristics of pedestrians fatally injured by motor vehicles in New York City is an example of the imaginative use of the case-control method to attack a serious and poorly understood problem (Haddon et al., 1961).

At the time of the study in 1959, little was known about pedestrian-associated, or *host,* factors related to being struck and killed by a car. Substantial funds were being expended for public education programs and other means of "pedestrian control," without much evidence that these were effective preventive measures. Previous findings that many fatally injured pedestrians had been drinking heavily had not been evaluated in comparison to the alcohol consumption of the population at risk or, more simply, to that of noninjured pedestrians. Likewise, the age distribution of killed pedestrians, with relatively high percentages of young children and elderly adults, had not been compared with the age distribution of all or of nonkilled pedestrians, to determine whether the *mortality rate,* or risk of being killed, is actually greater in very young and very old pedestrians. Thus, age and blood-alcohol concentration were included among several characteristics that were measured in fatally injured pedestrians and their matched controls in the study to be described.

Manhattan was an appropriate place for this investigation. Pedestrian deaths were relatively frequent, and they accounted for about 70 percent of all fatalities in motor vehicle accidents. The case series consisted of 50 adults (18 years of age or older) who were struck and killed by automobiles in Manhattan between May 3, 1959, and November 7, 1959. Autopsy confirmation of the cause of death was required. Of 57 cases initially considered, the 7 omissions consisted of 2 who were killed by bicycles, 1 who was purposely pushed into the path of a car, 1 with unknown site or time of the accident, 1 who died of a coronary occlusion while convalescing from the accident, and 2 who were omitted because of clerical errors.

Four matched controls were selected for each case by visiting each accident site at a later date but on the same day of the week and as close as possible to the time of day when the accident occurred. All but eight site visits for control selection were completed within 6 weeks of the accident. Thus, controls were matched to the cases for accident site and time. In addition, controls were matched to the accident cases for sex and were limited, as were the cases, to adults.

The practical problems involved in this form of "shoe-leather" epidemiology can best be communicated by the investigators' own description of the control selection and interview procedures.

The site visits were made by a team of two or three of the authors and one to four medical students working at each location with one or two uniformed members of the Police Department Accident Investigation Squad (A.I.S.).

In visiting each site one of three basic approaches was used. In the first type, that used in many busy neighborhoods, for example, opposite Grand Central Station on a weekday at 6:10 p.m., the entire team arrived and immediately stopped the *first* 4 adult pedestrians of the same sex as the deceased. At such busy sites the group arrived and accomplished its purposes in 15 minutes or less from start to finish.

When the accident site was in a neighborhood in which it

was suspected that the group might be seen and avoided, a second approach was used. Under such circumstances, for example, at sites in the Bowery, the group arrived and "swept the block" stopping successively the *first* 4 adult pedestrians of the required sex who were headed toward or away from the accident site. By pedestrian here and throughout this report is meant a person progressing by walking, not lounging stationary, sitting, or lying down.

In the third approach, used when pedestrian traffic was very light, for example at 108th Street and the East River (F.D.R.) Drive at 1:40 a.m., the group would lounge nearby or sit in a car at or near the site watching for approaching pedestrians, and as each of the *first* 4 of these came into view he, or, where appropriate, she, was quickly approached and stopped.

The site visited was the sidewalk point closest to the exact location of the accident as described on the police or medical examiner's report. For example, one report indicated that the deceased had been crossing the street 40 feet from a given corner. This was found to be directly in front of a "rathskeller," and it was at that point that the first 4 pedestrians were stopped.

Great care was taken to avoid any attempt at matching for the characteristics of the deceased, except in so far as sex and adulthood were concerned. In addition, for methodologic uniformity, at all sites the same investigator pointed out to the accompanying police each individual to be stopped. Although the exact details varied with the circumstances, the person was immediately approached and told by the policeman, "Please step over for a minute while the doctors ask you a few questions." A nearby member of the team immediately stepped up and began talking uninterruptedly: "I don't want to know your name; I merely want to ask you a few questions. Do you live in Manhattan?" The interview was usually easily begun in this manner, although 12 refusals occurred (for each of which the next pedestrian was substituted). . . .

This investigation was carried out without publicity of any kind. With one exception it was invariably possible to stop the members of each pedestrian sample prior to the formation of the substantial group of watchers which sometimes formed thereafter. The exception, in a "tough" neighborhood at 2:30 a.m., involved the only site at which 2 persons had been fatally injured in the same accident. On arrival, it was possible to obtain quickly the first 7 but not the eighth interview and specimen of breath, a small, hostile crowd quickly forming from an adjacent bar. As a result, only the first 4 of the 7 interviews and specimens obtained at this site were used, being counted twice in the analysis of the data.

The interview included questions as to: place and length of residence; place of birth; age; present occupation; and marital status. Sex, apparent race, appearance and apparent sobriety, date, location, time of interview, and weather were also recorded.

Immediately on finishing the interview the interviewer stated approximately as follows, "I only have one more thing for you to do (and then you can go) and that is to blow up this bag for me." Simultaneously he removed a Saran bag from an envelope and showed the pedestrian how to place one of its two ends in his mouth and blow until told to stop. This finished, the pedestrian was thanked and told that the interview was over.

A large percentage of those interviewed were foreign-born, and many of these admitted to no knowledge of English. Rather than weaken the investigation by omitting these pedestrians when no member of the team knew a common language, passersby were stopped and asked to serve as interpreters. Apparently because those walking in the same neighborhoods or, in some cases, accompanying those stopped (many of the latter being interviewed themselves) tended to know the same languages, this procedure proved very satisfactory. With its use no one failed to be interviewed because of a language barrier and interviews were completed in Armenian, German, Greek, Spanish, and other languages and dialects (pp. 657–659).

As implied above, blood-alcohol concentrations were measured by analysis of breath specimens and the other data concerning the controls were recorded as described. Data concerning the cases were obtained chiefly from official records describing the accidents. Postmortem blood-alcohol measurements were studied in those cases who survived fewer than 6 hours after the accident.

Data analysis for the case-control comparison revealed that fatally injured pedestrians were indeed older than the controls, their mean ages being 58.8 years and 41.6 years, respectively. Additional data collected later showed nonfatally injured pedestrians to be intermediate in age, with a mean of 48.4 years. Thus, advancing age appeared to increase the pedestrian's risk both of being struck by a car and of dying once struck.

Regarding the effects of alcohol, significantly higher blood-alcohol concentrations were found in cases than in controls. Appreciable increases in risk were noted even at the relatively low levels of 10 to 40 mg/100 mL. Putting together the age and alcohol data, it appeared that there were two relatively discrete high-risk groups: the elderly who had been drinking little if any alcohol and the middle-aged who had been drinking heavily.

It was also found that the case group was less often married and more often foreign-born and of lower socioeconomic status than were the controls. However, these differences could be explained by age differences between the case and control groups. Weather conditions, rain in particular, did not appear to be associated to any substantial degree with traffic deaths.

In addition to the case-control comparisons, information about the fatally injured group itself was of interest and importance. Only a small percentage lived outside Manhattan, either as commuters or out-of-town visitors. While the accidents were scattered about the city, most occurred outside of major business and shopping areas. The accidents occurred most frequently in the evening and night hours, suggesting the importance of having emergency care available during this time.

Example 3: Estrogens, Progestogens, and Endometrial Cancer

Estrogen preparations are commonly taken by women to treat menopausal symptoms and prevent complications of the menopause such as osteoporosis. Unfortunately, they also greatly increase the risk of endometrial cancer. It was proposed that if a progestogen (a compound with progestational activity) were also taken for several days per month, this would counteract the tendency of estrogens to cause endometrial cancer, because progestogens stop estrogen-induced proliferation of the endometrium, promote differentiation of endometrial glands, and lead to sloughing of the endometrium. Investigators at the Fred Hutchinson Cancer Research Center in Seattle, Washington, undertook a population-based case-control study to measure this promising protective effect of progestogens (Voigt et al., 1991).

The cases for this study were identified through the cancer surveillance system covering residents of King County, Washington. They consisted of all English-speaking women, age 40 to 64 years, diagnosed with endometrial cancer in the years 1985, 1986, and 1987. Of the 192 eligible cases, 158 (82 percent) were interviewed. Controls were recruited by random digit dialing with sampling stratified by age. As is not often appreciated until one gains experience with random digit dialing, this procedure requires considerable time and effort. A total of 6880 telephone numbers had to be called to obtain the final control group of 182 women.

Here is what happened: 2302 calls were to nonworking numbers; 1631 calls went to nonresidential numbers, mostly businesses. An additional 310 numbers were dialed at least nine times each at different times—at least three each on weekdays, evenings, and weekends. For these, there was either no answer or a repeated busy signal, making it impossible to tell whether the telephone was at a residence. Calls to 2637 numbers were answered at residences, but 2155 of these proved to be ineligible because the potential control either was not a resident of King County or did not meet the study's requirements for age stratification. Eligibility could not be determined for another 134 numbers because the answerer refused to provide eligibility information or could not understand or respond in English or because all that could be reached after nine attempts was an answering machine. An additional 16 respondents were eligible but refused to receive a letter describing the study. This left 332 women who agreed to receive the letter. However, 111 proved to be ineligible because of past hysterectomy, 37 refused the study interview, and 1 was lost to follow-up. Of the 183 women who were finally interviewed, one refused to answer the question about hysterectomy, leaving the final 182 available for analysis. These investigators calculated their overall response rate for controls to be 73.3 percent, computed by multiplying a 94.9 percent screening response (based on 2503 residential numbers screened/2637 reached) by a 77.2 percent interview response (based on 183 interviews/237 eligible) (L. Voigt, personal communication).

Almost all interviews of the cases and controls were conducted in person. Recall was assisted by a calendar of major life events and by photographs of oral contraceptives and hormone preparations. The time period of interest was before 1 month prior to diagnosis of the cases and a corresponding reference date for controls.

Data analysis employed mainly logistic regression to determine odds ratios while controlling for the confounding variables, age and weight, which tended to be higher in cases than in controls, and parity—cases were more often nulliparous. (Control of confounding variables is explained in Chap. 11 and logistic regression in Chap. 12.)

As in previous studies, the relative risk of developing endometrial cancer was found to be markedly elevated—5.7—in women who had taken estrogens alone for at least 3 years. If progestogens were also taken, the elevated relative risk was greatly reduced to 1.6. Of women who took both types of hormone, those who took progestogens for at least 10 days per month had almost no relative risk elevation, their odds ratio being only 1.1. Use of progestogens for less than 10 days per month was associated with an odds ratio of 2.4—better, certainly, than the 5.7 with unopposed estrogens but not as favorable as with longer use.

This investigation exemplifies the modern well-conducted case-control study of cancer. Note that it was population-based, only incident cases were used, and controls were identified and recruited by random digit dialing. The interviews were carefully conducted using visual aids to promote accuracy of recall. Multivariate analysis employing logistic regression was used to estimate relative risk while controlling for confounding variables.

One limitation, acknowledged by the investigators, was the possibility that hormone use differed in those who refused to participate. Another was the relatively small numbers of subjects in certain important subgroups, permitting substantial variation due to chance. For example, the women who took estrogen for at least 3 years and progestogens for at least 10 days per month numbered only 6 cases and 9 controls. Thus, the 95 percent confidence interval (see Chap. 11) around their relative risk estimate of 1.1 was wide: 0.4 to 3.6. The upper limit of 3.6 is compatible with much less protection from estrogen-induced endometrial cancer than the primary estimate of 1.1 would suggest.

Evidence for this protective effect of progestogens continues to accumulate, and they are now prescribed frequently along with estrogens to postmenopausal women who have not had a hysterectomy. Research continues to better define their potential adverse effects and the optimal timing of their administration.

Evaluation and Role of the Case-Control Method

Case-control studies are usually the most readily and cheaply carried out of all analytic epidemiologic studies. For rare diseases they may be the only practical approach. Yet the problems involved in locating a representative group of cases, selecting appropriate control groups, and collecting comparable information on cases and controls are often of such magnitude that the results of case-control studies are open to a variety of legitimate questions and objections, generally more so than the results of cross-sectional and cohort studies.

Case-control studies have played a vital role in the development of many fruitful lines of study. For example, the relationship of cigarette smoking to lung cancer was demonstrated in case-control studies before any cohort studies of this question were carried out. Because of their relatively low cost, case-control studies should often be the first approach to the testing of a hypothesis. They are also useful for an exploratory study of a variety of variables (sometimes referred to as a "fishing expedition") to find clues and leads for further study.

Another cost-saving application is the *nested* case-control study. In a large cohort study, difficult, expensive, or not-originally-thought-of data collections can be applied to the cases that develop and to only a subset of those that remain free of disease. For example, a nested case-control study was carried out in the Evans County cohort (described in Chap. 6) to determine whether vitamin A (retinol) level in the blood was related to the development of cancer (Peleg et al., 1984). Measurements of the concentration of vitamin A were made on the previously frozen serum specimens of the 135 persons who developed cancer and a sample of 237 cohort members who remained free of cancer through 1981. The high cost of measuring vitamin A in the entire cohort of 3102 persons was not justified by the small gain in statistical reliability that would have resulted. As found in several other studies, vitamin A level was not a useful predictor of cancer development.

A related cost-saving approach is the so-called *case-cohort* study (Prentice, 1986). As in a nested case-control study, cases are derived from a defined cohort but instead of controls who remain free of the disease studied, a representative sample of the entire cohort is chosen. Although initially free of the disease, some members of this sample will have become cases. The analysis of data from a case-cohort study depends on comparisons of each case with persons who are still free of disease at the time the case's disease begins or is diagnosed. Thus, cases who are part of the representative sample of the cohort serve as controls for other cases whose disease occurs earlier. A suitable analytic method, which takes into account the time at which disease occurs, is a modification of the Cox proportional hazards model, discussed in Chap. 12.

PROBLEMS

7-1 A case-control study of myocardial infarction gave results for prior alcohol consumption as shown in Table 7-3. Using the odds ratio method, estimate the relative risk of the "two or less" drinkers, the "three to five" drinkers, and the "six plus" drinkers as compared to the nondrinkers. Does the table show a positive or negative association between alcohol consumption and myocardial infarction?

7-2 In the study of oral contraceptives described in Example 1 in this chapter, there were 175 cases and 175 controls. Within 1 month before admission to the hospital, 67 cases and 23 con-

Table 7.3
Reported Daily Alcohol Consumption by Myocardial Infarction Cases and Controls

Drinks per day	Cases Number	(percent)	Controls Number	(percent)
0 (nondrinkers)	136	(34.8)	110	(26.3)
≤ 2	202	(51.7)	238	(56.9)
3–5	42	(10.7)	46	(11.0)
6+	11	(2.8)	24	(5.7)
Total	391	(100.0)	418	(100.0)

Source: Adapted from Klatsky et al., 1974.

trols had used oral contraceptives. Of the 175 matched pairs, both members used oral contraceptives in 10 pairs, only the case used them in 57 pairs, only the control used them in 13 pairs, and neither used them in 95 pairs. Estimate relative risk by both the odds ratio and the matched-pair method.

7-3 List the usual advantages and disadvantages of case-control studies of etiologic factors in disease.

7-4 Consider a case-control study to determine whether coffee drinking leads to cancer of the urinary bladder.

a For which of the following variables should the controls be matched to the cases: age, sex, strength of coffee used, addition of sugar to coffee, addition of saccharin to coffee, and cigarette smoking? State your reasons.

b If interview data are to be used, would you ask about current coffee consumption?

c Would you bother to review the pathology report of each case?

d If hospital controls are used, should patients with any specific diseases be avoided?

7-5 a To gain proficiency in understanding and using two types of fourfold tables found in case-control studies, show how the paired data in Table 7-2 can be converted to the unpaired data in Table 7-1. Verify this with the numbers given. (*Hint:* Which letter in Table 7-1 = $a + b$ in Table 7-2?)

b Produce some other sets of findings for pairs that could be put in Table 7-2 and still be consistent with the unpaired data in Table 7-1. What relative risk estimates would be obtained from these new sets of paired data?

BIBLIOGRAPHY

Breslow NE, Day NE: *Statistical Methods in Cancer Research. Volume I. The Analysis of Case-Control Studies* (Lyon: International Agency for Research on Cancer, 1980).

Cole P, MacMahon B: Attributable risk percent in case-control studies. *Br J Prev Soc Med* **25:**242–244 (1971).

Cornfield J: A method of estimating comparative rates from clinical data: Applications to cancer of the lung, breast, and cervix. *J Nat Cancer Inst* **11:**1969–1975 (1951).

Greenberg ER: Random digit dialing for control selection: A review and a caution on its use in studies of childhood cancer. *Am J Epidemiol* **131:**1–5 (1990).

Haddon W, Jr, Valien P, McCarroll JR, Umberger CJ: A controlled investigation of the characteristics of adult pedestrians fatally injured by motor vehicles in Manhattan. *J Chron Dis* **14:**655–678 (1961).

Klatsky AL, Friedman GD, Siegelaub AB: Alcohol consumption before myocardial infarction: Results from the Kaiser-Permanente epidemiologic study of myocardial infarction. *Ann Intern Med* **81:**294–301 (1974).

MacMahon B, Pugh TF: *Epidemiology: Principles and Methods* (Boston: Little, Brown, 1970), chap. 12.

Mantel N, Haenszel W: Statistical aspects of the analysis of data from retrospective studies of disease. *J Nat Cancer Inst* **22:**719–748 (1959).

Peleg I, Heyden S, Knowles M, Hames CG: Serum retinol and risk of subsequent cancer: Extension of the Evans County, Georgia, Study. *J Nat Cancer Inst* **73:**1455–1458 (1984).

Prentice RL: A case-cohort design for epidemiologic cohort studies and disease prevention trials. *Biometrika* **73:**1–11 (1986).

Rodrigues L, Kirkwood BR: Case-control designs in the study of common diseases: Updates on the demise of the rare disease assumption and the choice of sampling scheme for controls. *Int J Epidemiol* **19:**205–213 (1990).

Rothman KJ: *Modern Epidemiology* (Boston: Little, Brown, 1986), pp. 237–250.

Sartwell PE, Masi AT, Arthes FG, Greene GR, Smith HE: Thromboembolism and oral contraceptives: An epidemiologic case-control study. *Am J Epidemiol* **90:**365–380 (1969).

Schlesselman JJ: *Case-Control Studies: Design, Conduct, Analysis* (New York: Oxford University Press, 1982).

Voigt LF, Weiss NS, Chu J, Daling JR, McKnight B, van Belle G: Progestagen supplementation of exogenous oestrogens and risk of endometrial cancer. *Lancet* **338:**274–277 (1991).

Waksberg J: Sampling methods for random digit dialing. *J Am Stat Assoc* **73:**40–46 (1978).

Chapter 8

Cohort Studies

Of the various types of observational epidemiologic studies, *cohort,* or *incidence,* studies are generally thought to provide the most definitive information about disease etiology. They do provide the most direct measurement of the *risk of disease development.* However, if carried out prospectively, they can be expensive and time-consuming, requiring a long-term commitment of funds and dedicated personnel. Furthermore, as will be discussed, they are not free of potential biases and other scientific problems.

How Cohort Studies Are Carried Out

Defining the Study Population Initially, a study population, or cohort, is identified. This population is to be followed up over a period of time for the development of the disease(s) under investigation. In a *prospective cohort study* the population is defined and characterized as it exists at the start of the study and followed up into the future. In a *retrospective,* or *historical, cohort study* the population is defined and characterized as it existed in the past, based on data already recorded, and followed up toward the present to some cutoff time.

The cohort chosen may be a rather general population group, such as the residents of a community, or a more specialized population that can readily be studied, such as an occupational group or a group of insured persons. Or, the cohort may be selected because of a known exposure to a suspected etiologic factor, such as a source of ionizing radiation, a drug, or a pesticide. If exposure to the suspected factor characterizes all or virtually all cohort members, then a similar but unexposed cohort or some other standard of comparison is required to evaluate the experience of the exposed group.

The cohort study focuses on disease *development.* In order for a disease to develop, it must, of course, be absent initially. Thus the study population must be shown, in some way, to be free of the disease, that is, to be a population at risk for disease development. For a rare, rapidly fatal disease such as acute leukemia, a few cases initially present in the population will probably be self-evident. For a more common disease such as coronary heart disease in middle-aged men, an initial examination of the potential study population may be required to find and exclude existing cases of disease. As illustrated by the Evans County study (Chap. 6), this initial examination may be part of a cross-sectional study.

An initial examination may serve another important purpose, that is, to measure some or all of the potential etiologic factors and other pertinent study variables. However, some cohort studies with certain specific objectives do not require an initial examination since the data necessary to characterize the study subjects are available from other sources.

Follow-up   Once the population is initially defined and the appropriate characteristics of its members have been assessed, the population must be followed up for the development of the disease. Follow-up procedures vary from study to study both in intensity and completeness, depending on the disease manifestations to be measured.

Simple, relatively complete follow-up is available for life insurance company investigations of factors affecting mortality. For their purposes, death is the only end point of importance, and it must be reported to the company in order for the policy benefits to be paid.

However, follow-up to detect all new cases of coronary heart disease or stroke may require several different procedures, including periodic reexaminations, surveillance of deaths, hospitalizations, and physicians' office visits, and correspondence with subjects who have moved from the area. However, limitations on available resources may dictate that only some of all possible follow-up procedures be used, perhaps just hospitalizations and deaths, for example. Even though incomplete, such partial follow-up may be perfectly adequate for the purposes of the study.

The duration of follow-up required is determined primarily by the number of disease cases needed to provide reliable, statistically significant answers to the specific questions under study. This can usually be determined in advance, once the study population size and the disease incidence rate are known. For example, if the study population contains 1000 persons and the incidence rate is 1 percent per year, about 10 new cases may be expected during each year of follow-up. If 100 cases are needed to provide answers with a certain degree of reliability, then the study may be expected to last about 10 years.

This example is somewhat oversimplified and does not take into account such factors as a possible reduction over the years in the number of new cases per year due to losses of subjects to follow-up, or a possible increase in new cases per year as the population ages if the incidence increases with age. Although it is often most practical to keep follow-up as short as possible, a study may be designed specifically with a long follow-up period in mind to assess factors which cause or predict disease in the distant future. This is necessary for diseases, including many cancers, with a long *induction period* between exposure to a causal factor and the resulting increase in incidence. [The induction period between exposure and disease onset is commonly referred to as *latency,* although, more precisely, latency refers to a period when the disease is already present but not symptomatic or detected (Rothman, 1986; Walker, 1991).]

During the follow-up period it may be possible to repeat the initial measurements of population characteristics. In this way disease development may be studied in relation both to initial characteristics and to *changes* in these characteristics. For example, it is of interest to know not only whether serum cholesterol level is related to subsequent coronary heart disease but also whether a *rising* level or a *falling* level adds additional predictive information.

There are other reasons for reassessing population characteristics in the follow-up period. During a long-term study there may be technological improvements in the measuring devices that were used initially. Also, new scientific information about the disease may indicate the importance of measuring additional variables that were not included at first.

Data Analysis   As in a cross-sectional study, the population is subdivided or classified according to the variables that are to be related to the disease. The disease incidence rate is determined for each subgroup, and the rates are compared to see whether the presence or absence (or differences in level, if quantitative) of the variable is related to subsequent disease development. If the study population is a special cohort exposed to a suspected etiologic factor, then its disease incidence is compared to that in a similar nonexposed cohort or to that in the general population.

If all or virtually all study population members are followed up for the same period of time, then a simple cumulative incidence rate can be used. For example, if the period is uniformly 3 years, then the 3-year incidence rate may be computed for each subgroup. If there are substantial differences among study subjects in length of follow-up, these will have to be taken into account in the data analysis. Follow-up durations may differ markedly when subjects are lost to follow-up before the study is complete—if, for example, they move out of the area or die. Also, some investigations require that new subjects be added to the study population over a relatively long period of time (resulting in a so-called *open cohort,* as contrasted with a *closed cohort,* in which a forever-fixed study group is defined when observation begins). As a result, if disease incidence is determined up to a specific point in time, subjects will have been followed up for different durations from their time of entry into the study.

The standard method of handling variable follow-up periods involves the use of *person-years* of observation in the denominator of the incidence rate (or person-months or person-days, etc., if more appropriate or convenient). With this approach, each subject contributes only as many years of observation to the population at risk as he or she is actually observed; if the subject leaves after 1 year, he or she contributes 1 person-year; if after 10, 10 person-years.

A valuable feature of the person-year method is that one person may contribute person-years of observation to more than one subgroup. Suppose, for example, that in a 5-year study, disease incidence is determined for age-decade subgroups. A person entering the study population at age 48 will contribute 2 person-years of observation to the 40- to 49-year-old subgroup and 3 person-years of observation to the 50- to 59-year-old subgroup. This may also happen with other measurements if they change over time. A person may spend a few years in a particular quartile of serum cholesterol and then shift to a higher or lower quartile.

Follow-up time must be limited to that during which persons are truly at risk of developing the study outcome(s). It is obvious that time following the outcome, death, would no longer be time at risk for a study subject. However, it is easy to fall into the trap of erroneously including time *before* the subject is at risk of dying, time during which survival is guaranteed by the eligibility criteria for inclusion in the study or in a particular category of subjects. Problem 8-5 provides an illustration.

Interpretation and Evaluation of Cohort Studies

The emphasis in cohort studies is on the prediction of disease development. This type of investigation clearly demonstrates the time sequence between the presence or absence of a factor and the subsequent occurrence of the disease. However, even the prediction of disease does not necessarily imply a cause-and-effect relationship, as will be discussed in Chap. 11. Furthermore, as has been pointed out, factors associated with a disease can be shown to precede and thus predict the disease in cross-sectional and case-control studies as well.

A problem that has been emphasized with cross-sectional studies is the likelihood of overrepresentation of cases of long duration. This will not be a problem with cohort studies that have complete and comprehensive follow-up; the full spectrum of the disease should be available for study.

Despite their good reputation, cohort studies can be subject to important biases. We have mentioned how, in a cross-sectional or case-control study, the presence or absence of disease may affect the factor under investigation or the measurement of that factor, using the example of cancer and its effects on one's emotional state. Conversely, in a cohort study, the presence or absence of a study factor may affect the subsequent assessment of disease. In a stroke study, for example, it is clearly possible for knowledge of a subject's prior blood pressure to influence, consciously or unconsciously, the investigator's decision as to whether or not a stroke has occurred. If this happens, the study will have a built-in correlation between blood pressure and stroke incidence. Similarly, in a study of cancer, if disease detection depends partly upon the initiative or cooperation of the subjects in seeking an examination, those with a family history of cancer or those who smoke might be especially motivated to have a checkup. This can result in bias or in a built-in correlation of the disease with a family history of cancer or with smoking. Thus, every effort should be made to ensure that disease development is detected or decided upon independently of the possible etiologic factors under investigation.

Cohort studies are also subject to possible biases due to loss of study subjects. Such losses may occur initially if a portion of the target study population does not participate, or later on as members of the study population are lost to follow-up. Marked losses of either type do not necessarily invalidate the study. However, the investigators should consider whether the reasons for loss of subjects might reasonably have affected the study outcome. Sometimes it is possible to gather outside information concerning lost subjects, particularly whether they left due to illness or death or for any reason that might be related to the variables and the disease under investigation.

Example 1: The Framingham Study

Considering the barrage of information about "coronary risk factors" to which the public has been subjected, it may come as a surprise to health care personnel now in training that only a few decades ago atherosclerosis and its clinical consequences were generally viewed by the medical profession as degenerative changes that were an inevitable consequence of aging. However, by the late 1940s, descriptive epidemiologic findings and clinical observations were beginning to convince public health authorities that environmental factors and life-style might be playing an important role in the disease and that, as a result, prevention was a real possibility. Because of the major importance of coronary heart disease as a cause of disability and death in this country, the U.S. Public Health Service decided to undertake a major long-term cohort study to better define the factors producing this disease.

When the Framingham Study began, around 1950, Framingham, Massachusetts, was a town of about 28,000 inhabitants. There were several reasons for selecting this location for the study. At the time, it was a relatively self-contained community with both industrial and rural areas. In this and other ways it was not obviously atypical. There were sufficient numbers of residents in the desired age range to provide an adequate study group. There was evidence, both from a successful previous study of tuberculosis in the community and from discussions with medical and lay residents, that the townspeople would be cooperative. The area of the town was small enough to allow residents to come to one central examining facility. Follow-up of hospitalizations would be relatively easy since most occurred at one central hospital in the town. Furthermore, Framingham was only 20 miles from major medical centers in Boston; thus medical and scientific consultation would be readily available. The study was planned to last 20 years, in view of the slow development of atherosclerosis and its consequences.

The lower and upper age limits of the study population were set at 30 and 60 years. It was felt that older persons should be excluded since many of them already had extensive coronary atherosclerosis and, as a result, to study them could reveal only immediate precipitating factors for clinical events. Persons under 30 were excluded primarily because their incidence of coronary heart disease would be very low and because their mobility would make follow-up difficult.

In selecting the study sample, the goal was a group of about 5000, since this size sample in the 30- to 60-year range would produce adequate numbers of cases over the 20-year follow-up period. Knowing that there would be some nonresponse, the investigators selected a larger systematic sample comprising two-thirds of the 10,000 residents of the appropriate ages. The list of town residents was arranged according to precinct, and within each precinct by family according to family-size groups (one member, two members, three or more members, ages 30 to 60). Two out of every three families were selected. Selection of *families* rather than individuals was a wise decision since (1) one member of a family in the study's age range would not be denied an examination service offered to another member of the same family, (2) many reluctant men received examinations because they were "persuaded" by their more cooperative wives to go to the clinic at the same time, and (3) studies of spouse pairs and familial aggregation of characteristics would be fostered.

The 6507 members of the sample were invited to participate in the study by town residents who recruited subjects living in their own neighborhoods. These recruiters were part of a group of volunteers who were given a cardiovascular examination at the clinic before the study officially began. Having experienced the examination that was to be given in the study, the volunteer recruiters would be able to describe it to the invited subjects on the basis of personal experience.

Despite this personal approach, only 4469, or about two-thirds of the sample, participated. A group of 740 volunteers was added, yielding a total of 5209 subjects. The initial examination revealed that 82 subjects already had clinically evident coronary heart disease. These were excluded from the population at risk, leaving a total of 5127.

This study population has been offered a relatively complete examination every 2 years since the study began. The examination has included a medical history, physical examination, and pertinent laboratory tests such as electrocardiogram, chest x-ray, and serum lipid levels. It has been directed primarily at detecting the development of coronary heart disease and other atherosclerotic conditions such as stroke and peripheral vascular disease. Variables to be related to disease development have also been measured every 2 years. As new types of measurements have acquired importance in this area of research, they have been added to the examination. Thus the investigators have not been limited to the first examination as their only source of information about possible etiologic variables.

Every effort has been made to maintain rapport with the community and with the medical profession in the town. Subjects are kept waiting as little as possible during the examination. A complete report of the examination findings has been sent to each subject's personal physician. No medical care or advice is given by the study's examination physicians except that persons with newly discovered serious abnormalities are advised to contact their own physicians.

Although the biennial examinations at the clinic have been the chief source of follow-up information, disease development has been detected by other means as well. These additional sources include records of hospitalizations and of local physicians' office visits, and information about deaths from death certificates, coroner's reports, and reports of relatives. The diagnosis of any disease studied has been made according to strict criteria so as to include only definite cases in the diseased group.

Maintaining a continuing program of biennial examinations for a few thousand persons has involved a major investment in the operation of the study clinic. A staff of physicians, nurses, laboratory technicians, receptionists, clerical personnel, and others has been necessary for the smooth operation of the clinic and to ensure the collection of complete and accurate data. Epidemiologically oriented physicians and statisticians located both on site and at the National Heart, Lung, and Blood Institute headquarters in Bethesda, Maryland, have carried out the research analyses of data and the preparation of scientific papers.

The study findings, which have emerged in a large series of reports over the years since 1951, can only be summarized briefly here. Several representative papers are listed in the references under the first authors, Castelli, Dawber, Eaker, Feinleib, Friedman, Gordon, Hubert, Kannel, Wilson, and Wolf.

The study has been able to confirm in great detail that atherosclerotic diseases do not strike persons at random as they age and that highly susceptible individuals can be indentified in advance of any definite clinical manifestations. Indications of susceptibility, or "risk factors," that have been found in the Framingham Study and other epidemiologic investigations include male sex, advancing age, high serum lipid concentrations, high blood pressure, cigarette smoking, diabetes mellitus (or even milder degrees of carbohydrate intolerance), obesity, low vital capacity, enhanced blood clotting factors, and certain electrocardiographic abnormalities. Other risk factors that have been emphasized more by other studies include certain psychosocial factors, family history of coronary heart disease, and physical inactivity.

The detailed information and large population available at Framingham have permitted more intensive investigation of the unique role of each risk factor. For example, it was found that obesity is not related equally to all manifestations of coronary heart disease. It did appear to predispose to angina pectoris and to sudden unexpected death, but it showed a much weaker relationship to myocardial infarction, particularly in men. Also, sufficient numbers of cases emerged to permit the study of interrelationships of several risk factors. One important finding was that persons with combinations of risk factors (for example, hypertensive male smokers with high serum lipid levels) are at especially high risk of developing coronary heart disease.

As the study population aged, more emphasis was placed on diseases of the elderly such as stroke and senile dementia. Furthermore, the wide scope of information collected in Framingham has permitted the epidemiologic study of other nonatherosclerotic diseases as well, for example, cancer, rheumatic heart disease, gout, gallbladder disease, glaucoma, and cataracts. The adult offspring of the original cohort have now been brought under surveillance, permitting the study of cardiovascular disease and its risk factors as related both to familial and genetic influences and to the effects of long-term changes in life-style that have occurred. In addition, several studies of epidemiologic methods have been carried out in Framingham.

At present the major research efforts in the epidemiology of coronary heart disease are being switched more and more from observational studies, of which Framingham has been one of the most important, to experimental trials that actually attempt to lower the risk of disease. The predictive value of serum lipids, blood pressure, and cigarette smoking has been repeatedly demonstrated. Many have felt it necessary to prove that actively changing these characteristics by diet, drugs, and other means will safely lower risk and prevent or postpone atherosclerotic disease before widespread measures are applied to the general public or to high-risk individuals. Thus, the National Institutes of Health has carried out large-scale controlled experimental trials (see Chap. 9) to evaluate active preventive measures. The largest of these studies were (1) the Hypertension Detection and Follow-up Program, or HDFP (1982), which showed that a special program of treatment for hypertension, applied to members of the general community, lowered their mortality rate and their incidence of stroke, (2) the Multiple Risk Factor Intervention Trial, or MRFIT (1982), which did not demonstrate a statistically significant reduction in mortality from coronary heart disease in high-risk men treated with a three-pronged approach aimed at reducing serum cholesterol level, blood pressure, and cigarette smoking, and (3) the Coronary Primary Prevention Trial of the Lipid Research Clinics, or LRC (1984), which showed that cholesterol-lowering drug treatment of hyperlipidemic men reduced their incidence of coronary heart disease. To compensate for the relative neglect of women in these trials, a huge 13-year Women's Health Initiative was started in 1993. In it dietary, hormonal, and other factors will be studied, both experimentally and observationally, in relation to cardiovascular disease, cancer, osteoporosis, and other diseases.

While it is generally accepted, then, that enough has been learned about factors predisposing to coronary heart disease to justify serious attempts at prevention, this does not mean that observational epidemiologic studies and other efforts to identify causal factors are no longer needed. There are many individuals developing the disease who by present criteria are at low risk. Conversely, many persons in the apparent high-risk groups remain free of clinical coronary heart disease. Thus, our power to predict coronary heart disease is limited, and further studies are needed to identify pertinent risk factors. The recognition that a portion of the blood cholesterol (the fraction that circulates in the high-density lipoproteins, or HDL-cholesterol) is protective illustrates the advances provided by further observational studies. This, in turn, has led to studies of the relationship of more specific components of circulating lipoproteins to coronary disease risk. Similarly, new investigations are focusing on the factors in childhood, adolescence, and early adulthood that lead to the high-risk state in middle age that was so clearly demonstrated in the Framingham Study.

Example 2: Mortality in Radiologists—Does Radiation Shorten Their Lives?

As the use of synthetic sources of ionizing radiation has increased, so has the concern that these may be producing a variety of adverse effects on life and health (Boice and Land, 1982; Phillips, 1992). While intense acute exposures have clearly proved to be quite harmful or even fatal, the evidence is less obvious regarding the consequences of chronic exposure to relatively low levels of radiation. Experimental animals subjected to chronic exposure have died sooner than expected, but findings in animals are not always applicable to human beings.

The effects on the human life span are clearly a matter requiring epidemiologic study. Laboratory investigations of radiation effects on animals, cells, and other biological or biochemical systems, however important and illuminating, do not answer the basic question: *Does exposure to low and moderate levels of radiation actually shorten human lives?*

Since the intentional exposure of human beings to radiation for the sole purpose of answering this question is ethically unthinkable, one problem for the epidemiologist is to locate human groups who have been or are being exposed for other reasons, so that their mortality experience may be investigated. Groups already studied for a relationship between ionizing radiation and overall mortality or cancers of various types include uranium miners, residents of Hiroshima and Nagasaki who survived the atom bomb, patients receiving radiation therapy for noncancerous conditions such as enlargement of the thymus gland or ankylosing spondylitis, and children exposed in utero to diagnostic x-rays of their mothers' abdomen and pelvis.

Radiologists have also been studied for possible life-shortening effects. Since the findings of some earlier studies of radiologists were inconclusive, either because of small numbers of subjects or because of questionable comparison groups and measures of outcome, Seltser and Sartwell (1965) undertook a study of all members of an organization of radiologists compared to members of other medical specialty societies.

The Radiological Society of North America was the radiologists' organization studied. Founded in 1915, it existed during some of the early years of radiology when many radiologists were much less concerned and self-protective about radiation exposure than they have been more recently. (Some of the old-time radiologists even placed their own hand next to the patient routinely, so that its image on the x-ray photograph would help in judging the exposure time.) It was hypothesized in advance that the radiologists were the high-exposure, *high-risk* medical specialty group. The American College of Physicians is composed largely of internists and was studied as a probable *intermediate-risk* group, since some physicians in this group have fluoroscoped patients to aid in diagnosis. The hypothesized *low-risk* specialty society was the American Academy of Ophthalmology and Otolaryngology, whose membership contains only a few persons exposed routinely to radiation.

This investigation is described here as an example of a *retrospective,* or *historical,* cohort study, contrasting greatly with the Framingham Study in scope and expense. In this study, all the events to be studied had already taken place and the required data were already recorded. Also different, the three cohorts compared were *open,* whereas that in the Framingham Study was *closed.*

Because all the information was already recorded does not mean that preparing the data for analysis was an easy task. Several years of work were required to extract the necessary information from the files of the specialty societies and the American Medical Association's Directory Department. All specialists studied were traced from the time of joining their societies in or after 1915 until the end of 1958, and the time and place of death for all deceased members were noted. The cause of death was determined for over 99 percent of the deceased subjects by obtaining death certificates or reviewing other death records. The study was limited to men.

The end point of this study was, of course, mortality. The data were analyzed in terms of person-years of observation. Each physician was considered to have contributed ½ person-year of observation during the year he joined—a convenient approximation which represents the average—plus a full person-year for each subsequent calendar year survived through 1958. Subjects dying before the end of 1958 were credited with ½ year during the year they died, again a convenient approximation. All told, there were 16,339 physician specialists studied, of whom 3521 were radiologists. Person-years of observation totaled 232,708, of which the radiologists contributed 48,895.

Mortality rates were summarized for three age groups, 35 to 49 years, 50 to 64 years, and 65 to 79 years, as well as for the total group. Similarly, mortality experience was looked at in three separate time periods, 1935 to 1944, 1945 to 1954, and 1955 to 1958.

As hypothesized, the death rate was highest among radiologists, intermediate for internists, and lowest for ophthalmologists and otolaryngologists. The differences were larger in the earlier time periods than in later ones and more apparent in older than in younger men. In fact, after 1944, radiologists in the 35- to 49-year group showed no increase in mortality over the other specialists of the same age.

The authors interpreted these age and time relationships as consistent with a cumulative harmful effect of x-ray exposure becoming manifest in later life and a decreasing or disappearing effect in more recent years due to improvements in equipment, techniques, and safety measures.

It was of interest that the radiologists' death rates were similar to those of all United States white males. Since physicians are, on the average, of higher socioeconomic status and probably receive better medical care, they would be expected to show a lower mortality rate than all males. This illustrates the importance of selecting appropriate comparison groups when special cohorts, such as radiologists or other occupational groups, are followed up. Comparison with all men would have revealed no mortality difference. The more appropriate comparison, with other medical specialists, *did* reveal a difference.

Putting the age-specific death rates into one cross-sectional analysis of life expectancy starting at age 40 (see Chap. 5, page 68) was another way of looking at the data. This revealed a similar relationship to medical specialty. The median ages at death for 40-year-olds starting in the three successive time periods, 1935 to 1944, 1945 to 1954, and 1955 to 1958, respectively, were radiologists—71.4, 72.0, and 73.5 years; internists—73.4, 74.8, and 76.0 years; and otolaryngologists and ophthalmologists—76.2, 76.0, and 76.4 years.

Recognizing the limitations of death-certificate diagnoses, the investigators noted that the causes of death for each medical specialist group would probably have been recorded with reasonably equal accuracy. They compared the rates for major causes such as cardiovascular disease and cancer. The mortality ratios for major causes in radiologists as compared to ophthalmologists and otolaryngologists were relatively close to the overall ratio of 1.4 for all deaths.

Leukemia showed a higher mortality ratio—2.5, based on 19 *observed* leukemia deaths in the radiologists as compared to the 7.7 *expected* if the eye-and-ear group's mortality rates had applied to the radiologists. This is consistent with the results of other studies showing that radiation increases the risk of developing leukemia. It was pointed out, though, that the approximate 11 excess deaths from leukemia (19 observed minus 7.7 expected) constituted only a small fraction of the 228 total excess deaths. Thus, the higher death rate in radiologists appeared to be largely a nonspecific across-the-board increase.

The studies were updated in 1975, based on mortality in the specialty societies through 1969 (Matanoski, 1981; Matanoski et al., 1975*a*, 1975*b*). The apparent life-shortening effects of radiation again showed a decrease in recent years, particularly among radiologists who joined the society in the 1940s and 1950s. Nevertheless, radiologists continued to experience an excess cancer death rate.

In evaluating the findings, the investigators considered other possible sources of the mortality differences among the specialties, such as place of residence and initial self-selection of a medical specialty on the basis of health. The additional information available suggested that these factors did not account for the relatively shorter life expectancy of radiologists and that occupational exposure to ionizing radiation was the most likely explanation.

The investigators stressed, rightfully, that their findings were enhanced by the fact that they had predicted the outcome in advance. This deserves special emphasis because epidemiologists and other scientists can be trapped by the so-called *post hoc,* or after-the-fact, explanation. Given a set of findings or measurements, the human mind is usually ingenious enough to produce a reasonable theory or explanation as to why they occurred. This is accomplished with special ease in fields like medicine or psychology, which deal with systems of great complexity. Quite plausible explanations can be brought forth to explain diametrically opposite observations, and almost any result can be made to appear consistent with someone's pet theory. A much better test of a theory is whether it will predict specific outcomes of a study *in advance.*

This is not meant to detract from the importance of exploring data in order to develop new hypotheses or theories for further study. However, once such hypotheses are arrived at, they sooner or later will have to be tested to see whether they *predict* study outcomes.

Role of Cohort Studies

It should be clear from the description of the Framingham Study why prospective cohort studies of general populations are infrequently carried out. They are difficult and expensive and require an initial willingness to make a long-term commitment and continuing patience on the part of both the sponsoring agencies and the study personnel. Yet the investment may well prove its worth in the depth and variety of information that such a study can produce. Note how the cohort study permits the investigation of many outcomes in relation to base-line exposures and other characteristics. A case-control study starts with cases having only one disease or end point and investigates only this single outcome.

The need for either a long-term follow-up or a very large study population, or both, rests fundamentally on the fact that most diseases studied in this manner have surprisingly low incidence rates. Coronary heart disease is the leading cause of death in the United States, and coronary atherosclerosis is well known to be common in middle-aged men at autopsy. Yet the incidence of new *clinically identified* cases of coronary heart disease in middle-aged men is only about 1 percent per year. Similarly, although hypertension is a highly *prevalent* condition in United States adults, many hypertensives seem to have drifted gradually to their present state, making it difficult both to define and to find *new* cases in a population for a cohort study.

Retrospective cohort studies, of course, can be accomplished relatively quickly if suitable cohorts can be identified and if adequate data about them are available. Epidemiologic evaluations of occupational hazards frequently employ this approach. Nevertheless, many diseases of interest are so rare that case-control studies currently represent the only practical epidemiologic inquiry into their etiology.

It now appears that technological changes will increase the feasibility of cohort studies in the future. Storage of medical and demographic information in computer data banks is becoming an accepted approach to improving the efficiency and quality of medical care. A by-product will be the increased availability of information about a variety of cohorts that can be studied both retrospectively and prospectively. Ongoing efforts in the area of *record linkage* (that is, the combination of a variety of records about each person, such as birth, physical examination, drug prescription, illness, and death records) will increase the number of different relationships that can be studied—relationships between a variety of initial characteristics and a variety of disease outcomes.

PROBLEMS

8-1 In 1957 a study was conducted in which persons employed in a large tobacco company during the previous 4 years were followed up to the end of 1956 to assess their mortality (Haag and Hanmer, 1957). It was found that the death rates from all causes, from all cancers (except lung cancer), and from cardiovascular diseases were lower than, and lung cancer death rates were equal to, those in the corresponding age-sex-race groups of the general United States population. Noting a previous survey that showed that these employees contained a higher proportion of both cigarette smokers and heavy cigarette smokers than did the general United States population, the authors concluded that "the existence of such a population [the employees] makes it evident that cigarette smoking *per se* is not necessarily or invariably associated with a higher risk of lung cancer or cardiovascular diseases or with diminished longevity."

a   What type of study was this?

b   What comparison group was used? Was this appropriate? Explain your answer.

c   Using the same study population, how could the investigation be made more pertinent to the question under study (that is, the relation of smoking to mortality) without using the same comparison group?

d   Does it follow logically from the authors' conclusion (in quotation marks) that cigarette smoking could not be a cause of increased mortality?

8-2   You wish to determine whether diabetes mellitus in adults is a precursor of pancreatic cancer. A biostatistician informs you that to be reasonably certain of detecting a twofold increase in risk among diabetics as compared to a nondiabetic comparison group a cohort study will require the occurrence of 60 cases of pancreatic cancer in the observed diabetic group. About 2 percent of the adult population has diabetes mellitus, and the incidence of pancreatic cancer in the general adult population is about 1 per 10,000 per year. You want to complete the study after 5 years of follow-up.

a   Assuming complete follow-up, how many diabetics will have to be followed for 5 years to observe the required 60 cases if the twofold excess rate of pancreatic cancer actually holds true for diabetics?

b   If this study requires the identification of diabetics in a general population sample, how large a general adult population sample will be required initially?

c   Is this a practical approach?

8-3   Each of the following phrases or statements except one is most characteristic of one or two types of study—cross-sectional, case-control, retrospective cohort, or prospective cohort. Select the appropriate study type(s) for each.

a Generally most expensive

b Involves a population at one point in time

c Generally least expensive

d Time required to conduct the study generally less than the duration of follow-up observed

e Presence of disease may have changed the characteristic under study

f Interview data subject to recall bias—ill persons may remember past events better or differently than do well persons

g Least likely to be a medical student's summer elective research project

h Most apt to include all types of cases of the disease under study

i Permits study of many diseases in relation to a single causal factor

j Proves cause-and-effect relationship

8-4 A physician in an isolated rural area believes that eating substantial amounts of refined sugar during early adulthood may lead to easy fatigability and premature loss of sexual function in middle-aged men. She decides to test this hypothesis in her practice. She asks her healthy male patients in their thirties about their sugar consumption and classifies them into high- and low-sugar eaters. Ten years later, she spends her free time during one month visiting the high-sugar eaters, asking them to describe their energy level and sexual function. The following month she repeats this process with the low-sugar eaters. She finds a higher relative frequency of fatigue and impotence in the high-sugar eaters. Do you see any pitfalls in this prospective cohort study?

8-5 Someone suggested that the person-year mortality follow-up for the radiologists, described in Example 2 in the chapter, should have started earlier—at the beginning of their residency training rather than when they joined their specialty society. The reason given was that they might already have been receiving considerable x-ray exposure during residency. What problem do you see with this suggestion?

BIBLIOGRAPHY

Boice JD, Jr, Land CE: Ionizing radiation, in D Schottenfeld and JF Fraumeni, Jr (eds.), *Cancer Epidemiology and Prevention* (Philadelphia: Saunders, 1982), pp. 231–253.

Castelli WP: Epidemiology of triglycerides: A view from Framingham. *Am J Cardiol* **70:**3H–9H (1992).

Dawber TR: *The Framingham Study: The Epidemiology of Atherosclerotic Disease* (Cambridge: Harvard University Press, 1980).

Dawber TR, Kannel WB: Atherosclerosis and you: Pathogenetic implications from epidemiologic observations. *J Am Geriat Soc* **10:**805–821 (1962).

Eaker ED, Pinsky J, Castelli WP: Myocardial infarction and coronary death among women: Psychosocial predictors from a 20-year follow-up of women in the Framingham Study. *Am J Epidemiol* **135:**854–864 (1992).

Feinleib M, Kannel WB, Garrison RJ, McNamara PM, Castelli WP: The Framingham offspring study: Design and preliminary data. *Prev Med* **4:**518–525 (1975).

Friedman GD, Kannel WB, Dawber TR: The epidemiology of gallbladder disease: Observations in the Framingham study. *J Chron Dis* **19:**273–292 (1966).

Gordon T, Kannel WB: Predisposition to atherosclerosis in the head, heart, and legs. *J Am Med Assoc* **221:**661–666 (1972).

Haag HB, Hanmer HR: Smoking habits and mortality among workers in cigarette factories. *Ind Med Surg* **26:**559–562 (1957).

Hubert HB, Feinleib M, McNamara PM, Castelli WP: Obesity as an independent risk factor for cardiovascular disease: A 26-year follow-up of participants in the Framingham Heart Study. *Circulation* **67:**968–977 (1983).

Hypertension Detection and Follow-up Program Cooperative Group: Five-year findings of the Hypertension Detection and Follow-Up Program. III. Reduction in stroke incidence among persons with high blood pressure. *J Am Med Assoc* **247:**633–638 (1982).

Kannel WB, Anderson K, Wilson PW: White blood cell count and cardiovascular disease: Insights from the Framingham Heart Study. *JAMA* **267:**1253–1256 (1992).

Kannel WB, Castelli WP, McNamara PM: The coronary profile: 12-year follow-up in the Framingham Study. *J Occup Med* **9:**611–619 (1967).

Kannel WB, Dawber TR, Kagan A, Revotskie N, Stokes J: Factors of risk in the development of coronary heart disease: Six-year follow-up experience: The Framingham study. *Ann Intern Med* **55**:33–50 (1961).

Lipid Research Clinics Program: The Lipid Research Clinics Coronary Primary Prevention Trial results. *J Am Med Assoc* **251**:351–374 (1984).

Matanoski GM: Risk of cancer associated with occupational exposure in radiologists and other radiation workers, in JH Burchenal, HF Oettgen (eds.), *Cancer, Achievements, Challenges, and Prospects for the 1980s* (New York: Grune & Stratton, 1981).

Matanoski GM, Seltser R, Sartwell PE, Diamond EL, Elliott EA: The current mortality rates of radiologists and other physician specialists: Deaths from all causes and from cancer. *Am J Epidemiol* **101**:188–198 (1975*a*).

————: The current mortality rates of radiologists and other physician specialists: Specific causes of death. *Am J Epidemiol* **101**:199–210 (1975*b*).

Multiple Risk Factor Intervention Trial Research Group: Multiple Risk Factor Intervention Trial—Risk factor changes and mortality results. *J Am Med Assoc* **248**:1465–1477 (1982).

Phillips TL: Radiation injury, in JB Wyngaarden, LH Smith, Jr, JE Bennett (eds.), *Cecil Textbook of Medicine*, 19th ed. (Philadelphia: Saunders, 1992) pp. 2351–2356.

Rothman KJ: *Modern Epidemiology* (Boston: Little, Brown, 1986), pp. 14–15.

Seltser R, Sartwell PE: The influence of occupational exposure to radiation on the mortality of American radiologists and other medical specialists. *Am J Epidemiol* **81**:2–22 (1965).

Walker AM: *Observation and Inference: An Introduction to the Methods of Epidemiology* (Newton Lower Falls, MA: Epidemiology Resources Inc., 1991), p. 48.

Wilson PW, Cupples LA, Kannel WB: Is hyperglycemia associated with cardiovascular disease?: The Framingham Study. *Am Heart J* **121**: 586–590 (1991).

Wolf PA, D'Agostino RB, Belanger AJ, Kannel WB: Probability of stroke: A risk profile from the Framingham Study. *Stroke* **22**:312–318 (1991).

Chapter 9

Experimental Studies

Experimental studies resemble cohort studies in that they require follow-up of the subjects to determine outcome. However, the essential distinguishing feature of experiments is that they involve some *action* or *manipulation* or *intervention* on the part of the investigators; that is, something is done to at least some of the study subjects. This contrasts with cohort and other observational studies, where the investigators take no action, but only observe.

Experiments are believed to be the best test of a cause-and-effect relationship. Something is done to an *experimental group,* and the observed outcome is presumed to be the effect of that action, provided that the same outcome did not occur in an equivalent *control group* that was not acted upon. A cause-and-effect relationship can also be demonstrated by *removing* or *reducing* the alleged causal factor in the experimental group and showing a disappearance or reduction in the effect while no change is observed in the control group.

The latter approach is especially relevant to epidemiologic experiments in preventive medicine (Hutchison, 1981). If a factor is removed or reduced and the disease incidence declines as a result, the factor is, for practical purposes, a causal one.

Although great value is placed on experimental evidence, experimental studies are often exceedingly difficult to carry out. In addition, they raise some ethical issues that must be considered.

Ethical Problems

In observational studies, the investigator's chief ethical problem, aside from the need for objectivity and conscientious work, is to maintain the confidentiality of records about each person studied. Harm might come to an individual if some characteristics, recorded in confidence for medical or scientific purposes, were made available to others or were communicated to the individual in an inappropriate manner. In the main, though, the observational epidemiologist is a passive observer of nature whose studies involve few ethical problems.

The ethical position of experimenters is quite different, since they take it upon themselves to do something to people. They must have good reason to believe that what they propose to do has an excellent chance of being helpful. At the same time, they must also have ample doubt about the value of what is to be done, compared to doing nothing or doing what had been done in the past. Otherwise they could not, in good conscience, subject the control group to no action or the traditional action.

Thus, medical experiments can be carried out only in a situation of uncertainty. Unfortunately, some potential investigators are so convinced of the benefits of a treatment or preventive measure that they are unwilling to carry out a controlled experimental test of its effects. Their *feeling* of certainty, even if based on inadequate evidence, makes them reluctant to withhold the treatment from a control group. Similarly, the unreasonable skeptic, convinced of the superiority either of the traditional treatment or of doing nothing, may be unwilling to try new methods on an experimental basis. Both types of "believers" should realize that the failure to carry out a controlled experiment, when it is needed and feasible, is also unethical (Hill and Hill, 1991).

Sensitivity to the ethical aspects of human experimentation has resulted in the formation of committees in universities and other research institutions to review and approve all proposed studies of human subjects. It is now commonly believed that, whenever possible, the potential subject should share in the decision about whether he or she should participate in the study. This decision should be made with adequate understanding of the potential risks and benefits involved. Accordingly, informed consent is generally required from experimental subjects or from appropriate relatives or guardians.

Even so, patients' autonomy may be compromised if they cannot receive their preferred treatment unless they participate in a study in which they might be randomly assigned to a different one (Kodish et al., 1991). This must be weighed against society's need for prompt and accurate evaluation of a treatment before it becomes generally available.

How Experiments Are Carried Out

Experimental epidemiology is concerned primarily with testing the efficacy of measures to *prevent* disease. The preventive measure to be tested is applied to a group of persons. The incidence of the disease or disease-related outcome, such as disability, is measured in this experimental, or treated, group.

In order for the experiment to be informative, it must be controlled; that is, the outcome must be compared to some standard to determine whether any benefit has resulted. The standard may be the outcome in another similar group who do not receive the preventive measure. This control group may receive, instead, either no preventive measure or whatever is currently being applied.

Experiments may involve comparisons among several groups. For example, different amounts or dosages of the treatment may be tested. Or, there may be two or more aspects or elements in a preventive program. In this case, each experimental group may receive a different element or combination of elements. Experiments may be designed in an even more complex fashion so that each group receives a variety of treatments in sequence, possibly including periods of time with no treatment (Smart, 1970; Friedman et al., 1985; Fleiss, 1986; Spilker, 1991).

Randomized Control Groups   The traditional and most accepted means of defining the treated and control groups is to identify one group of all eligible study subjects and then divide them randomly into two or more groups. If only chance determines who gets into one group or another, then the usual tests of statistical significance can be applied to see whether chance could have produced the observed outcome. Also, randomization helps to equalize the treated and control groups with respect to unknown as well as known factors that might affect the results.

Ordinarily, random assignment to groups should be done after the subjects are shown to be qualified and willing to participate. This will minimize subsequent losses from one or more groups. However, randomization before establishing that subjects are willing, or "prerandomization," has been proposed as a way to reduce refusals to participate in the study, because each subject would not be asked to consent without knowing what treatment he or she would be given. Unfortunately, this approach can accentuate the problem of "crossing-over" by the subjects to the nonassigned treatment. Crossovers make it harder to discern differences between the treatments, since all subjects must be retained in their initially assigned treatment groups for data analysis no matter what treatment they actually received. Thus, prerandomization has been little used and needs further evaluation (Zelen, 1979; Ellenberg, 1984).

If it is crucial that the treated and control groups be equivalent with regard to certain characteristics that might affect the outcome, the entire study population can be divided, or stratified, into subgroups, and each subgroup can then be randomly divided into treated and control subjects. For example, stratification into age subgroups can be accomplished to ensure that the treated and control groups have similar age distributions. Practical advice on methods of randomization may be found in Zelen, 1974; Friedman et al., 1985; Shapiro and Louis, 1983; Meinert, 1986; and Spilker, 1991.

If, after randomization, the experimenter would like to be sure that some nonstratified crucial characteristic is similar in the treated and control groups, he or she should examine the distribution of this characteristic in the two groups. If crucial characteristics differ appreciably, then the experimenter had bad luck in the randomization process. Randomization may have to be repeated, if possible, or the results of the experiment will have to be analyzed in a way that takes into account the differences in these important characteristics. Appropriate analytic methods are discussed in Chaps. 11 and 12.

Nonrandom Control Groups   Randomized control groups are not always available for epidemiologic experiments. The reason may be economic. Funds may not be adequate for careful follow-up of both a treated and control group of adequate size. Or, the extra assurance that can be provided by this more ideal method may be judged to be not worth the cost involved. Also, there may not be enough subjects available for the two groups.

Even if there are enough subjects and enough money, randomization into subgroups may be impossible or may fail in actual practice. Randomization is impossible if the preventive measure can be applied only to the entire population, as when something is added to the water supply of a total community. Or, learning of the preventive measure through conversations with members of the treated group or through publicity campaigns, the control group may adopt the preventive measure to almost the same extent as does the treated group.

If randomized control groups are not used, alternative standards of comparisons are available. A comparison group may be selected from persons known to be similar to the experimental group with respect to several pertinent characteristics such as age, sex, occupation, and social class. Or if the preventive program is applied to an entire community, a similar untreated community may be used as a control.

Another approach is to have the experimental group serve as its own control. That is, a before-after comparison is made, in which there is a base-line period of observation on the experimental group before any preventive program is applied. The disease experience during this period can be compared with what happens after the program is put into effect. Similarly, although the same individuals may not be involved, the previous experience of the same community or another defined population can be compared with that which occurs after the preventive measure is introduced. Persons observed in the prior period are often referred to as *historical* controls.

Even when a distinct comparison group is observed concurrently, a base-line observation period is helpful. If systematic differences between the groups are noted during the base-line period, these can be taken into account in comparing the groups after the preventive measure is applied.

Possible biases or underlying group differences should always be considered when nonrandom control groups are used. Having a group serve as its own control seems especially attractive, since this appears to eliminate virtually all group differences. However, the control and experimental observations are made during different time periods. Thus, there is the real danger that changes in the study group over time might lead to the appearance of benefit from the preventive measure when none exists or, conversely, might mask true benefits. Rapid changes in diagnostic and treatment methods or even in ways of life are the order of the day; these may result in real or apparent changes in disease incidence that have nothing to do with the preventive methods being tested.

Subject Cooperation   Many preventive measures require the cooperation or active participation of the study subjects. Experimental evaluations of these measures must take into account the failure of many subjects to cooperate. Even after initially agreeing to participate, persons drop out of the study for a variety of reasons. Also, in the treated group there will be those who take none or only part of the treatment. Similarly, in the control group there may be some who openly or surreptitiously obtain the treatment on their own.

Study of outcomes should not be limited to the cooperators in each group since they represent a self-selected subgroup, often characterized by higher educational level, higher socioeconomic status, more concern about health, and better health habits. Furthermore, if the preventive measure is eventually adopted, it will be applied in the "real world," which also has its full share of noncooperators.

Thus, the most important comparison to be made is that of the *entire* study group versus the *entire* control group, a so-called *intention-to-treat analysis*. This will provide the best estimate of the overall benefit to be obtained from the preventive measure if it is put into practice. If, in addition, the cooperators are compared, their special characteristics should, to the extent possible, be accounted for in the analysis and the results should be interpreted with caution.

Blind Experiments If possible, experimental subjects should be kept unaware of whether they are treated or control subjects. Then, their own prejudices or enthusiasms will not result in behavior that promotes or inhibits the recognition of disease outcomes. Often, however, the nature of the treatment makes it impossible to keep the subjects "blind" to their assignment to treated or control groups.

More important is that the *assessment* of outcome be blind. Whenever possible, the physicians or others who determine whether the disease outcome has occurred should be unaware of whether the individual is a treated or control subject. The use of objective tests and criteria for diagnosis will help prevent any bias in favor of the treated or control group.

Even when experiments are designed to be blind, the subjects or their evaluators often become aware of their status. If drugs are involved in the treatment, characteristic side effects may reveal their identity. Also, unbeknown to the investigator, medical personnel involved in the care of the subjects may have access to the code or other information which identifies treated and control groups.

Thus, blind experiments are often desired but less often achieved. As for any type of study, a careful evaluation of methods and results for possible bias is necessary.

The term *double-blind* is frequently encountered. Some authors use it to refer to experiments where both the assignment to treatment or control group and the assessment of results are blind. Others use it to refer to experiments in which neither the patient nor the physician knows whether the patient is in the experimental or control group.

Sample Size Considerations and Sequential Analysis Statistical methods are available for determining in *advance* how large the treatment and control groups must be to obtain answers of the desired precision (Cohen, 1977; Friedman et al., 1985; Meinert, 1986; Shuster, 1990). In general, the more subjects, the greater assurance that the results of the experiment are accurate and not subject to chance variation.

The desirability of having large numbers of subjects is counterbalanced by practical considerations of cost and difficulty. Ethics also enter into decisions about sample size. The more subjects included, the more who will have received the inferior treatment if either the experimental or control regimen proves to be better.

Sometimes subjects are brought into an experiment over a relatively long period of time rather than all at once. The results for the subjects who started early may be available before the experiment is completed as planned. It is tempting to peek at early results for a few subjects and end the experiment if a difference between experimental and control groups is apparent. Unfortunately, these preliminary findings will not have the accuracy that was originally planned and agreed upon for the experiment. Stopping the experiment at this point may seem economically or ethically justified, but unless the differences noted are striking and compelling, the investigators may later regret reaching a conclusion on the basis of incomplete data. However, treatment-control differences may be much greater than originally expected and therefore be accurately demonstrable on a smaller number of subjects. The investigators certainly would not wish to continue the experiment if they could be sure that this were the case.

Sequential analysis is a statistical method that allows an experiment to be ended as soon as an answer of the desired precision is obtained. The result of the comparison of each pair of subjects, one treated and one control, is looked at as soon as it becomes available and is added to all previous results. A criterion for deciding in favor of either the experimental or the control treatment is specified in advance with the desired degree of accuracy. The comparison of a relatively small number of pairs may show sufficient differences to permit the decision to be reached. If not, the results for each additional pair are added as soon as they become available until the decision criterion is met or until it becomes apparent that there is no appreciable difference. As soon as any conclusion is reached, the experiment is stopped. The use of sequential analysis in medical experiments is described further by Armitage (1960), Smart (1970), Colton (1974), Friedman et al. (1985), Whitehead (1983), and Simon (1991).

Example 1: Controlled Field Trial of Poliomyelitis Vaccine

The first poliomyelitis vaccine widely used in the United States was the injectable vaccine containing inactivated virus, which was developed by Dr. Jonas Salk. By 1953, evidence had accumulated that this vaccine could be safely administered to humans and that it stimulated the production of antibodies that protected against the three known types of poliomyelitis virus. What was needed next was an experimental trial of the vaccine to demonstrate whether it was safe and effective when put into general use.

A large-scale cooperative field trial was undertaken in 1954, coordinated by the Poliomyelitis Vaccine Evaluation Center at the University of Michigan (Francis et al., 1955). Through the cooperation of state and local health authorities, over 200 areas participated. These were selected partly because they had experienced higher-than-average poliomyelitis incidence rates in previous years.

The initial plan was to inoculate schoolchildren in the second grade and observe the first and third graders as a control group. Although this would not permit a blind assessment of outcome, many states had agreed to participate on this basis, and this procedure was carried out in 127 counties or towns in 33 states (called *observed areas*). Eleven states were willing to cooperate in a blind experiment with a randomized control group. In the 84 counties and towns in this latter group (called *placebo areas*), participating children in the first through third grades would all receive a series of three injections, but half would receive the vaccine and half would receive an inactive *placebo,* or *dummy.*

All children in the first through third grades of the participating schools were first identified by means of a "registration form" on which were also recorded birth date, sex, race, and previous history of poliomyelitis or disability. Each child was to give a "participation request" form to his or her parents. This form described either the observed or the placebo study and provided space for the parents to sign a request that their child participate in the study. A vaccination record form was used to record all inoculations given to each participant.

Unique identification of each child on all the forms, plus cross-checking and editing of the information, was carried out to ensure a high degree of accuracy. In this study there were 200,745 vaccinated and 201,229 receiving placebo among the 1,829,916 first- to third-grade children in the placebo areas, and 221,998 vaccinated second graders and 725,173 first- and third-grade controls among the 1,080,680 first to third graders in the observed areas.

The vaccination phase took place between April 26 and June 15, 1954. Participating children in each classroom received vaccine or placebo from numbered vials in such a way that all three injections would be of the same material. In the placebo areas, there were vaccinated and placebo children in virtually every class. The vial code numbers could be interpreted as representing vaccine or placebo only at the evaluation center. Preinoculation and postinoculation blood specimens were obtained from a sample of children to assess antibody response.

During follow-up, through the rest of the year, uniform procedures were instituted to detect and investigate all suspected cases of poliomyelitis among first- to third-grade children, regardless of their participation or vaccination status. The evaluation center was notified of all suspected cases plus all deaths from any cause. Each local health department arranged for the complete investigation of each case. The data collected included (1) a complete clinical report including history, physical examination, and spinal fluid findings; (2) laboratory specimens, including stool and blood samples for viral and antibody studies; (3) examinations by a physical therapist to classify the patient according to physical disability; and (4) autopsies, when obtainable for fatal cases.

Checking systems plus a good deal of correspondence with physicians and other persons involved were required to make certain that the data collected were complete. By December 31, 1954, 290 case records of the total of 1103 reported were still incomplete. A campaign of telegrams, telephone calls, letters, and field visits reduced the number of incomplete reports to 78 by the end of January, but the last delinquent report was not received until March 9, 1955.

Criteria were drawn up for interpreting the laboratory and clinical findings, and on the basis of these, the investigated cases were classified as *not polio, doubtful polio, nonparalytic polio,* or *paralytic polio*. Paralytic cases were further divided into spinal, bulbar, bulbospinal, and fatal. These decisions were all made without knowledge of the vaccination status of the children.

The experiment clearly established the benefits of the vaccines. In the placebo areas the cumulative incidence of poliomyelitis during the 7½-month follow-up period was less than half as great in those who were vaccinated (28 per 100,000) as in those who were given placebo (71 per 100,000). Similarly, in the observed areas the incidence was 25 per 100,000 in the vaccinated second graders and 54 per 100,000 in the first- and third-grade controls. These differences were highly significant statistically. The protection appeared to be only against paralytic poliomyelitis, since there were no appreciable differences between vaccinated and controls in the incidence of nonparalytic disease.

Supporting evidence for the vaccine's effectiveness was obtained from the antibody studies. Furthermore, cases among the vaccinated tended to occur in children who received vaccine which was independently judged less effective on the basis of antigenic response. Other detailed analyses revealed that the vaccine conferred greater protection against more severe forms of paralysis and that older children appeared to benefit more than younger ones.

No ill effects of the vaccine could be demonstrated. School absenteeism for 6 weeks after the inoculations did not differ significantly among the vaccinated, placebo, and noninoculated populations. Nor was there any difference in the occurrence of rashes or other allergic manifestations, which were very rare despite the presence of small amounts of penicillin in the vaccine and the placebo. Other symptoms and illnesses at the time of the injection series were quite unusual and occurred no more often in the vaccinated than in the placebo group. The minute quantities of kidney protein in the vaccine caused some concern about possible side effects on the kidney, but none could be demonstrated in the study, nor could any deaths be reasonably attributed to the vaccine.

This study represents a major achievement in experimental epidemiology. The low incidence of poliomyelitis required that a very large population be studied to provide adequate cases to reliably demonstrate the vaccine's effectiveness. Coordinating a large-scale field trial of this nature is a difficult undertaking. This summary has emphasized study design and data collection efforts, but major problems of a logistical nature should not be forgotten. For example, hundreds of thousands of children all over the country had to be supplied with the right vaccines at the right times, and thousands of blood specimens had to be drawn and transported to 28 different laboratories.

Example 2: Fluoride and Tooth Decay

Experimental studies to test the effects of adding fluorides to community water supplies were begun around 1945. The expectation that raising the fluoride concentration of drinking water to 1 part per million would safely lower the incidence of tooth decay was based on a number of previous observational studies. These studies had demonstrated that ingestion of water containing large amounts of fluorides during the years of tooth enamel calcification resulted in discoloration and even pitting of the teeth. However, these "mottled" teeth appeared to be quite resistant to decay. Comparisons of dental status in communities with differing fluoride concentrations in their drinking water showed that the decay rates were relatively low and that no disfiguring mottling of the enamel was apparent in areas where the fluoride level was about 1 part per million.

On the basis of these findings the water supply of certain low-fluoride communities was treated on an experimental basis to bring the fluoride level up to the desired 1-part-per-million concentration. Since randomized control groups could not be obtained for these studies, the experiment was controlled by concurrently measuring dental health status in similar but untreated low-fluoride communities. Furthermore, the dental health of children in the treated communities was assessed before the addition of fluoride to provide a before-after comparison. Still another comparison was made of each treated community with Aurora, Illinois, where the naturally occurring concentration in water was 1.2 parts per million and where relatively little tooth decay was observed. One of these investigations, the Newburgh-Kingston Caries-Fluorine Study (Dean, 1956; Hilleboe, 1956; Schlesinger et al., 1956; Ast et al., 1956), will be described here.

The cities studied, Newburgh and Kingston, New York, are located on the Hudson River about 35 miles apart. Each had a population of about 30,000. Newburgh agreed to serve as the treated community, and beginning on May 2, 1945, sodium fluoride was added to its drinking water to raise the fluoride content from about 0.1 part per million to 1.0 to 1.2 parts per million. Kingston agreed to serve as the control community, and its water supply with a fluoride concentration of about 0.1 part per million was left unchanged.

During the year prior to adding fluoride, base-line dental examinations were carried out on the public and parochial school children, ages 6 to 12, in both communities. Base-line pediatric examinations were performed on smaller samples. Kingston and Newburgh children were, at first, similar regarding both general health and the prevalence of tooth decay.

Periodic assessments of both dental and other health measures were made subsequently. Although the caries experience in Kingston children remained relatively stable, a continuing improvement was noted in Newburgh.

A final evaluation was carried out after the experiment had gone on for 10 years. Over 2000 children, ages 6 to 16, were given dental examinations in each community. They were selected by taking every second schoolchild who weas present on the day of the examination. Although the clinical dental examinations were not conducted in a blind fashion, x-rays were taken and were randomized at the state health department so that the interpreters would not know whether they were reading Kingston or Newburgh films.

The data analysis was carried out for separate age groups. The Newburgh subjects aged 6 to 9 had used fluoridated water all their lives. The older age groups had been exposed to fluoridation starting at later periods in their dental development and thus might be expected to show less benefit.

The efficacy of fluoridated water in preventing dental decay was clearly shown in this experiment. One of the indexes of the prevalence of tooth decay was the number of decayed, missing, or filled (DMF) permanent teeth per 100 erupted permanent teeth. For the 6- to 9-year-olds, this measure was 23.1 in Kingston and

10.0 in Newburgh, a relative reduction of 57 percent of the Kingston rate. The reduction in Newburgh was present in all age groups but was relatively less in older children. Thus the DMF rates in 16-year-olds were 58.9 in Kingston and 34.8 in Newburgh, a relative reduction of 41 percent of the Kingston rate. The Kingston-Newburgh differences were found in both the clinical and x-ray examinations.

Dental-caries prevalence rates in Newburgh and other communities with experimental water fluoridation programs were reduced to levels very similar to those noted in Aurora, Illinois. Thus, artificially fluoridated water was shown to have the same benefit as observed for the naturally occurring fluoride.

Adverse effects of fluoridation were also looked for. There were no instances of disfiguring dental fluorosis, or mottling. About 18 percent of the Newburgh children were found to have questionable or mild fluorosis when examined by an expert trained in detecting the effects of fluoride. The mild changes noted would have been hardly noticeable to the average dentist. However, 19 percent of the children in Kingston had nonfluoride opacities or circular patches in the enamel which would have been obvious even to the untrained eye. These were found in only 8 percent of Newburgh children.

The medical examinations, x-ray estimates of bone maturation, measures of growth and development, eye and ear tests, blood counts, and quantitative studies of urinary excretion of albumin, red blood cells, and casts, all revealed no significant differences between Kingston and Newburgh children. Vital statistics data showed no consistent differences between the two communities in cancer and cardiovascular-renal death rates or in infant mortality, maternal mortality, or stillbirth rates. Later studies in several countries (U. S. Department of Health and Human Services, 1991) that compared large numbers of areas with and without fluoridated water supplies showed no excess in death rates associated with fluoridation, confirming the safety of this simple public health measure.

The Newburgh-Kingston studies present rather convincing evidence of the benefits of water fluoridation. They illustrate how well-designed preventive medical experiments can be carried out even when randomized control groups are not available.

Example 3: Evaluating the Periodic Multiphasic Health Checkup

An experiment to evaluate the long-term effects of periodic multiphasic health checkups was recently conducted by the Kaiser Permanente Medical Care Program in northern California. This experiment is described to introduce the reader to studies of preventive medical services that go beyond the prevention of single diseases.

Until recently, it was widely accepted in the United States that annual physical examinations are an important means of maintaining good health. The rationale for annual checkups is that the physician may detect early or asymptomatic disease and initiate treatment before serious consequences develop.

Because of this belief, many persons request and expect annual checkups as part of the medical care services they receive. Providing checkups to large numbers of patients can consume a substantial portion of a physician's time—time that might otherwise be used to provide more care of the sick. Because of the growing awareness in this country of the high costs and limitations of physician time and medical care resources, efforts to simplify the checkup are being developed and evaluated. Along these lines, paramedical personnel and automated instruments are being used to assist in examinations in order to save physician time.

Yet the basic question still remains as to just how much overall benefit periodic checkups actually offer. While common sense supports the value of early disease detection and treatment, physicians must also conclude that at least some aspects of checkups (such as listening to the heart and lungs of a young healthy patient every year, year after year) are almost always a waste of time.

The available scientific data on this question are surprisingly limited. A few studies have shown reductions in mortality and in other unfavorable outcomes in groups who received periodic health examinations. However, the comparison groups have not been randomly selected but have been superficially similar populations not receiving examinations. Persons who receive examinations have been shown to be like volunteers and other "cooperators" in that they tend to be more educated, more health-conscious, less apt to smoke cigarettes, and so on. Thus, serious questions can be raised about the comparability of the examined and nonexamined populations in these earlier studies.

In the Kaiser Permanente experiment, the control group is quite comparable to the examined, or "study," group. The over 5000 subjects in each group were selected on the basis of having certain digits in their medical record numbers, a systematic sampling method that is equivalent to random sampling, since these numbers are assigned in sequence with no relationship to any personal characteristics. These two samples were drawn from a large pool of Kaiser Foundation Health Plan members living in Oakland, Berkeley, and San Francisco, California, and aged 35 to 54 when the study started in 1964. To minimize losses to follow-up, another selection criterion was membership in the Health Plan for at least 2 years, since persons quitting the plan tend to do so soon after joining.

For almost 16 years, each study-group subject was telephoned and urged to have a multiphasic health checkup every year. Control-group subjects were not urged or reminded to have these checkups, but, of course, they were entitled to receive this service if they chose. On the average, 20 to 24 percent of the control group sought this service each year; the mean number of examinations received per subject was 2.8, with 36 percent of control subjects having received none. In contrast, 60 to 70 percent of the urged study group were examined annually, and the average number of examinations per subject was 6.8, with only 16 percent of the study group having had no examinations. Thus the urging resulted in a considerably larger "dosage" of multiphasic checkups for the study group.

Follow-up of the two groups consisted of a number of components to measure the development of morbidity, mortality, and disability and to assess the utilization and costs of all medical care services. Hospitalizations and outpatient visits were tabulated, and the names of all persons lost to follow-up were checked against death certificate lists at the state health department to see if they had died. A questionnaire survey was sent to both groups at approximately 2-year intervals to learn of the development of disability and other pertinent problems.

Whenever possible, assessment of various outcomes was made in such a way as to avoid bias in favor of the study or the control group. For example, subjects' recent addresses were not submitted to the state health department to aid in the search for deaths, since the annual telephone contact with the study group led to more accurate and up-to-date information about addresses than was available for the control group.

Initially, of course, the urging and additional health examinations led to the discovery and diagnosis of a variety of conditions. By the time that follow-up ended, in 1980, the study group appeared to have experienced some benefits from this effort, but not as many as was hoped. There was a statistically significant reduction in mortality from a group of "potentially postponable" conditions that had been expected to be influenced by early detection and therapy. Prominent among these were hypertension and cancer of the large bowel. However, the difference in total mortality was smaller and not statistically significant. Although an early reduction in self-reported disability in one subgroup attracted attention, this was not borne out by subsequent experience, and the investigators had to conclude that, overall, there was no difference in disability between the two groups (Friedman et al., 1986).

An unavoidable problem with carrying out this study was the matter of crossovers. The study group was diluted with a substantial number of subjects who chose to undergo few or no checkups, and the control group was diluted with subjects who sought and had several checkups. This commonly happens in clinical and epidemiologic experiments, and it makes the effects of the intervention more difficult to discern. Ignoring the randomized assignment and comparing the participators with the nonparticipators is not the answer, because this introduces the self-selection bias mentioned earlier.

Although the reduction in potentially postponable mortality noted in the Kaiser Permanente study strongly suggests that health examinations are beneficial, they continue to be controversial. Another controlled trial failed to show any health benefit from a series of two multiphasic screening examinations in the setting of general practice patient groups in southeast London, England (The South-East London Study Group, 1977). Much remains to be learned about the value, optimal content, and optimal frequency of health checkups.

The Kaiser Permanente experiment did lead indirectly to a case-control study that provided strong evidence for the value of one component of the checkup. Although the investigators had interpreted the findings with caution, authorities in cancer prevention concluded that the study group's relative reduction in colorectal cancer mortality was randomized-trial evidence that sigmoidoscopy, a recommended but not required part of the checkup, was effective in preventing death from colorectal cancer. A new investigator joined the Kaiser Permanente research group, questioned this interpretation, and performed additional analyses of data collected in the experiment. These showed that sigmoidoscopy could not reasonably be responsible for the mortality reduction, particularly since the study group underwent this unpleasant procedure so little more than the control group (Selby et al., 1988). Even though good clinical judgment suggested that early detection and removal of colorectal cancers and premalignant polyps should be beneficial, there was little epidemiologic evidence to support routine sigmoidoscopic screening.

It was recognized that the northern California Kaiser Permanente setting would be very suitable for a case-control study of the efficacy of sigmoidoscopy since this health maintenance organization's subscriber population of over 2 million persons (1) would yield many persons who died of colorectal cancer—the cases, (2) would yield as many matched controls as desired, (3) would contain persons who did and did not receive sigmoidoscopic screening, and (4) would have all the necessary information about screening and subsequent cancer in their medical records. A case-control study based on medical record review was conducted. It showed that persons who died of colorectal cancer had received considerably fewer screenings by sigmoidoscopy than the controls. After control for confounding variables (see Chap. 11), this yielded a relative risk of 0.41 for fatal colorectal cancer for those who had received at least one screening sigmoidoscopy as compared to those who had received none. More persuasive, this 59 percent reduction in risk was confined to cancers potentially within reach of the sigmoidoscope; death from cancers higher in the colon was not prevented. This was a clear demonstration of the efficacy of screening sigmoidoscopy, to the extent possible in an observational study. The other good news was that performing the procedure every 10 years was about as efficacious as performing it at the generally recommended 3- to 5-year intervals (Selby et al., 1992).

PROBLEMS

9-1 Penicillin is currently the drug of choice for treating strepto-coccal pharyngitis if the patient is not allergic to it. Suppose that a new antibiotic is developed which appears in preliminary tests to be more effective than penicillin for this condition. In setting up an experimental trial of the new drug for streptococcal pharyngitis, which of the following randomly selected control groups would you prefer?
  a A control group that receives the standard dose of penicillin
  b A control group that receives a small dose of penicillin
  c A control group that receives a placebo
  d Two control groups, one receiving the standard dose of penicillin and one receiving a placebo

9-2 Two drugs for hypertension are to be compared. One is prepared as a tablet to be taken orally twice a day, and the other is to be injected subcutaneously once a day by the patient. Suppose that patients with hypertension are randomly assigned to one drug or the other in a clinical trial to compare the efficacy and side effects of the two therapies. At the time of evaluation, 6 weeks later, the investigators find that 10 percent of the tablet-takers have discontinued taking their medication for one reason or another and that 60 percent of those who were to inject their medicine have quickly discontinued doing so, mostly because they disliked giving themselves injections. The investigators rightly consider their trial a failure, since the majority of those who were to receive the injectable medication did not actually receive it and since those who did receive it were too few to provide reliable data on changes in blood pressure.

a   How could this unfortunate situation have been prevented?

b   Can you think of a way to make this a double-blind study so that neither the physician nor the patient would know which medication is being given?

9-3   During certain weather conditions the air in a town becomes polluted by the smoke produced by a large factory upon which the town's economic well-being depends. During these periods of air pollution, about 20 percent of the inhabitants complain of severe eye irritation and about 5 percent experience asthmatic attacks severe enough to bring them to the local hospital emergency room. A new pollution-control device becomes available whose installation requires a year. The device is claimed to remove the offending substances from the factory's smoke. By monitoring visits to the hospital emergency room, the county health officer would like to evaluate the efficacy of the device in preventing asthma attacks.

a   Is a randomized controlled study possible? Explain your answer.

b   What control group, or basis of comparison, should the health officer use?

c   What problems in interpreting study results might this basis of comparison lead to?

d   What additional control group(s) might the health officer seek?

BIBLIOGRAPHY

Armitage P: *Sequential Medical Trials* (Springfield, Ill.: Charles C Thomas, 1960).

Ast DB, Smith DJ, Wachs B, Cantwell KT: Newburgh-Kingston caries-fluorine study: XIV. Combined clinical and roentgenographic dental findings after 10 years of fluoride experience. *J Am Dent Assoc* **52:**314–325 (1956).

Cohen J: *Statistical Power Analysis for the Behavioral Sciences* (New York: Academic Press, 1977).

Colton T: *Statistics in Medicine* (Boston: Little, Brown, 1974), chaps. 4, 5, and 8.

Dean HT: Fluorine in the control of dental caries. *J Am Dent Assoc* **52**:1–8 (1956).

Ellenberg SS: Randomization designs in comparative clinical trials. *N Engl J Med* **310**:1404–1408 (1984).

Fleiss JL: *The Design and Analysis of Clinical Experiments* (New York: Wiley, 1986).

Francis T, Jr, Korns RF, Voight RB, Boisen M, Hemphill FM, Napier JA, Tolchinsky E: An evaluation of the 1954 poliomyelitis vaccine trials: Summary report. *Am J Public Health* **45**:(5)1–63 (1955).

Friedman GD, Collen MF, Fireman B: Multiphasic health checkup evaluation: A 16-year follow-up. *J Chron Dis* **39**:453–463 (1986).

Friedman LM, Furberg CD, Demets DL: *Fundamentals of Clinical Trials,* 2d ed. (Littleton, Mass.: PSG Publishing, 1985).

Hill AB, Hill ID: *Bradford Hill's Principles of Medical Statistics,* 12th ed. (London: Arnold, 1991), chap. 23.

Hilleboe HE: History of the Newburgh-Kingston caries-fluorine study. *J Am Dent Assoc* **52**:291–295 (1956).

Hutchison GB: Experimental trial and program review, in DW Clark, B MacMahon (eds.), *Preventive and Community Medicine* (Boston: Little, Brown, 1981), pp. 81–95.

Kodish E, Lantos JD, Siegler M: The ethics of randomization. *Ca-A Cancer J Clinicians* **41**:180–186 (1991).

Meinert CL: *Clinical Trials: Design, Conduct, and Analysis* (New York: Oxford University Press, 1986).

Schlesinger ER, Overton DE, Chase HC, Cantwell KT: Newburgh-Kingston caries-fluorine study: XIII. Pediatric findings after ten years. *J Am Dent Assoc* **52**:296–306 (1956).

Selby JV, Friedman GD, Collen MF: Sigmoidoscopy and mortality from colorectal cancer: The Kaiser Permanente multiphasic evaluation study. *J Clin Epidemiol* **41**:427–434 (1988).

Selby JV, Friedman GD, Quesenberry CP, Jr, Weiss NS: A case-control study of sigmoidoscopy and mortality from colorectal cancer. *N Engl J Med* **326**:653–657 (1992).

Shapiro SH, Louis TA (eds): *Clinical Trials: Issues and Approaches* (New York: Marcel Dekker, 1983).

Shuster JJ: *CRC Handbook of Sample Size Guidelines for Clinical Trials* (Boca Raton, Fla.: CRC Press, 1990).

Simon R: A decade of progress in statistical methodology for clinical trials. *Stat Med* **10**:1789–1817 (1991).

Smart JV: *Elements of Medical Statistics,* 2d ed. (London: Staples, 1970), chaps. 5, 8, 10–12.

Spilker B: *Guide to Clinical Trials* (New York: Raven Press, 1991).

The South-East London Study Group: A controlled trial of multiphasic screening: Results of the South-East London screening study. *Int J Epidemiol* **6:**357–363 (1977).

U. S. Dept. of Health and Human Services, Committee to Coordinate Environmental Health and Related Programs, Ad Hoc Subcommittee on Fluoride: *Review of Fluoride Benefits and Risks: Report of the Ad Hoc Subcommittee on Fluoride of the Committee to Coordinate Environmental Health and Related Programs* (Washington: Public Health Service, DHHS, 1991).

Whitehead J: *The Design and Analysis of Sequential Clinical Trials* (Chichester: Ellis Horwood, 1983).

Zelen M: A new design for randomized clinical trials. *N Engl J Med* **300:**1242–1245 (1979).

———: The randomization and stratification of patients to clinical trials. *J Chron Dis* **27:**365–375 (1974).

Chapter 10

Clinical Studies of Disease Outcome

Just as some questions relating to disease occurrence and disease etiology are best answered by studying population groups, clinical problems often require the study of *groups of patients*. Many methods for studying patient groups are similar to the epidemiologic methods for studying populations, discussed in previous chapters. Although some authorities define it more broadly (e.g., Fletcher et al., 1982), the term "clinical epidemiology" has been applied by others (e.g., Weiss, 1986) to the studies of disease outcome to be described here.

The process by which healthy people become sick and the factors that determine who will become sick and who will stay healthy are the primary concern of epidemiology. Many clinical studies, on the other hand, aim at sick people and try to identify the factors that determine what the outcome of illness will be. This difference in focus between the two types of studies is illustrated in Fig. 10-1. Note that illness or disease can have several outcomes, including recovery, improvement, no change, worsening, complications, disability, and death.

The ultimate goal of epidemiology is to learn how to prevent disease. The ultimate goal of clinical studies is to learn how to cure or successfully treat disease.

The purpose of this chapter is to demonstrate some of the parallels between clinical studies of disease outcome and epi-

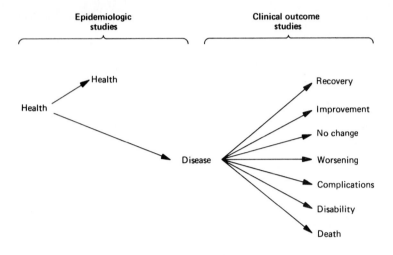

Figure 10-1   Areas of concern of epidemiologic studies and clinical-outcome studies.

demiologic studies and to describe the analytic methods commonly used to measure disease outcome.

Natural History of Disease

Studies of the *natural history of disease* are analogous to descriptive studies in epidemiology. The outcomes of a particular disease are observed, and the proportions of the affected patients developing each outcome are measured. This information is the basis of *prognosis,* that is, predicting a patient's future. As in descriptive epidemiologic studies, disease outcomes are generally determined for major subgroups of patients such as males versus females, various age groups, and so on.

   A good example of a study of the natural history of disease is Bland and Jones's (1951) 20-year study of 1000 children and adolescents with rheumatic fever or chorea. These patients, initially hospitalized at the House of the Good Samaritan in Boston, were carefully followed up into adulthood. Among the findings were that 65 percent of the children had signs of rheumatic heart disease when they recovered from their acute illness but that 16 percent of those with such signs had no evidence of heart disease 20 years later. However, of those without apparent heart disease initially, 44 percent had valvular disease when they were examined as adults. Also described were the recurrent rates of acute rheumatic fever, the evolution of murmurs, and the frequency of deaths and other sequelae of the disease.

Analytic Studies

The clinical investigator usually wishes to go beyond general descriptions of prognosis and to determine what factors lead to improvement, worsening, death, and other outcomes. Such factors include patient characteristics and environmental influences. One of the main environmental factors that is investigated is, of course, therapy.

Analytic clinical investigations of prognostic factors may be carried out in a fashion quite analogous to cross-sectional, case-control, and cohort studies in epidemiology. A physician is conducting what amounts to an informal cross-sectional study by noting during rounds on two wards for paralyzed stroke patients that in one ward several patients have decubitus ulcers (bedsores) and in the other ward the patients are ulcer-free. He or she will probably conclude that some factor in the first ward is conducive to the development of this complication of paralytic stroke and will make appropriate comments to the nursing staff.

Analytic studies of factors affecting prognosis are usually similar to cohort studies. That is, attributes of a group of patients are assessed early in the course of the illness. Then, the patients are followed up to determine outcome.

The clinical investigator can adopt this prospective follow-up approach much more readily than can the epidemiologist. The rates of development of many disease outcomes are relatively high, compared to the incidence of most diseases in a population. Thus, a relatively small patient group can be observed in one clinic or hospital until the various outcomes are noted.

Consider, for example, the follow-up study by Stahlman et al. (1967) to determine characteristics predicting the outcome of hyaline membrane disease in the newborn. Of 115 affected newborns studied, 33, or 29 percent, died in the neonatal period. A number of measurements taken within 12 hours of birth, such as arterial-blood oxygen tension, birth weight, and respiratory rate, all proved to be related to mortality, and statistical-significance tests showed that these relationships could not reasonably be attributed to chance. Thus, the predictive value of these measurements was demonstrable in this study of only several dozen patients.

However, some analytic follow-up studies of prognosis deal with events that develop relatively slowly and infrequently, so that large numbers of patients must be followed for years. This is particularly true of chronic diseases. For example, the Health Insurance Plan of Greater New York (HIP) investigated the prognosis of patients with angina pectoris and myocardial infarction. The study demonstrated a relationship of blood pressure in these patients to the probability of subsequent myocardial infarction and cardiac death—the higher the blood pressure, the worse the prognosis. This study was based on 275 cases of angina pectoris and 881 cases of a first myocardial infarction found among 55,000 men during a 4-year case-finding period. The cases were followed up for 4.5 years (Frank et al., 1972).

When an analytic follow-up study cannot be carried out, it may be practical to use an approach analogous to the case-control method in epidemiology. That is, a group of patients with one particular outcome may be compared with a group showing another outcome, to see whether the two groups differ in any characteristic that might have affected or predicted the outcome. An example is Ellenberg's (1971) study of sexual impotence in patients with diabetes mellitus. Forty-five impotent diabetic men (*cases*) were compared with thirty male diabetics who were not impotent (*controls*). the potent diabetics were selected to match the impotent group with respect to age distribution and duration of diabetes. The striking difference between the two groups was in the percentage showing evidence of neuropathy affecting the autonomic system—82 percent of the impotent versus 10 percent of the potent. Thus it could be concluded that most cases of impotence in diabetics were due to diabetic neuropathy rather than to endocrine or other abnormalities.

Therapeutic Trials

The therapeutic trial is an experiment as applied to clinical medicine. In it, a drug, a surgical procedure, or other therapy is applied to patients and the outcome is compared with that observed in a suitable control group.

It is essential that alternative therapies be evaluated in a well-controlled fashion, using, whenever possible, the techniques of random allocation and blind assignment and assessment described in Chap. 9. The influence of the therapist's personality and the placebo effect (or tendency of patients to respond favorably even when a drug has no active ingredients) are potent determinants of outcome and should not be allowed to bias the experiment. Furthermore, because of wide variations in the way individual patients respond to treatment, large groups of patients are often required. Large groups will help ensure that an observed relationship between a treatment and an outcome is not due to chance and that the relationship has some general applicability.

The value of large patient series is apt to be forgotten by clinicians working with patients on an individual basis. A physician's use or avoidance of a particular therapy is often guided by his or her experience with a few patients. The physician's view of the values or dangers of a particular treatment may be exaggerated just because, as luck would have it, the first two or three patients treated happened to respond unusually well or unusually poorly.

There is a widespread belief that the individual physician is the best judge of the value of a drug or other treatment. Through knowledge of the patient, the physician may well be the best judge of what is most appropriate for that patient's particular problems. However, the average physician's limited experience with a few patients does not usually provide enough information to state a general principle or conclusion that one therapy is better than another. It may be possible to demonstrate in just a few patients dramatic effects such as the value of penicillin versus no antibiotic in treating lobar pneumococcal pneumonia. But conclusions as to less-striking differences between therapies should be based on good-sized and representative series of patients with observations controlled as well as possible.

Medical history is full of examples of therapies that become accepted or popular in an epidemic of enthusiasm based on uncontrolled observations. Feeding this epidemic is the preference of authors and journals for reporting positive findings over negative findings. If the treatment is either not helpful or actually harmful, its use may eventually diminish or end, as its deficiencies become recognized. Unfortunately, during the period of general acceptance, withholding the treatment from some individuals, as is required in a well-controlled experiment, may be considered unethical. Thus it is important to perform a good therapeutic trial as early as possible after the therapy is developed.

Nevertheless, controlled trials are better carried out late than never. For example, the Boston Inter-Hospital Liver Group (BILG) carried out a well-controlled therapeutic trial that failed to confirm the long-term value of a widely accepted surgical treatment (Resnick et al., 1969). Portacaval shunt operations had been performed as an elective prophylactic measure on patients with cirrhosis of the liver to relieve the excess pressure in esophageal varices and prevent serious bleeding episodes. Acceptance of the procedure by the medical profession was based on uncontrolled observations that cirrhotic patients who received this operation did better and lived longer than those who did not. What is often forgotten is that surgeons naturally prefer to operate on the relatively healthy or good-risk patients and reject the poor-risk patients as operative candidates.

In the BILG study, 93 cirrhotic patients with esophageal varices and no prior major bleeding episodes were randomly divided into a surgical group and a medical group. To avoid selection of the better-risk candidates for shunt surgery in this experiment, each patient was randomly assigned *after* the physicians and surgeons agreed that he or she was a candidate and *after* the patient had consented to have surgery. Both groups were followed up for several years.

The operation apparently did prevent bleeding episodes, as there were significantly more patients with subsequent hemorrhages in the medical group (12/45) than in the surgical group (1/48). However, the mortality of the surgical and medical patients was quite similar. Although the surgical patients were less apt to die of bleeding, they were more apt to die of the hepato-renal syndrome. They were also more prone to develop hepatic encephalopathy.

Another controlled therapeutic trial did confirm the value of a much-used but still-debated treatment. For many years, even the individual practitioner could reliably observe that antihypertensive drug therapy brought about a dramatic improvement in the progno-sis of severe and malignant hypertension. However, the value of drugs for mild to moderate hypertension was less easy to recognize and subject to considerable debate. As a result, the Veterans Ad-ministration (1967, 1970) carried out a cooperative study in which 523 men with diastolic blood pressures of 90 to 129 mmHg were assigned randomly to active drug therapy or placebo. Before ran-dom assignment there was a trial period during which the poten-tially uncooperative subjects—those who did not attend clinic regu-larly or take at least 90 percent of a marked placebo—could be excluded. (Because most hypertensives feel well, there is little immediate gratification for them in following a regular therapeutic program.)

Therapeutic benefit to the drug-treated group was apparent after only 20 months of follow-up of those starting with diastolic levels of 115 to 129 mmHg. Only 1 of 73 treated patients developed a major cardiovascular-renal complication, as compared to 27 of 70 control subjects, of whom 4 died. One other treated patient exhib-ited drug toxicity and had to be removed from the study therapy.

Longer follow-up of more subjects was required to demon-strate the benefits of treating milder hypertension—90 to 114 mmHg diastolic pressure. A total of 380 patients were followed up for an average of 3.3 years. Major complications were observed in 56 of 194 controls, as compared to only 22 of 186 treated subjects. Some complications, such as stroke, showed a markedly lower incidence among the treated group.

Concomitant with the reporting of controlled observations such as these has been a growing awareness that hypertension is serious and that large numbers of persons in this country are hyper-tensive and not aware of it. Moreover, many persons who are aware of hypertension are not treated adequately or consistently. Thus the detection and sustained treatment of hypertension has become a major public health effort.

Commonly Used Measures of Disease Outcome

Rates Just as incidence rates are used in epidemiology to measure the development of disease in healthy persons, the outcomes of illness can be measured similarly in groups of sick persons. Thus one may speak of recovery rates, disability rates, death rates, and so on, referring to the proportion of the ill that recover, become disabled, or die per unit of time. Again, the proportion of the sick who manifest a particular outcome at one point in time is analogous to a point prevalence rate of disease in a general population.

Survival Measures of mortality outcome are often expressed in terms of *survival* rather than death. For comparative purposes, it is not particularly important whether one focuses on successes or failures. However, the data from clinical studies are so often analyzed and presented in terms of survival that it is desirable to be familiar with the approaches used. It should be remembered, also, that these measures need not be restricted to life and death. They can be applied to any mutually exclusive alternatives. Thus, in a study of the development of congestive heart failure in cardiac patients, remaining free of failure can be considered analogous to survival.

One of the most common measures of outcome is the proportion surviving for a particular duration. Any duration may be chosen—5 years is frequently used in studies of the surgical treatment of cancer, because, for many types of cancer, a patient who survives for 5 years is likely to have been cured. Thus the *5-year survival rate* or *5-year cure rate* merely refers to that proportion of the original patient group still alive after 5 years of follow-up.

Another measure of survival is the *mean duration of survival.* As mentioned in Chap. 2, the mean duration should be used for comparative purposes only when all patients have died. When some are still living, it is preferable to compare *median duration of survival* or some other *quantile* of *survival durations* because once the stated percentage have died, their survival cannot change. For example, after 75 out of 100 patients have died, the survival duration of the seventy-fifth person becomes the 75th percentile of survival durations for the entire group. This cannot change no matter how much longer the other 25 live. The mean, on the other hand, is not finally determined until all 100 have died.

One of the most common and probably the most informative measures of survival is the survival curve. Starting initially at 100 percent, it shows the proportion still surviving at each subsequent point in time for as long as information is available. This picture of survival through time is much more revealing and is usually more reliable than a single measure such as the median duration of survival or the 5-year survival rate. Figure 10-2 shows the curves for the medical and surgical patients in the BILG study of portacaval shunt. The similarity in their survival experience is apparent.

Another graph, Fig. 10-3, shows marked differences in survival for several subgroups of patients with scleroderma, from the study by Medsger et al. (1971). The proportions of scleroderma patients surviving at the end of each year after entry into the study

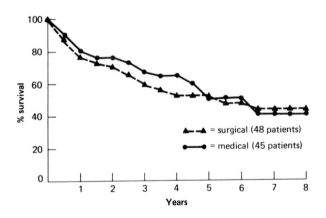

Figure 10-2 Survival of surgical and medical patients in the Boston Inter-Hospital Liver Group's controlled therapeutic trial of portacaval-shunt surgery for esophageal varices. *(Reproduced, by permission, from Resnick et al., 1969.)*

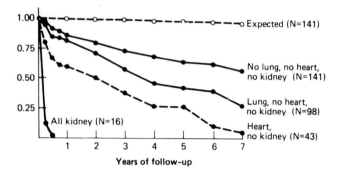

Figure 10-3 Survival of scleroderma patients according to organ involvement. Ordinate shows proportion surviving. *(Reproduced, by permission, from Medsger et al., 1971.)*

are shown by solid black circles. Those who had no involvement of their lungs, heart, or kidneys did the best, with 56 percent still alive after 7 years. Subgroups with poorer survival rates were: next, those with lung involvement; then, those with heart involvement; and finally, those with kidney involvement, all of whom died within the first half year. For comparison, the expected survival curve is shown on top with clear circles. This is the survival that would have been expected for a group of this age, sex, and racial composition if the overall United States mortality rates for the study years had been applicable.

Construction of survival curves for a certain duration following a specific event or time does not require that all patients be observed for that entire duration. Consider an example in which persons are to be followed for 10 years starting at the time their disease was first diagnosed. The experience of a person who moves away and is lost to follow-up after 5 years is still helpful in determining survival rates for the first 5 years. Similarly, someone who is diagnosed and enters the study 1 year before follow-up observations are to be completed can usefully be included among those persons observed during the first year after diagnosis.

Thus, all persons who are observed during each unit of time measured from the starting event can contribute their experience to the survival-rate computation for that time unit. The so-called *actuarial,* or *life-table,* approach takes advantage of all these observations by computing survival rates for each time unit and combining these rates into one composite survival curve. For details on life-table methods, which are not difficult to carry out, see Berkson and Gage (1950), Cutler and Ederer (1958), Hill and Hill (1991), or Colton (1974). The *product-limit,* or *Kaplan-Meier,* method is frequently used to measure survival in small- to medium-size clinical studies (Kaplan and Meier, 1958). In it, each person's survival time is viewed separately rather than grouped into intervals, as is commonly done in life tables. A simple statistical analysis for comparing life-table survival curves in clinical trials has been described by Peto et al. (1976, 1977). A comprehensive presentation of survival analysis may be found in Lee (1980).

Importance of Starting Times   When survival curves (or mortality rates) of two groups are to be compared, it is important that both have the same starting point. The starting time may be placed at the onset of symptoms, the first diagnosis, the beginning of therapy, discharge from a hospital, or some other landmark in the course of the disease.

Failure to follow this principle has led to many conflicting claims and erroneous conclusions about the benefits of therapy. For example, two equally good surgical treatments will appear to have different results if survival is measured from the hospital discharge date for one and from the date of operation for the other. Measuring from the date of discharge excludes operative and immediate postoperative mortality.

Although the inclusion or exclusion of operative mortality makes for an obvious error, more subtle and hard-to-recognize biases may result when follow-up of two groups does not begin at strictly comparable times. Consider a study to evaluate the efficacy of a new procedure for the early diagnosis of a disease. Even if detecting the disease early does not prolong life, it might appear to do so if survival is measured from the date of *early* diagnosis instead of from the usual diagnosis date resulting from traditional methods. Procedures for estimating this "lead-time" bias are discussed by Hutchison and Shapiro (1968), Feinleib and Zelen (1969), and Morrison (1992).

Similarly, treatment measures for rapidly fatal diseases may appear more effective than they really are if they are initiated after a short delay. Part of the apparent improvement in in-hospital mortality from myocardial infarction experienced by patients in coronary-care units may be related to the fact that many heart attack victims die soon after the onset of the attack. Patients in coronary-care units have already survived the short delay between admission to the hospital and admission to the unit.

Disease or Treatment Outcomes Centered on Patients' Preferences

During the 1980s and 1990s concern has been growing about the quality and costs of medical care, and there has been increased empowerment of patients in deciding among alternative treatments, including no treatment. These developments have led investigators of medical care to add to the traditional outcomes, such as survival and disability, newer measures such as costs of care, patient satisfaction, and quality of life. For example, survival is sometimes measured not merely in terms of years lived, but in *quality-adjusted life years (QALYs)* or *years of healthy life* afforded by different treatments of a condition. A year of life with a disability or illness is considered as some fraction of a year of healthy life. This fraction can simply be estimated in the evaluator's judgment or, preferably, determined by asking people how they rate the alternatives. For example, if on average a group of patients regarded 10 more years of life with frequent headaches as equal to living 8 years in good health without headaches, a year of life with headaches would receive a value of 0.8 of a year of healthy life.

Quality adjustment of years of life has been reviewed from the economic (Russell, 1986), statistical (Torrance and Feeny, 1989, and Schumacher et al., 1991), and ethical (La Puma and Lawlor, 1990) points of view. This approach raises vexing ethical questions such as concern over substituting community preferences, elicited in the interests of cost containment, for the desires of individual patients, and the implication that older and sicker patients have less capacity to benefit from treatment than the young and healthy.

PROBLEMS

10-1 **a** Define the 5-year survival rate.

     b Why is it often measured?

     c Can the 5-year survival rate be determined from survival curves such as those in Fig. 10-3?

     d If so, what was the 5-year survival rate for scleroderma patients with lung involvement but no heart or kidney involvement?

     e What was the 5-year survival rate for scleroderma patients with kidney involvement?

10-2 Surgeons at hospital A report that the mortality rate at the end of 1 year of follow-up after a coronary bypass operation is 15 percent. At hospital B the surgeons report a 1-year mortality rate of only 8 percent after the same procedure. What would you want to find out before concluding that the surgeons at hospital B perform the operation with greater skill?

10-3 Physicians practicing in the general community often find that, on the average, chronic debilitating conditions, such as multiple sclerosis or connective tissue diseases, lead to less disability and fewer complications than they were led to expect from reading reports in the medical literature on the natural history of these conditions. Why, do you suppose, is this the case?

BIBLIOGRAPHY

Berkson J, Gage RP: Calculation of survival rates for cancer. *Proc Staff Meet Mayo Clin* **25**:270–286 (1950).

Bland EF, Jones TD: Rheumatic fever and rheumatic heart disease: A twenty-year report on 1000 patients followed since childhood. *Circulation* **4**:836–843 (1951).

Colton T: *Statistics in Medicine* (Boston: Little, Brown, 1974), chap. 9.

Cutler SJ, Ederer F: Maximum utilization of the life table method in analyzing survival. *J Chron Dis* **8:**699–712 (1958).

Ellenberg M: Impotence in diabetes: The neurologic factor. *Ann Intern Med* **75:**213–219 (1971).

Feinleib M, Zelen M: Some pitfalls in the evaluation of screening programs. *Arch Environ Health* **19:**412–415 (1969).

Fletcher RH, Fletcher SW, Wagner EH: *Clinical Epidemiology—The Essentials* (Baltimore: Williams and Wilkins, 1982).

Frank CW, Weinblatt E, Shapiro S, Sager R: Prognosis of men with coronary heart disease as related to blood pressure. *Circulation* **38:**432–438 (1972).

Hill AB, Hill ID: *Bradford Hill's Principles of Medical Statistics,* 12th ed. (London, Edward Arnold, 1991), pp. 194–203.

Hutchison GB, Shapiro S: Lead time gained by diagnostic screening for breast cancer. *J Natl Cancer Inst* **41:**665–681 (1968).

Kaplan EL, Meier P: Nonparametric estimation from incomplete observations. *J Am Stat Assoc* **53:**457–481 (1958).

La Puma J, Lawlor EF: Quality-adjusted life years. *JAMA* **263:**2917–2921 (1990).

Lee ET: *Statistical Methods for Survival Data Analysis* (Belmont, Calif.: Lifetime Learning Publications, 1980).

Medsger TA, Masi AT, Rodnan GP, Benedek TG, Robinson H: Survival with systemic sclerosis (scleroderma): A life-table analysis of clinical and demographic factors in 309 patients. *Ann Intern Med* **75:**369–376 (1971).

Morrison AS: *Screening in Chronic Disease,* 2d ed. (New York: Oxford University Press, 1992).

Peto R, Pike MC, Armitage P, Breslow NE, Cox DR, Howard SV, Mantel N, McPherson K, Peto J, Smith PG: Design and analysis of randomized clinical trials requiring prolonged observation of each patient: I. Introduction and design; II. Analysis and examples. *Brit J Cancer* **34:**585–612 (1976); **35:**1–39 (1977).

Resnick RH, Chalmers TC, Ishihara AM, Garceau AJ, Callow AD, Schimmel EM, O'Hara ET, the Boston Inter-Hospital Liver Group: A controlled study of the prophylactic portacaval shunt: A final report. *Ann Intern Med* **70:**657–688 (1969).

Russell LB: *Is Prevention Better Than Cure?* (Washington: The Brookings Institution, 1986), pp. 66–70.

Schumacher M, Olschewski M, Schulgen G: Assessment of quality of life in clinical trials. *Stat Med* **10:**1915–1930 (1991).

Stahlman MT, Battersby EJ, Shepard FM, Blankenship WJ: Prognosis in hyaline-membrane disease: Use of a linear-discriminant. *N Engl J Med* **276**:303–309 (1967).

Torrance GW, Feeny D: Utilities and quality-adjusted life years. *Int J Technol Assess Health Care* **5**:559–575 (1989).

Veterans Administration Cooperative Study Group on Antihypertensive Agents: Effects of treatment on morbidity and mortality: Results in patients with diastolic blood pressures averaging 115 through 129 mmHg. *J Am Med Assoc* **202**:1028–1034 (1967).

————: Effects of treatment on morbidity in hypertension. II. Results in patients with diastolic blood pressure averaging 90 through 114 mmHg. *J Am Med Assoc* **213**:1143–1152 (1970).

Weiss NS: *Clinical Epidemiology: The Study of the Outcome of Illness* (New York: Oxford University Press, 1986).

Chapter 11

Making Sense Out of Statistical Associations

Positive findings of epidemiologic or clinical outcome studies are usually referred to as *statistical associations.* Having a proper perspective on the meaning and importance of statistical associations is essential, for all too frequently they are under- or overinterpreted. With regard to smoking, for example, at one extreme are those who discount the strong epidemiologic evidence relating cigarette smoking and lung cancer as being "only statistical." And at the other extreme are those who quickly blame a whole host of health problems on cigarette smoking on the basis of weak epidemiologic evidence, without considering the possible role of other characteristics of persons who smoke.

Statements and Measures of Statistical Association

In discussing the various types of epidemiologic and related studies in Chaps. 5 to 10, the usual methods of expressing the results of these studies have been mentioned several times. Typically, the findings would be that persons having one characteristic or environmental exposure have a higher or lower incidence of a disease than persons with a different characteristic or exposure. Or, the association may be expressed in terms of a greater or lesser proportion with the characteristic among the diseased as compared to the nondiseased. Similar statements may express the fact that there is an association between one characteristic and another or between one disease and another.

In addition to these easily understood statements of association in terms of differences in rates or proportions, epidemiologists sometimes employ other statistical tools to measure and describe associations. For example, data may suggest that there is a linear relationship between two quantitative variables. In a perfect linear relationship, for every unit of increase in one variable the other variable increases or decreases proportionally. A useful measure of association, the correlation coefficient (sometimes called *Pearson,* or *product-moment, correlation*) indicates the degree to which a set of observations fits a linear relationship. (For method of computation and more discussion, see Hill and Hill, 1991; Colton, 1974; or Moore and McCabe, 1993.) This coefficient, often represented by the letter *r,* can vary between $+1$ and -1. If $r = +1$, there is a perfect linear relationship in which one variable varies directly with the other. If $r = 0$, there is no association between the variables. If $r = -1$, there is again a perfect association, but one variable varies inversely with the other.

Plotted on a graph showing the relationship between two variables, data points would follow a slanted straight line if the correlation coefficient is $+1$ or -1. Where there is some, but not complete, correlation, the data points would not fall into line but would appear to cluster about a line. If there is no correlation at all, data points would form a regular or irregular clump with no underlying slanted line apparent. Note that the data points for the states in Fig. 11-1 show some degree of linear relationship between cigarettes sold per capita and coronary heart disease death rates. The correlation coefficient is $+.55$.

A related but more stringent measure of association is the *intraclass correlation,* which looks at the agreement of measurements within classes or categories. For an intraclass correlation to be $+1$ or perfect, the two series of measurements must not only be linearly related but must agree exactly. The intraclass correlation is thus a useful measure of validity, reliability, or interrater agreement, and in some situations yields the same results as Cohen's kappa (described in Chap. 3; for additional information, see Fleiss, 1981).

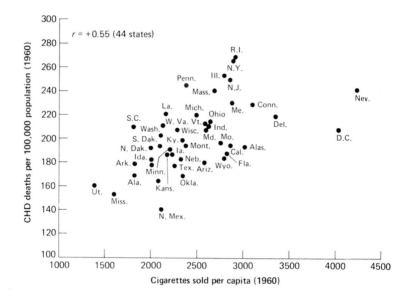

Figure 11-1 Relationship between the age-adjusted total death rate for coronary heart disease and per capita cigarette consumption in 44 states in 1960. *(Reproduced, by permission, from Friedman, 1967.)*

Other methods of measuring associations are also used, but as mentioned, contrasts in rates or proportions are most commonly employed. Regardless of how a statistical association is measured or expressed, the same problems of interpretation apply.

Associations Based on Groups of Groups

It has been emphasized in this book that, in epidemiology, the group is the unit of concern. Groups that provide the most useful and relevant information are *groups of individuals*. Nevertheless, it is also possible to study *groups of groups*. Statistical associations found in groups of groups may be useful, but they may also be quite misleading and not at all applicable to the individuals within the groups.

Consider, for example, the data shown in Fig. 11-1, relating per capita cigarette consumption to coronary heart disease mortality rates in 44 states in 1960. The statistical association, shown graphically and by the correlation coefficient of +.55, involves a group of states rather than a group of persons. Although the findings are suggestive of an association between cigarette smoking and coronary heart disease mortality in persons, we cannot be sure from these data alone that the persons who smoked in these states truly experienced a higher coronary heart disease mortality rate. (Actually, the association between smoking and coronary heart disease death rates had already been shown in groups of individuals when the study yielding Fig. 11-1 was done. This study's purpose was to cast some light on the striking geographic variation in coronary mortality in the United States.)

The potential for drawing fallacious conclusions about groups of individuals from associations observed in groups of groups was emphasized by Robinson (1950), who termed the latter "ecological correlations." He noted, for example, that among *persons* age 10 and over in the United States there was a moderate *positive* association between being foreign-born and being illiterate. However, looked at on the basis of *geographic regions* (i.e., groups), there was a stronger *negative* correlation. That is, those regions with the lowest percentages of foreign-born population had the highest percentages who were illiterate. Thus a conclusion about the relationship of nativity to literacy based solely on a study of geographic units would have been quite misleading.

Most epidemiologic observations showing that geographic differences in disease rates parallel geographic differences in possible causative factors are associations involving groups of groups. The same may be said of parallel time trends. As such, these correlations in space and time are interesting clues, but their limitations should be recognized (Morgenstern, 1982). Failure of investigators to respect the possible fallacies involved has contributed to the mistrust of epidemiologic or statistical data, as exemplified by Disraeli's famous reference to "lies, damn lies, and statistics."

Occasionally, causes of disease may be more clearly revealed by ecological correlations than by correlations based on individuals. Marked differences *among* populations with respect to certain characteristics may show a clear correlation with disease incidence, which cannot be readily demonstrated in studies of individuals *within* a population. This is thought to be particularly true of dietary characteristics such as fat consumption because marked day-to-day variation in most individuals' intake makes it difficult to discern relatively small differences among individuals within a relatively homogeneous population (Liu et al., 1978).

Evaluating Statistical Associations Involving Groups of Individuals

Fortunately, the main body of epidemiologic knowledge involves associations found in groups of individuals. When these associations emerge from a study, five basic questions usually require immediate attention:

1 Could the association have been observed just by chance?
2 Could the association be due to bias?
3 Could other *confounding* variables have accounted for the observed relationship?
4 To whom does the association apply?
5 Does the association represent a cause-and-effect relationship?

Evaluating the Possible Role of Chance

Regarding the first question, we have already mentioned in Chap. 3 (pp. 32–34) that chance may play a role in determining the outcome of a study. The fewer the subjects, the more the results may be influenced by chance sampling variation. Statistical significance tests are used to determine the probability that the observed association could have occurred by chance alone, if no association really exists. Selecting the appropriate test depends on the nature of the data and the method by which they are analyzed. For example, if the data analysis results in a fourfold table with subjects classified by presence or absence of a trait and of disease as illustrated by Table 3-2, the chi-square test may be most appropriate. Comparing the mean level of a quantitative attribute in a disease group with the mean level in a control group may involve a *t* test of the difference between two means. The reader is referred to medical statistics texts such as Hill and Hill (1991), Swinscow (1983), Glantz (1992), Colton (1974), Moore and McCabe (1993) for further details.

Unfortunately, the word *significant* in *statistically significant* is often misinterpreted as representing the medical or biological significance of an association. A slight difference in the mean hemoglobin concentration between two groups such as 0.1 g/100 mL may be statistically significant if the two groups are large—that is, it is most unlikely to be due to chance. However, this difference may be totally unimportant for health or longevity or in relation to a disease under investigation. Thus, to say that one group's mean level is significantly lower than that of the other group has connotations that should be avoided by stressing the fact that *statistical* and not *biological* significance is being discussed.

Confidence Intervals   Statistical significance tests are usually applied to the testing of hypotheses that certain associations exist and are not explained by chance sampling variation. A more general and more flexible way of evaluating the role of chance variation is to determine a *confidence interval* or the *confidence limits* around a finding such as a rate or a relative risk. The 95 percent confidence interval indicates the range of true values that could exist in an assumed underlying population, given the particular finding in the study sample. In other words, there is a 95 percent probability that the true value lies within the confidence interval or between the confidence limits. Thus, an association might be expressed as a relative risk of 1.2 with 95 percent confidence limits of 0.8 (lower limit) and 1.8 (upper limit). If the confidence interval includes a relative risk of 1.0, as in this example, the finding is quite compatible with there being no association at all. When the 95 percent confidence interval does not include 1.0, this is similar to finding that the association is statistically significant, with $p < 0.05$.

Examining the Possible Role of Bias

Statistical associations between exposures and diseases, as derived from epidemiologic studies, are subject to two main types of bias, *selection bias* and *information bias*. These encompass many of the possibilities for bias described in various contexts elsewhere in this book. Some authorities add a third kind of bias to these two major categories, that is, *confounding bias*. This bias, which involves the effects of additional variables on the exposure-disease association, is discussed in the next section of this chapter.

Selection bias occurs when study subjects are selected in a way that can misleadingly increase or decrease the magnitude of an association. For example, in a hospital-based case-control study of alcohol consumption in relation to a particular type of cancer, the investigator may decide to select patients admitted for traumatic injuries as the control group. Since alcohol use is strongly related to trauma, control selection will be biased in that controls will show a higher average level of alcohol consumption than would be shown by the general population free of the cancer. Thus, any true positive association of alcohol use with the cancer will be reduced or lost in this study. If the bias is strong enough, a true small positive association will appear to be a negative association, because the controls will report more alcohol use than the cases.

Similarly, consider a cohort follow-up study to determine whether persons who receive a particular screening test show a reduction in mortality. If the comparison group consists of persons who refuse the test, selection bias is almost guaranteed to make the test appear beneficial. This is because persons who cooperate with health testing generally take better care of themselves in many ways than those who do not.

Information bias results when the method of data collection makes the information obtained from two or more groups differ in some misleading way. This can occur, for example, in a case-control study of the relationships between prenatal workplace exposures or drug use and congenital anomalies in the newborn if exposure information is obtained by interviewing the mothers. Most mothers of malformed infants would have thought a lot about the possible causes of the anomalies and would be more apt to remember taking particular drugs or experiencing certain workplace exposures than would the usually contented mothers of normal babies. Similarly, a comparison of the degree of obesity of one group of persons who had been weighed with that of a group whose weights were obtained by questionnaire would almost certainly suffer from information bias.

Information bias can result in misclassification of subjects with respect to disease or possible causal factors. As noted at the end of Chap. 3, nondifferential misclassification always weakens an association whereas differential misclassification can either weaken or strengthen it.

Clearly, an important step in evaluating associations from epidemiologic studies is to consider whether selection bias or information bias could have occurred. [For those who wish to explore the matter of bias further, Sackett (1979) has provided an extensive compilation of its many forms.]

Evaluating the Role of Other Variables: The Problem of Confounding

In addition to chance and bias, it is important to rule out other variables as possible explanations for an association. To show in a very simple way how a third variable may account for part or all of a statistical association, an imaginary set of data is graphically plotted in Fig. 11-2. The figure shows, let us say, degree of coronary atherosclerosis measured by coronary angiography as related to hand-grip strength. Note that all eight data points form a pattern showing an association between the two variables. That is, on the average, those with stronger grips tend to have more coronary atherosclerosis.

However, also note that four of the data points are shown by open circles and four by solid black circles. The open circles happen to represent four women and the black circles, four men. Looking at each sex group separately by covering the other four points, it can be seen that there is no relationship between grip strength and amount of atherosclerosis. It is only because the two sexes have been combined in one set of data that the association appears. Thus, sex difference constitutes a third underlying, or *confounding,* variable that completely explains the apparent association between grip strength and coronary atherosclerosis, which is therefore considered a *spurious,* or *secondary,* association.

Another set of fictitious data, shown in Table 11-1, again illus-

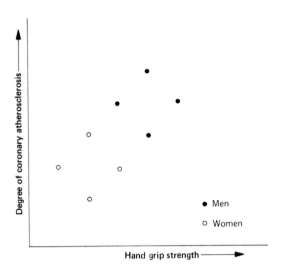

Figure 11-2 Relationship between hand-grip strength and degree of coronary atherosclerosis. Fictitious data showing spurious correlation resulting from combining the data for men and women.

trates how a confounding variable, age, can result in an apparent association between two other variables when no real association exists. A total of 600 persons aged 30 to 59 were asked whether they ever had been troubled by low-back pain and whether their parents were still living or whether either their mother or father had died.

The top section of the table shows the findings for the 200 subjects in their thirties. Twenty, or 10 percent, reported low-back pain. Also, half had both parents living and half reported at least one parent dead. Of the 100 in either parent-survival group, 10, or 10 percent, reported low-back pain. Thus, in this subgroup, death of a parent was not related to low-back pain.

The next section of the table shows the results for 200 subjects in their forties. At this later age a larger proportion had lost a parent (140/200), and a larger proportion reported low-back pain (20 percent), but parental death was again not related to low-back pain. In either parent-survival group, 20 percent reported low-back pain.

Table 11-1   Relationship between Parental Death and Low-Back-Pain History
(Fictitious Data Showing Spurious Association Due to Relation of Both Variables to Age)

	Total number	History of low-back pain	
		Number	Percent
Ages 30–39			
All subjects	200	20	10
Any parent dead	100	10	10
No parent dead	100	10	10
Ages 40–49			
All subjects	200	40	20
Any parent dead	140	28	20
No parent dead	60	12	20
Ages 50–59			
All subjects	200	60	30
Any parent dead	180	54	30
No parent dead	20	6	30
Total, all ages			
All subjects	600	120	20
Any parent dead	420	92	22
No parent dead	180	28	16

The results for 200 subjects in their fifties also showed no relationship between the two study variables. The proportion with at least one dead parent was still higher (180/200), and the prevalence of a low-back-pain history was higher (30 percent), but again the 30 percent low-back-pain prevalence held true for subjects both with and without a parent dead.

Now, look at what happens when the data for the three age groups are simply added together, as shown at the bottom of the table. A total of 22 percent of patients with a parent dead report low-back pain, whereas only 16 percent with both parents living have this complaint. The data for all ages combined appear to show that parental loss *is* related to low-back pain, whereas we know that in any age decade this is not the case.

The apparent relationship of low-back pain to parental loss in the total group is attributable to the difference in age distribution between those with and without a dead parent. Stated simply, those subjects with a dead parent tend to be older and, therefore, are more apt to report low-back pain. Actually, 180, or 43 percent, of the 420 subjects with at least one parent dead were in their fifties, whereas only 20, or 11 percent, of the 180 subjects with no parents dead were in their fifties.

Note that age, the confounding variable responsible for this spurious association, was related to both variables of interest, low-back pain and parental loss. This reflects an important principle: for a variable to confound, that is, to either increase or decrease an association between two others, it must be independently related to *both* of them, not just one.

Handling Spurious Association Due to Confounding Variables

Prevention   Knowledge of previous epidemiologic findings or of the pathophysiology of the disease under investigation will often suggest possible confounding variables. A study may be designed and carried out so as to prevent these confounding variables from producing misleading group differences. For example, cases and controls may be matched for age so that differences in age distribution will not lead to spurious associations such as the one described above.

It may not be possible to "control" all pertinent variables in this manner at the outset. Also, underlying variables may come to light or be thought of later, when the data are being analyzed. Fortunately, it is possible to analyze data in ways that take into account or control confounding variables.

Specification   The simplest method for controlling variables in the data analysis is *specification*. This involves examining the data separately for each subgroup of subjects who fall into one particular category or level of the variable to be controlled. In the foregoing example involving a relationship between hand-grip strength and coronary atherosclerosis, the fact that the correlation is spurious and is due to sex differences becomes obvious if we *specify* sex and look at the data separately for men and women. Similarly, if the parental-loss/back-pain association is examined in specific age groups, it is no longer apparent.

Actually, age and sex are so often related to disease occurrence and to other variables that it is customary to examine data in specific age-sex subgroups before combining them into an overall tabulation. This standard approach to data analysis in epidemiology is probably the reason that an epidemiologist has been defined as "a physician broken down by age and sex."

Just as specification can show associations to be spurious, it can also be used to show that suspected confounding variables are not explanations for an association. For example, in a study of smoking and the leukocyte count (Friedman et al., 1973), it was suspected that the higher mean leukocyte count in smokers compared with that in nonsmokers might really be due to chronic bronchitis, which is related both to smoking and to the leukocyte count. The data were analyzed separately for persons with and without evidence of chronic bronchitis. When this was done, large smoker-nonsmoker differences in mean leukocyte count were still present in each subgroup and were, thus, not attributable to chronic bronchitis.

Adjustment   Sometimes an investigator would like to compare two or more overall groups, knowing that they differ in a pertinent third variable. It is possible, by means of a procedure known as *adjustment,* or *standardization,* to make such comparisons, controlling for differences in a confounding variable. For example, in evaluating the parental-loss/back-pain association, it is possible through *age adjustment* to remove the effect of age as a confounding variable and compare subjects with and without parental loss to see if either group has a higher prevalence of a low-back-pain history.

Age adjustment by the *direct* method involves choosing a standard population and applying the rates observed for subjects in each specific age category to the corresponding members of the standard population. The choice of a standard population is fairly arbitrary. Often it is the population of a country at a particular time, such as the United States in 1980. Or, frequently, it is the total population involved in the study in question. Or, it may be one particular subgroup of that study population. In our low-back-pain study, for example, one might age-adjust the rates observed in the subgroup with no parental loss to the subgroup with loss of a parent or age-adjust the rates of both subgroups to the total study group.

To illustrate how this is accomplished, Table 11-2 shows the direct age adjustment of the rate of low-back pain in the subgroup without parental loss to the total study population used as a standard. The rate observed in each age category of the subjects with no parental loss is multiplied by the number of subjects in the same age category in the standard population. This yields the number that would be observed in the standard population if the low-back-pain rates in the group with no parental loss were applicable to the standard population. The numbers that would be observed in each age group of the standard population are then added together, and the total is divided by the total number in the standard population, yielding the age-adjusted rate of 20 percent. In this example, the same age-specific rates of low-back pain were observed in the subjects with parental loss; therefore, the age-adjusted rate for this subgroup would also be 20 percent. Thus, using age-adjusted rates, we would correctly conclude that parental loss was not related to low-back pain.

Table 11-2   Example of Direct Age-Adjustment: Observed Low-Back-Pain Rates Applied to Standard Population Consisting of All Study Subjects

Age	Observed low-back-pain rate	×	Total number in age subgroup of standard population	=	Number that would be observed in standard population
30–39	10%		200		20
40–49	20%		200		40
50–59	30%		200		60
		Total	600		120

Age-adjusted rate = 120/600 = 20%

The *indirect* method of age adjustment is somewhat different from the direct method. Instead of applying the study subgroup's age-specific rates to a standard population, the age-specific rates of the standard population are applied to the corresponding portions of the study subgroup. This procedure yields the number of cases that would be expected in each study subgroup if the age-specific rates in the standard population had been operative in the study subgroups. The overall expected rate in the study subgroup (total cases expected in subgroup divided by total population of a subgroup) is then compared to the overall rate in the standard population. Any difference must be attributable to the difference between the age distribution of the subgroup and that of the standard population.

The study subgroup's overall observed or crude rate is then corrected proportionally to make up for this difference in age distribution. For example, if the standard population's overall rate is 80 percent of the expected rate in the study subgroup, then the observed rate in the subgroup is reduced by multiplying it by 80 percent. After the overall rates in various subgroups have been modified in this manner, they are then compared with one another. More detailed examples of age adjustment by the direct and indirect methods are given by Hill and Hill (1991, Chap. 20).

Indirect adjustment can distort comparisons, particularly when the groups compared differ greatly in their distribution of the variable that is adjusted (Breslow and Day, 1987; Rothman, 1986). For this reason, indirect adjustment has fallen into disfavor among many epidemiologists. In this author's experience, comparisons based on direct and indirect adjustment have usually given similar results; the numerical examples others have used to show how indirect adjustment can yield biased comparisons involve gross differences between groups in the distribution of the variable to be adjusted—differences much larger than those usually encountered in practice. An advantage of indirect adjustment is that it suffers less from random sampling variation than does direct adjustment when there are small numbers of people in some categories of the adjusted variable. Rates used in direct adjustment would be based on these small numbers and would thus be subject to substantial sampling variation. With indirect adjustment the rates are more stable since they are usually based on a large standard population. To sum up, in comparing groups, direct adjustment is generally preferable to indirect because it is less likely to introduce bias, but indirect adjustment is often more reliable.

Note that the expected rate or the expected number of cases computed by the indirect method is used in the ratio of observed/ expected, which constitutes the standardized morbidity (or mortality) ratio (SMR) mentioned in Chap. 2. Similarly, the ratio comparison of two rates, directly standardized to the same standard population, is referred to as a standardized rate ratio (SRR).

It must be remembered that an age-adjusted rate is an artificial rather than an actual rate. Its value is that it permits one population to be compared with another, with age "controlled." It should not be substituted for the *crude* rate if what is wanted is an accurate description of a population rather than a comparison. The age-adjusted rate is a convenient summary of age-specific rates. The age-specific rates themselves are most informative and should be compared whenever possible.

This discussion of adjustment has focused on age adjustment because age is the variable that is most commonly controlled in this manner. However, direct or indirect adjustment may be applied to any variable suspected of confounding an association between two study variables.

Adjustment of Relative Risks So far, we have considered adjustment as applied to rates. It is often necessary to adjust relative risk estimates for confounding variables. As with rates, it is desirable first to divide the study group into subgroups, or strata, according to the level or category of the confounding variable. One should then examine the relative risk in each stratum, as determined by the rate ratio or risk ratio in a cohort study or as estimated by the odds ratio in a case-control study. There are methods for calculating a summary relative risk that combines the results from all of the strata in a way that eliminates confounding by the stratified variable. Probably the most commonly used is the method of Mantel and Haenszel. These statisticians also developed a related procedure known as the Mantel-Haenszel test, which is commonly used to determine whether the summary relative risk differs to a statistically significant degree from the no-association relative risk of 1.0 (Mantel and Haenszel, 1959). Instructions for use of these methods, including the calculation of confidence intervals, may be found in advanced texts (e.g., Breslow and Day, 1980, 1987; Kelsey et al., 1986; Rothman, 1986; and Schlesselman, 1982).

Variables That Link a Possible Causal Factor with a Disease Variables that are intermediate between the causal factor of interest and the disease of concern must be handled with care. Suppose, for example, that one wants to determine whether consuming large amounts of alcohol predisposes to stroke and that the suspected biological mechanism is a blood pressure–raising effect of alcohol. Although blood pressure is associated with both alcohol drinking and stroke, it is a mediating rather than a confounding variable, and if it is adjusted or controlled in the analysis, the relationship between alcohol intake and stroke incidence will be partially or completely hidden. Thus, it is advisable not to adjust for variables believed to lie in the causal pathway between the exposure to be evaluated and the disease, unless the aim is to determine whether the exposure is connected to the disease by some other causal pathway.

The controversy over whether obesity is a causal factor for coronary heart disease is due partly to the fact that, in many studies of this question, coronary risk factors that are made worse by obesity, particularly lipid levels and blood pressure, have been controlled in the analysis. When this is done, the relationship between obesity and coronary heart disease often appears small or absent. Analytical control for lipids and blood pressure is appropriate only if the question asked is whether obesity increases risk of coronary heart disease over and above its effects on these risk factors.

Other Considerations Concerning Confounding Variables Some other general rules about adjusting confounding variables will be mentioned briefly.

There is no reason, and it is probably counterproductive regarding study reliability, to adjust for variables related to the potential causal variable of interest, but not to the disease. These are not true confounders.

In addition to variables that link a possible causal factor with a disease, those which are a consequence of the factor should not be controlled. For example, one should not control for presence or absence of cough in a study of smoking and lung cancer.

Confounders previously established by other studies or by knowledge of the biological or clinical processes involved should be controlled.

Judging whether a potential confounder exists in a particular set of data should be based on the strength of its associations with the possible causal factors and the disease, not on the statistical significance of these associations.

If a variable could be a confounder according to the suspected biological mechanism and controlling for it affects the strength of the exposure-disease association under consideration, then for all practical purposes it is a confounder.

Positive confounding exaggerates or creates spurious associations. *Negative confounding* decreases or obscures associations and may even reverse their direction.

For a confounding variable to explain an association of a given strength, it must have a much stronger association with both the possible causal factor and the disease.

Misclassification of confounding variables makes it difficult to adequately control for them.

Again, the reader is referred to advanced texts for further discussion of these principles (e.g., Breslow and Day, 1980, 1987; Kelsey et al., 1986; Rothman, 1986; Schlesselman, 1982).

Other Methods of Adjustment   More complex statistical procedures are also available for removing the effects of one or more confounding variables on statistical associations. Some of these, including multiple regression analysis, multiple logistic regression analysis, and the Cox proportional hazards model, are now frequently used and often appear in medical journal articles. Thus, health professionals should have a basic understanding of how they work (see Chap. 12).

Interaction

When the strength of an association varies from one subgroup of a study population to another, *interaction* or *statistical interaction* is said to occur. Epidemiologists frequently call this phenomenon *effect modification*. To this author, this is often inappropriate because it seems to imply causality even when none is involved. An example of interaction would be the association between cigarette smoking and myocardial infarction, which is much stronger in young adults, who have relative risks of 3 or more, than in the elderly, who have relative risks of 1.5 or less. Cigarette smoking is said to interact with age in influencing the risk of myocardial infarction.

Interaction can be recognized and described in simple cross-classification tables. For example, in Table 11-3 (fictitious data) it is clear that there is an interaction between educational level and urban versus rural residence in determining the prevalence of alcoholism. The urban/rural ratio of alcoholism prevalence is 2.5 (0.05/ 0.02) among those with elementary education, 1.2 (0.06/0.05) among those with high school or trade school education, and 0.5 (0.04/0.08) among those who attended college.

To fully characterize epidemiologic associations, it is useful to determine whether interaction exists and, if it does, which subgroups show strong and weak exposure-disease relations. Also, if there is considerable variation in relative risk from stratum to stratum, summary measures of relative risk, such as the standardized rate ratio or the Mantel-Haenszel summary estimate, become less informative, and emphasis should be placed on the stratum-specific data.

Interaction in the context of multivariate analysis is discussed in Chap. 12.

General Applicability of an Association

In evaluating observed statistical associations one must always consider to whom they apply. The study in which the association is observed was conducted on a finite group of persons with certain characteristics. Would the association also hold true for other groups? Obviously, the more different groups that show the asso-

Table 11-3 Prevalence of Alcoholism in Urban and Rural Areas of a State, by Educational Level (Fictitious Data)

Education	Urban areas			Rural areas			Entire state		
	Total number	Alcoholic No.	Alcoholic Prevalence	Total number	Alcoholic No.	Alcoholic Prevalence	Total number	Alcoholic No.	Alcoholic Prevalence
Elementary only	40,000	2,000	0.0500	60,000	1,200	0.0200	100,000	3,200	0.0320
High school or trade school	70,000	4,200	0.0600	80,000	4,000	0.0500	150,000	8,200	0.0547
At least some college	110,000	4,400	0.0400	40,000	3,200	0.0800	150,000	7,600	0.0507
Total	220,000	10,600	0.0482	180,000	8,400	0.0467	400,000	19,000	0.0475

ciation, the more certain one can be that it is widely applicable. Where a variety of studies are lacking, it becomes a matter of judgment to determine whether an association observed in one group is applicable to another.

Questions of generality might be raised, for example, regarding the association between serum cholesterol level and coronary heart disease found in the Framingham Study. The study population is virtually all white. Thus it can legitimately be asked whether the same association holds true for blacks and Asians. Fortunately, other studies provide a positive answer to this question.

More subtle is the fact that the Framingham Study and similar studies have as subjects volunteers or cooperative people. Does the cholesterol-coronary disease association apply also to uncooperative individuals? While volunteers do differ from others in certain characteristics, it is difficult to imagine that these characteristics would produce this observed relationship. Thus, one might reasonably judge that cholesterol is related to coronary heart disease in the uncooperative as well.

If a study's findings are generalizable to persons not studied, they are said to have *external validity*. This is to be distinguished from *internal validity*. If a study has the latter, its findings are true of the study's subjects, but nothing is implied about generalizability.

Statistical Associations and Cause-and-Effect Relationships

It is common knowledge that statistical associations do not necessarily imply causation. The "price of tea in China" is a frequently cited example of a variable which can be related statistically to some other variable but has no causal relation to it.

Statistical associations derived from well-controlled experimental studies can usually be interpreted to represent cause-and-effect relationships. Something is done and a result is observed. In epidemiology, however, most studies are observational, and an experiment to establish a cause-and-effect relationship may be difficult or impossible to carry out. Vital decisions affecting public health and preventive medicine must be made on the basis of observational evidence. It is important, therefore, to have some basis for deciding whether a statistical association derived from an observational study represents a cause-and-effect relationship.

A number of authors have grappled with this philosophical problem. Certain criteria seem to be universally accepted, while others remain controversial. The reader wishing to explore this question in greater depth should refer to Chap. 2 of MacMahon and Pugh (1970), Chap. 28 of Hill and Hill (1991), Yerushalmy (1962), Larsen and Silvette (1968), Susser (1973, 1986), and Chap. 2 of Rothman (1986).

Strength of the Association   In general, the stronger the association, the more likely it represents a cause-and-effect relationship. Weak associations often turn out to be spurious and explainable by some known, or as yet unknown, confounding variable. As noted above, in order for an association to be spurious, the underlying factor that explains it must have a stronger relationship to the disease than does the suspected causal factor (Bross, 1966). When the causal factor under consideration is strongly related to the disease, it is likely, although not certain, that the underlying variable with the necessarily even stronger relationship to the disease would be recognizable.

Strength of an association is usually measured by the *relative risk* or the ratio of the disease rate in those with the factor to the rate in those without. The relative risk of lung cancer in cigarette smokers as compared to nonsmokers is on the order of 10:1, whereas the relative risk of pancreatic cancer is about 2:1. This difference suggests that cigarette smoking is more likely to be a causal factor for lung cancer than for pancreatic cancer.

Time Sequence   In a causal relationship the characteristic or event associated with the disease must *precede* the disease. This time relationship should be clear in cohort studies. In cross-sectional and case-control studies it may not always be obvious which came first.

Consistency with Other Knowledge   If the association makes sense in terms of known biological mechanisms or other epidemiologic knowledge, it becomes more plausible as a cause-and-effect relationship. Part of the attractiveness of the hypothesis that a high-saturated-fat, high-cholesterol diet predisposes to atherosclerosis is the fact that a biological mechanism can be invoked. Such a diet increases blood lipids, which may in turn be deposited in arterial walls. A correlation between the number of telephone poles in a country and its coronary heart disease mortality rate lacks plausibility as a cause-and-effect relationship partly because it is difficult to imagine a biological mechanism whereby telephone poles result in atherosclerosis.

Failure to Find Other Explanations   When a statistical association is observed, the thoughtful investigator will consider possible explanations for the relationship *other* than the associated variable's causing the disease. The data already collected may be used to learn whether these other possible explanations might hold true. Or, additional data may have to be obtained to answer such questions.

Failure to find an alternative to the cause-and-effect hypothesis despite conscientious searching does not prove that there is no alternative. But it does strengthen the evidence for a cause-and-effect relationship.

An interesting example of a search for other explanations comes from a case-control study showing an association between oral contraceptives and thromboembolic disease (Vessey and Doll, 1968). Since it is easy to overlook the diagnosis of deep-vein thrombosis or pulmonary embolism, the investigators considered the possibility that a history of oral contraceptive use would alert the physician to these conditions, resulting in a spurious association. They reasoned that a spurious association of this type would be strongest among patients with the least evident disease, since this group would contain women whose condition was diagnosed only because they were known to have taken oral contraceptives. Cases were therefore classified by degree of certainty as to the presence of thromboembolism. It was found that the association with oral contraceptive use was actually less marked among the less certain and milder cases than among the definite and severe cases. Thus, this alternative explanation could reasonably be rejected, lending greater credence to the idea that thromboembolism was actually caused by oral contraceptives.

Other Criteria Although stressed by some authorities, the following criteria seem less valuable, to this author, as yardsticks for assessing a cause-and-effect relationship per se.

Gradient of Risk It has been stated that a dose-response relationship argues for a cause-and-effect relationship. For example, the fact that moderate cigarette smokers have a lung cancer death rate intermediate between nonsmokers and heavy smokers is considered evidence that cigarette smoking causes lung cancer.

This criterion would appear less satisfactory. Threshold phenomena are well known in nature whereby no effect is seen until a causal stimulus reaches a certain level, above which a response is seen. In this situation a gradient of response might well be absent if two different dosages of the causal factor are well below the threshold level. Conversely, a spurious correlation could easily show a nice gradient. A spurious correlation of cigarette smoking with a disease caused by alcohol consumption might show an apparent dose-response relationship of disease incidence to amount smoked, due to a correlation between amount smoked and amount of alcohol consumed.

Consistency in Several Studies Finding the same association in several different studies provides assurance that the association *exists* and is not an artifact based on the way one particular study was carried out or based on an unusual group of study subjects. In this sense, consistency across studies is reassuring, but it does not argue strongly that an association is one of cause and effect.

Specificity By specificity is meant that the possible causal factor is observed to be associated with one or just a few diseases or effects rather than with a wide variety of diseases. One of the arguments that has been used against cigarette smoking as a cause of lung cancer is that in epidemiologic studies, smoking also appears to be associated with an assortment of seemingly unrelated diseases such as coronary heart disease, peptic ulcer, bladder cancer, and cirrhosis of the liver. Thus, it is argued either that smokers differ from nonsmokers in a biological characteristic that leads health to break down in a variety of ways or that the studies were affected by some kind of hidden bias or artifact that falsely incriminates smoking.

Although finding specificity *is* reassuring and although an apparent lack of specificity *should* lead to some suspicion of an artifact, the importance of a lack of specificity as negative evidence has been overemphasized. This can readily be seen when one considers other recognized disease agents such as the tubercle bacillus and applies the lack of specificity argument to them. How, it might have been asked, can the tubercle bacillus cause an increased rate of lung lesions when it also has been associated with scrofula, meningitis, collapsed vertebrae, peritonitis, bleeding from the kidney, marked wasting, and so on. We now know that the tubercle bacillus can produce a variety of effects, and we have some understanding of the mechanisms by which these occur. Cigarette smoke has a variety of active constituents that get carried throughout the body; therefore, a lack of specificity is not surprising.

Statistical Associations between Diseases

Epidemiologic and clinical studies may reveal statistical associations between two or more diseases. Two diseases are associated in a population if the incidence or prevalence of one disease is higher when the other is present than when it is absent.

A true association between diseases may occur because one disease predisposes to another (e.g., diabetes mellitus and coronary heart disease) or because both diseases share a common etiologic factor (head injuries and cirrhosis of the liver, both due to alcoholism). Thus, discovery of disease associations may provide valuable information if the etiology of one disease is obscure.

Disease associations may be more apparent than real. Two diseases may produce similar signs, symptoms, or laboratory findings, thus leading to a greater chance of *diagnosis* of one disease if the other is present. Also, diseases are detected in the clinic, in the hospital, or at autopsy, and the presence of more than one disease may make it more likely for a person to be seen at one of these diagnostic facilities. Due to this and other selective factors, diseases may appear to be associated at a medical facility even when they are not associated in the general population—the so-called *Berkson's bias*. Further discussion of disease associations and the potential fallacies involved may be found in Berkson (1946), Mainland (1953), Wijsman (1958), and Friedman (1968).

Even false associations due to selection may be useful to the clinician. For example, an association between inguinal hernia and colon cancer has been noted on the surgical ward by some (Terezis et al., 1963) but not all investigators (Brendel and Kirsh, 1971). Even if this association is not present in the general population, it still may be wise for surgeons in some settings to look for colon cancer in their patients with hernias.

Absence of Association

The emphasis in much of this chapter has been on the factors—chance, bias, and confounding—that produce false associations and how they can be surmounted. It should not be forgotten that the absence of an association may be of great interest and that the same factors may reduce or conceal an association which is truly present.

A study should have sufficient subjects to reduce to acceptable levels the chance variation that could lead to a conclusion of no association when there actually is one. We apply the term *power* to a study's ability to demonstrate an association that is truly present. If a study has a power of 50 percent, it has a 50-50 chance of detecting the association. Most studies aim for a power of at least 80 or 90 percent, since it would be unfortunate if there were more than a 10 or 20 percent chance of missing a true association. If the association is especially important to detect, it may be worth spending the extra resources to study more people and raise the power to 95 percent or more. [For more discussion of study size and power, see Cohen (1977); Colton (1974); Schlesselman (1982); Glantz (1992); or Moore and McCabe (1993).]

Studies can confirm that associations exist by disproving the absence of association, that is, by "rejecting the null hypothesis." Unfortunately, it is essentially impossible to prove that an association is not present. Because of chance sampling error, data apparently showing no association may be obtained when an association actually exists. The best we can do is to apply statistical procedures to such data to determine confidence limits (described earlier in this chapter). For example, in a particular study the relative risk may be shown to be 1.0, with 95 percent confidence interval of 0.7 to 1.5. This means that, with the degree of sampling error present in this study, the probability is 95 in 100 that the true relative risk could be as low as 0.7 or as high as 1.5, even though the data show no association. If the sample can be enlarged, the confidence limits will be narrowed and may be brought closer to, but never exactly equal to, 1.0.

A finding of no association may be of great practical importance. If an inexpensive therapy for a serious common disease can be shown to be as safe and effective as an expensive therapy (for example, home care versus hospital care for myocardial infarction), millions of dollars in medical care costs may be saved if the cheaper method is universally adopted. A decision to adopt the cheaper method should be based on studies of large numbers of subjects, so that a small difference in mortality will fall outside the confidence interval around "no difference" and can thus be distinguished from it. Just 1 or 2 extra deaths per 100 patients treated would probably be, if recognized, a price that society is unwilling to pay for the monetary savings provided by the cheaper treatment.

Many experimental clinical trials have failed to show a statistically significant degree of benefit from the therapy being evaluated. However, because of the relatively small numbers of subjects in some of these studies, the confidence limits around "no effect" were wide enough to encompass substantial benefit. Freiman et al. (1978) warned against prematurely discarding therapies on the basis of these inconclusive "negative" trials.

PROBLEMS

11-1 Suppose that in a cohort study of fractures 3 percent of persons who drank less than 1 pint of milk per day experienced a broken bone in a 6-year follow-up period. Among those who drank 1 pint per day or more, the average annual incidence was 0.5 percent per year. What can you conclude from this study about the statistical association of milk drinking and fractures?

11-2 The correlation coefficient (r) between two measurements in a group of children turned out to be $-.98$. Would it be correct to say that there was almost no association between the two measurements?

11-3 What is an ecological correlation? Which of the following statements expresses an ecological correlation? If the correlation is ecological, what corresponding study question would refer to groups of individuals?

    a Nations with little beef consumption have a low incidence of colon cancer.

    b The patient mortality rates are lower in hospitals that do not employ interns or residents than in those that do.

    c Persons who wear hats have lower rates of skin cancer than those who do not.

    d The suicide rate in black men has shown a steady increase during the same decade that the use of microwave ovens has become widespread.

11-4 Suppose that in a controlled trial of a pneumonia vaccine, 10,000 military recruits received the vaccine and 10,000 received a placebo. During the 1-year follow-up period there was a threefold excess risk of meningococcal meningitis among those receiving vaccine, based on three cases in that group versus one in the placebo group.

    a Is there a statistical association between receiving the vaccine and developing meningococcal meningitis?

    b What is the first noncausal explanation of the threefold difference you would attempt to rule out, and how would you do this?

11-5 The following statements or passages are from examples of studies presented in previous chapters. Indicate whether the procedure described was done primarily to prevent selection bias, to prevent information bias, or to prevent or control confounding.

    From the case-control study of pedestrians fatally injured by motor vehicles (Chap. 7):

    a "The site visited [for selecting controls] was the sidewalk point closest to the exact location of the accident as described on the police or medical examiner's report."

    b [When a control subject was approached] "a nearby member of the team [said], 'I don't want to know your name; I merely want to ask you a few questions.' "

    c "Rather than weaken the investigation by omitting [non-

English-speaking controls] when no member of the team knew a common language, passersby were stopped and asked to serve as interpreters."

d "The case group was less often married and more often foreign-born and of lower socioeconomic status than were the controls. However, these differences could be explained by age differences between the case and control groups."

From the experimental study to evaluate the effects of multiphasic health checkups (Chap. 9):

e "For example, subjects' recent addresses were not submitted to the state health department to aid in the search for deaths, since the annual telephone contact with the study group led to more accurate and up-to-date information about addresses than was available for the control group."

f "The over 5000 subjects in both groups were selected on the basis of having certain digits in their medical record numbers, [which] are assigned in sequence with no relationship to any personal characteristics."

From the case-control study of oral contraceptives and thromboembolic disease (Chap. 7):

g "Two matched controls were selected for each case. . . . Matching was based on several criteria: [hospital, sex, discharge date, discharge status, age, marital status, residence, race, parity, and hospital pay status]."

h "Cases and controls were interviewed at home."

11-6 Suppose you are performing a case-control study on the relation of gout to eating habits. For each case, a control subject is randomly selected among all residents of the same community whose sex and year of birth are the same.

a Would it be desirable to age-adjust the data when comparing all cases to all controls?

b Would there be any point in making the comparisons in specific age groups such as the forties, fifties, sixties, and seventies age decades?

c How would you handle the potentially confounding variable of race?

11-7 The fictitious data in Table 11-3 show the prevalence of alcoholism among men in urban and rural areas of a state. The crude prevalence rates are very similar: 0.0482 in urban areas and 0.0467 in rural areas.

   a Compute alcoholism prevalence rates for urban and rural men, adjusting for educational level by the direct method. As the standard population, use that of the entire state.

   b Compute alcoholism prevalence rates for urban and rural men, this time adjusting for educational level by the indirect method. Again, use the entire state as the standard.

11-8 In each of the following examples, which is more likely to be a causal factor, X or Y? Explain your selection.

   a Persons who eat food X show a twofold increase in stomach cancer incidence. Persons who drive car Y show a twofold increase in stomach cancer incidence.

   b Persons who eat food X show a twofold increase in stomach cancer incidence. Persons who eat food Y show a 3.5-fold increase in stomach cancer incidence.

   c The percentage of stomach cancer cases who now eat food X is twice as great as the corresponding percentage of controls. The percentage of stomach cancer cases who ate food Y in their twenties is twice as great as the corresponding percentage of controls.

   d Food X is shown to be associated with a twofold increase in risk of stomach cancer among Hawaiians of Japanese ancestry, residents of Helsinki, Finland, and certain Bantu tribes in Africa. Food Y is shown to be associated with a 2.3-fold increase in risk of stomach cancer in Helsinki but not in the other study populations mentioned.

BIBLIOGRAPHY

Berkson J: Limitations of the application of fourfold table analysis to hospital data. *Biom Bull* **2**:47–53 (1946).

Brendel TH, Kirsh IF: Lack of association between inguinal hernia and carcinoma of the colon. *N Engl J Med* **284**:369–370 (1971).

Breslow NE, Day NE: *Statistical Methods in Cancer Research. Vol. 1—*

The Analysis of Case-Control Studies (Lyon: International Agency for Research on Cancer, 1980).

Breslow NE, Day NE: *Statistical Methods in Cancer Research. Vol. II— The Design and Analysis of Cohort Studies* (Lyon: International Agency for Research on Cancer, 1987).

Bross IDJ: Spurious effects from an extraneous variable. *J Chron Dis* **19:**637–647 (1966).

Cohen J: *Statistical Power Analysis for the Behavioral Sciences* (New York: Academic Press, 1977).

Colton T: *Statistics in Medicine* (Boston: Little, Brown, 1974), chap. 6.

Fleiss JL: *Statistical Methods for Rates and Proportions,* 2d ed. (New York: Wiley, 1981).

Freiman JA, Chalmers TC, Smith H, Jr, Kuebler RR: The importance of beta, the type II error and sample size in the design and interpretation of the randomized controlled trial: Survey of 71 "negative" trials. *N Engl J Med* **299:**690–694 (1978).

Friedman GD: Cigarette smoking and geographic variation in coronary heart disease mortality in the United States. *J Chron Dis* **20:**769–779 (1967).

————: The relationship between coronary heart disease and gallbladder disease: A critical review, *Ann Intern Med* **68:**222–235 (1968).

Friedman GD, Siegelaub AB, Seltzer CC, Feldman R, Collen MF: Smoking habits and the leukocyte count. *Arch Environ Health* **26:**137–143 (1973).

Glantz SA: *Primer of Biostatistics,* 3d ed. (New York: McGraw-Hill, 1992).

Hill AB, Hill ID: *Bradford Hill's Principles of Medical Statistics,* 12th ed. (London: Edward Arnold, 1991).

Kelsey JL, Thompson WD, Evans AS: *Methods in Observational Epidemiology* (New York: Oxford University Press, 1986).

Larsen PS, Silvette H: *Tobacco: Experimental and Clinical Studies,* suppl. I (Baltimore: Williams and Wilkins, 1968), pp. 346–362.

Liu K, Stamler J, Dyer A, McKeever J, McKeever P: Statistical methods to assess and minimize the role of intra-individual variability in obscuring the relationship between dietary lipids and serum cholesterol. *J Chron Dis* **31:**399–418 (1978).

MacMahon B, Pugh TF: *Epidemiology: Principles and Methods* (Boston: Little, Brown, 1970).

Mainland D: The risk of fallacious conclusions from autopsy data of the incidence of diseases with applications to heart disease. *Am Heart J* **45:**644–654 (1953).

Mantel N, Haenszel W: Statistical aspects of the analysis of data from retrospective studies of disease. *J Natl Cancer Inst* **22:**719–748 (1959).

Moore DS, McCabe GP: *Introduction to the Practice of Statistics,* 2d ed. (New York: Freeman, 1993).

Morgenstern H: Uses of ecologic analysis in epidemiologic research. *Am J Pub Health* **72:**1336–1344 (1982).

Robinson WS: Ecological correlations and the behavior of individuals. *Am Sociol Rev* **15:**351–357 (1950).

Rothman K: *Modern Epidemiology* (Boston: Little, Brown, 1986).

Sackett DL: Bias in analytic research. *J Chron Dis* **32:**51–63 (1979).

Schlesselman JJ: *Case-Control Studies: Design, Conduct, Analysis* (New York: Oxford University Press, 1982).

Susser M: *Causal Thinking in the Health Sciences: Concepts and Strategies of Epidemiology* (New York: Oxford University Press, 1973).

———: The logic of Sir Karl Popper and the practice of epidemiology. *Am J Epidemiol* **124:**711–718 (1986).

Swinscow TDV: *Statistics at Square One* (London: British Medical Journal, 1983).

Terezis LN, Davis WC, Jackson FC: Carcinoma of the colon associated with inguinal hernia. *N Engl J Med* **268:**774 (1963).

Vessey MP, Doll R: Investigation of relation between use of oral contraceptives and thromboembolic disease. *Br Med J* **2:**199–205 (1968).

Wijsman RA: Contribution to the study of the question of associations between two diseases. *Hum Biol* **30:**219–236 (1958).

Yerushalmy J: Statistical considerations and evaluation of epidemiological evidence, in G James, T Rosenthal (eds.), *Tobacco and Health* (Springfield, Ill.: Charles C Thomas, 1962), pp. 208–230.

Chapter 12

Introduction to Multivariate Analysis

A disease generally has many causes. Thus, investigators frequently examine the relationship of a disease to several causal factors simultaneously or take into account several other known or suspected causes in evaluating one potential cause. For example, to determine whether oral contraceptive use contributes to the development of uterine cervical cancer, an investigator would need to consider at least two confounding factors that are related to both oral contraceptive use and cervical cancer: early onset of sexual activity with multiple partners and cigarette smoking. Thus, the investigator would want to examine the three factors—sexual behavior, cigarette smoking, and oral contraceptive use—simultaneously to identify the independent contribution of each to the risk of cervical cancer.

Cross-classification and Adjustment

Using the important example of age, we have seen in Chap. 11 how to take into account one additional factor in studying disease etiology. The age range studied was broken down into several portions, or *strata,* and the relation of a possible causal factor to a disease was evaluated within each stratum and in a summary fashion by an overall adjustment for age.

To adjust for additional factors, the simplest approach is to subdivide the age groups further. So, for example, to adjust an analysis for both age and cigarette smoking, we might subdivide each age decade into three smoking groups: current smokers, former smokers, and persons who never smoked. This cross-classification will obviously increase the number of subgroups threefold. But, by brute force (or more simply, by computer, which is ideal for repetitive arithmetic), we can perform the calculations needed for direct or indirect adjustment for both age and smoking just as we adjusted solely for age.

One problem with this approach commonly occurs when adjustment is made for several factors. The subgroups can then become very small or even nonexistent. Let us say that a study population includes 100 people in the 50- to 59-year age group, a respectable number if we intend to adjust only for age. Suppose that we also wish to adjust for sex (female or male), race (Asian, black, or white), cigarette smoking (current, former, or none), and socioeconomic status (high, medium, or low). This requires subdividing by two for sex and by three for each of the other variables, yielding $2 \times 3 \times 3 \times 3 = 54$ possible subcategories within the one age group. On the average, we could expect about two persons in each subcategory, or *cell,* which would yield very imprecise and unreliable results. (For example, in a two-person cell, the disease rate could only be: 0 if no one had the disease, 50 percent if one person had it, or 100 percent if both persons had it.) Even worse, there would undoubtedly be many totally empty subcategories. For example, in a typical sample of 100 persons aged 50 to 59 years in the United States, there would often be no Asian female smokers of low socioeconomic status, since Asian females constitute a small minority and few of them smoke. Thus, in a study of an effect of smoking, one might have only nonsmokers in this age-sex-race-socioeconomic status subgroup and thus no smokers with whom they could be compared.

For this reason and others, epidemiologists now frequently employ the statistical methods of multivariate analysis. These usually provide an accurate view of the relationships between possible causal factors and disease while adjusting simultaneously for many variables and smoothing out the irregularities that tiny or nonexistent subgroups can introduce into ordinary adjustment procedures or stratified analysis.

In the following simple introduction to multivariate analytic methods, the discussion will begin with the basic concept of regression and will lead up to and include the multiple logistic and proportional hazards models. As two of the most frequently used methods, they are commonly encountered in medical journal articles. The purpose is to give the reader a basic understanding of how these methods work and of the concepts and terms used to discuss them. For a more mathematical and detailed discussion of multivariate analysis in epidemiology, more advanced texts should be consulted (Breslow and Day, 1980, 1987; Kelsey et al., 1986; Kleinbaum et al., 1982; Rothman, 1986; and Schlesselman, 1982).

Regression

Most multivariate methods are based on the concept of regression. In high school we learned its most basic form, simple linear regression, where the dependent variable, y, is considered a function of one independent variable, x, and the relationship between them can be portrayed graphically as a straight line, as in Fig. 12-1. The

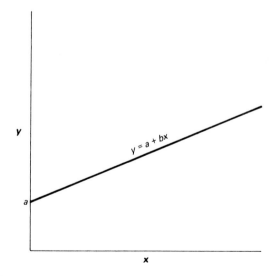

Figure 12-1   Simple linear regression.

formula for this relationship is $y = a + bx$, where a is a constant that indicates what y would be when x is 0, and b (often referred to by the Greek letter β, beta) is a coefficient that tells how strongly y is related to x. On the graph, a greater b is seen as a steeper slope of the regression line.

A medical example of this simple linear regression is the relationship of the secretion of a pituitary gonadotrophic hormone, luteinizing hormone, to the amount of body fat in eight teenage girls with Turner's syndrome (Boyar et al., 1978). (Since girls with this group of congenital anomalies lack significant ovarian production of estrogen, which could influence pituitary function, the effects of body fat could be more readily discerned.) The relationship is depicted in Fig. 12-2. In this case, $b = -3.40$, and the relationship is inverse, as shown by the downward slope of the regression line to the right. That is, the more body fat, the lower the luteinizing hormone secretion. The data points for each girl are

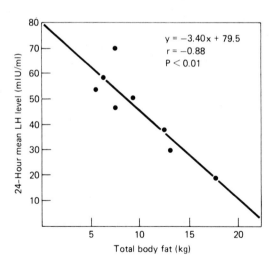

Figure 12-2   Example of simple linear regression fitted to actual data showing the relationship between the 24-hour mean luteinizing hormone level and the total amount of body fat in eight teenage girls with Turner's syndrome. *(Reproduced, by permission, from Boyar et al., 1978.)*

shown as dots on the graph. The regression line was calculated to best fit the points by the method of least squares. This method yields the regression line that is closest to all the points in the sense that it has the smallest total of squared vertical distances, or squared differences, from all of them. The fitting to a set of data points of a regression equation that expresses a relationship between independent and dependent variables is the basic process in all the multivariate analyses to be described.

Multiple Linear Regression

A dependent variable, y, can also be viewed as being explained by several independent variables, x_1, x_2, x_3, and so on. The formula becomes $y = a + b_1 x_1 + b_2 x_2 + b_3 x_3 +$ and so on. Each coefficient, b, tells how strongly its particular independent variable, x, is related to the dependent variable, y. Although this relationship was easily portrayed for one independent variable on a two-dimensional graph, as in Fig. 12-1 or 12-2, and could be depicted for two independent variables in three dimensions, we can no longer visualize it in this conventional manner as the number of independent variables increases beyond two. However, the logic is the same and does not require visualization for understanding.

Multiple linear regression is useful when we want to know how strongly each of several independent variables is related to a continuous dependent variable. For example, we might want to study how height, weight, chest circumference, and age affect the vital capacity of the lungs. We can analyze this in the form of multiple linear regression. By using standard computer programs, we would determine the multiple regression equation that best fits the data on these variables that were collected from our subjects. In this way, we construct a *mathematical model* (or just *model*). There are statistical tests to see if our model, in this case multiple regression, fits our data well. If it does, we can feel confident that the b's probably express the true degree of relationship between each independent variable and vital capacity when all the other variables are taken into account.

It is interesting to note that a characteristic related to the dependent variable in a univariate analysis can show little or no relationship to that variable in a multivariate analysis. This situation is no different from that described in Chap. 11 in which a simple adjustment for age removed the relationship between a history of parental death and low-back pain.

Table 12-1 shows some of the findings of a multiple regression analysis of the relationship between the consumption of three beverages and systolic blood pressure in 20,171 white men (adapted from Klatsky et al. 1986). For simplicity, the regression coefficients (i.e., the b's) of other personal characteristics that were also included in the model are not shown. For coffee, the regression coefficient was -0.38, indicating that the greater the coffee consumption, the lower the blood pressure, amounting to an average decrease of 0.38 mmHg per additional cup per day. The coefficient for tea was also negative and small. For alcohol we see a positive relationship, with a regression coefficient of 1.08. For each additional drink per day the blood pressure averaged 1.08 mmHg higher. Although the larger b for alcohol might suggest a stronger relationship to blood pressure, we must remember that the magnitude of b depends on the units used to measure the variable. If alcohol consumption were expressed in milliliters instead of "drinks," its b would be much smaller. However, if we consider a cup as a "drink" of coffee or tea, we can say that on a per-drink basis, alcohol is more strongly related to blood pressure than are the other two beverages.

The low p value for each beverage indicates statistical significance. For example, there was less than one chance in ten thousand that the b for alcohol could have arisen from chance sampling

Table 12-1 Multiple Regression Analysis of the Relationship of Consumption of Certain Beverages to Systolic Blood Pressure in 20,171 White Men

Beverage consumption	Regression coefficient	p value for difference from zero
Coffee (cups per day)	-0.38	0.0002
Tea (cups per day)	-0.29	0.0242
Alcohol (drinks per day)	1.08	<0.0001

Source: Adapted from Klatsky et al., 1986.

variation if there were truly no relation between alcohol use and blood pressure. Note that the p value would be the same no matter what units were used to measure alcohol intake.

When alcohol consumption was not included in the regression equation, cigarette smoking (not displayed in Table 12-1) showed a positive relationship to blood pressure, with $b = 0.43$ and $p = 0.11$, fairly close to statistical significance. (Here the b indicates that the mean blood pressure was 0.43 mmHg higher in smokers than in nonsmokers.) However, when alcohol use was added to the equation, the b for cigarette smoking dropped to 0.16 and its p value rose to 0.56. On the other hand, the presence or absence of the cigarette smoking variable in the regression had virtually no effect on the b for alcohol. These observations may be explained as follows: Without consideration of alcohol consumption, cigarette smoking appeared to be more positively related to blood pressure because smoking and alcohol drinking are correlated in the study population. Of the two habits, alcohol drinking is more directly associated with blood pressure.

Multiple Logistic Regression

In epidemiology the outcome studied, or dependent variable, is often the presence or absence of disease or some other dichotomous (yes-or-no) variable. In multiple logistic regression analysis the outcome variable is the *probability* or *odds* of this dichotomous outcome, either of which are, conveniently, continuous rather than dichotomous variables. Logistic regression is most easily understood if we consider the outcome variable to be the *odds*. The odds of having a disease are the chances of having it divided by the chances of not having it. The odds can thus vary from 0 if there is no chance of having it, up through 1 if there is a 50-50 chance of having it, up to infinity if it is certain that the disease is present. Logistic regression does not use the odds itself as the dependent variable, but rather the *log odds,* that is, the natural logarithm of the odds. (The base of natural logarithms is e, which is approximately 2.71828.) As the odds themselves can range from 0 to infinity, the log odds can range from minus infinity when the odds are 0, through 0 when the odds are 1, up to infinity when the odds are infinity. (The log odds is also known as the *logit,* hence the term *logistic.*)

The multiple logistic regression equation thus reads:

$$\text{log odds} = a + b_1x_1 + b_2x_2 + b_3x^3 + \text{and so on}$$

In a particular study, a computer is used to calculate the a and the b's that best fit the data. This is usually accomplished by the so-called *maximum likelihood method,* which means that the a and the b's are computed to be those that have the highest likelihood of having produced the observed set of data in that study. As with other models, statistical tests can then be applied to determine how well the calculated multiple logistic regression equation fits the data. Even though the a and the b's are selected to be the best possible, they still might not be very good. In such case, a different model or different variables may be tried. Sometimes changing the way the variables are expressed will improve the fit. For example, if one of the x variables is age, and the increase of disease risk with age is very great, the model may fit better if age squared (x^2) is used instead of, or in addition to, just age (x).

The multiple logistic regression model has a very interesting and useful property. When a particular x changes by a certain amount and is multiplied by its coefficient, b, the log odds also changes. By virtue of the nature of logarithms, adding to the log odds is equivalent to multiplying the odds themselves. A particular b then determines how much the odds are multiplied when the x that goes with that b changes by a given amount. By exponentiating b, that is, taking e^b, one can get an odds ratio, which, as we saw earlier (pages 118–119), gives an estimate of relative risk. Thus, if we consider the b that goes with the x that represents age in years in the logistic equation, e^b tells us how much risk is multiplied as age increases by 1 year.

One of the first epidemiologic studies in which multiple logistic regression analysis was employed was the Framingham Study (described in Chap. 8). Using 12-year follow-up data, Truett et al. (1967) examined the independent contribution of seven personal characteristics to risk of coronary heart disease. The results for men are shown in Table 12-2. The constant term α, which is part of the fitted equation that tells what the log odds would be if all x's were 0, need not concern us here. The first characteristic shown, age, had a β coefficient of 0.0708, which when exponentiated equaled 1.07. This indicates that, holding all other independent variables in the model constant, for each additional year of age the risk is multiplied by a factor of 1.07. The p value of less than 0.001 indicates that this relationship is most unlikely to have been due to chance. In the same way we can interpet the findings for the next four variables shown, cholesterol, systolic blood pressure, relative weight, and hemoglobin; for hemoglobin, note that chance could more readily explain the association, the p value being 0.124. The unit shown next to each variable (for example, mg/dl for cholesterol) indicates what difference in the variable gives rise to the relative risk shown. Thus, for cholesterol the relative risk of 1.01 applies to the tiny increase of 1 mg/dl. The last two characteristics, cigarettes per day and electrocardiographic abnormality, were entered as categorical variables—four different categories for smoking (defined in a footnote to the table) and two categories, normal

Table 12-2   Multiple Logistic Regression Analysis of Risk of Coronary Heart Disease, Framingham Study, Men, 12-year Follow-up Data

Risk factor	Constant term (α) and regression coefficients (β)	Relative risk (Odds ratio)	Probability (p) value
Constant	-10.8986		
Age (years)	0.0708	1.07	<0.001
Cholesterol (mg/dl)	0.0105	1.01	<0.001
Systolic blood pressure (mmHg)	0.0166	1.02	<0.001
Relative weight (%)*	0.0138	1.01	0.007
Hemoglobin (g/dl)	-0.0837	0.92	0.124
Cigarettes/day†	0.3610	1.43	<0.001
Electrocardiogram‡	1.0459	2.85	<0.001

* Percent of median for sex/height group.

† Coded 0 for never smoked, 1 for less than one pack per day, 2 for one pack per day, and 3 for more than one pack per day.

‡ Coded 0 for normal and 1 for abnormal.

Source: Adapted from Truett et al., 1967.

versus abnormal, for the electrocardiogram. For these categorical variables, the relative risk tells how much the risk is multiplied when subjects in one category are compared to those in the adjacent category. Thus, having an abnormal electrocardiogram entailed a 2.85 times greater risk of coronary heart disease than having a normal one.

Multivariate methods also allow the estimation of risk for individuals. For example, in the Framingham Study analysis just described, the coronary disease risk of any particular man may be estimated by plugging his values into the multiple logistic equation. Consider, for example, a man aged 52 years who has a cholesterol of 240 mg/dl, a systolic blood pressured of 145 mmHg, a weight that is 110 percent of the median weight for his height group, a hemoglobin of 15.0 g/dl, who smokes one pack of cigarettes per day (smoking category = 2) and has a normal electrocardiogram (electrocardiographic category = 0). His multiple logistic equation, based on the constant term and the coefficients in Table 12-2, would be:

$$
\begin{aligned}
\log \text{odds} = \\
-10.8986 + (0.0708 \times 52) + (0.0105 \times 240) + (0.0166 \times 145) \\
+ (0.0138 \times 110) - (0.0837 \times 15) + (0.3610 \times 2) + (1.0459 \times 0) \\
= -1.3055
\end{aligned}
$$

Exponentiating,

$$
\text{odds} = e^{-1.3055} = 0.271
$$

The probability (cumulative incidence) of developing disease is smaller than the odds of developing disease. In fact, probability = odds/(1 + odds). In this case, probability = 0.213.

We estimate then, from Framingham Study data, that over the next 12 years this man has a 21.3 percent chance of developing coronary heart disease. This illustrates a commonly used application of multiple logistic analysis, the estimation of an individual's risk of a disease. This is being employed increasingly in health risk appraisal, an educational tool for health counseling.

Another logistic analysis from the Framingham Study illustrates the value of any regression analysis in smoothing out the haphazard chance variation that is apparent when the number of

Table 12-3 Average Annual Incidence of Stroke by Level of Systolic Blood Pressure. Men, Age 55–64 Years. The Framingham Study

Systolic blood pressure	Person-years	No. of strokes	Incidence per 10,000 person-years	
			Directly calculated	Estimated by logistic model
<110	578	1	17	9.1
110–119	1284	2	16	12.3
120–129	1908	3	16	16.6
130–139	1972	4	20	22.3
140–149	1566	2	13	30.0
150–159	1082	6	55	40.4
160–169	734	6	82	54.3
170–179	496	1	20	72.9
180–189	300	3	100	97.9
190+	434	8	184	131.1

Source: Shurtleff, 1974, Table 8-1.

subjects is small in the various subgroups studied. Table 12-3 shows the number of cases of stroke and the average annual incidence of stroke in men aged 55 to 64 years, categorized according to systolic blood pressure. Note that there were only one to six strokes in any category and that the directly calculated incidence in the 170 to 179 mmHg blood pressure subgroup (where there was only one stroke) was much lower than that in the adjacent categories. It is much more reasonable to conclude that stroke risk rises continuously as blood pressure rises and that the drop in the 170 to 179 group was an artifact due to chance variation than to conclude that somehow the 170 to 179 group was specially protected. Thus, the smoothed incidence rates, estimated by fitting a logistic regression equation, are probably much closer to the truth.

The multiple logistic method can be used in any type of epidemiologic study—cross-sectional, case-control, or cohort. Since it is a method for dealing with a yes-or-no, disease-or-no-disease outcome variable, we must understand that it would have limitations if applied to a cohort study with variable lengths of follow-up. Consider, for example, a simple situation in which half the people in a cohort are followed up for 1 year and half are followed up for 2 years. A person observed for only 1 year who remains free of disease during that time may or may not remain disease-free during a second year. So persons observed to be disease-free for just 1 year are not equivalent to persons observed to be disease-free for 2 years. Thus, we now have two categories of disease-free people to compare with those who develop the disease, and we have already departed from the simple yes-or-no dependent variable suitable for multiple logistic regression analysis. Clearly, this method should be applied to cohort studies only when all subjects have equal follow-up time.

Proportional Hazards Model

The proportional hazards model, sometimes referred to as the Cox model (developed by D. R. Cox, 1972), is applicable to the situation of unequal follow-up times, mentioned above, in which multiple logistic regression falls short. As shown below, the form of the regression equation in the proportional hazards model is very similar to the form used in multiple logistic regression analysis.

$$\log \text{ rate } = a(t) + b_1 x_1 + b_2 x_2 + b_3 x_3 + \text{ and so on}$$

Two differences between the proportional hazards equation and the multiple logistic equation should be noted. First, the dependent variable is not the logarithm of the odds of disease but the logarithm of the incidence rate—here, the instantaneous incidence, or hazard, rate. Second, instead of the constant term a, the proportional hazards model uses the variable term $a(t)$, where t stands for time. Thus, the incidence of disease can vary with time in this model, irrespective of the effects of the independent variables, or x's. Each b indicates the effect of the accompanying x on the log of the incidence rate at any point in time. The term *proportional hazards* indicates that the model is based on the assumption that the effect of each independent variable will be in a specified proportion, regardless of time. Thus, if a change in the independent variable increases the incidence rate, or hazard, by 50 percent at the end of the first year of follow-up, it will also increase it by 50 percent at the end of the fifth year of follow-up even if the incidence is much greater at the fifth year than at the first. To the extent that the actual data are not consistent with this proportionality rule, this model will not fit well.

Computer programs are generally needed to perform the necessary calculations. Just as with multiple logistic analysis, the b's indicate the strength (per unit of x) of the relationship between the independent variables and the dependent variable. Exponentiating each b provides an estimate of the relative risk (technically, the rate ratio), that is, the factor by which the incidence rate is multiplied for each unit change in the x under consideration.

How a variable length of follow-up can be accommodated is illustrated by the following example. Consider a study of oral contraceptive use and cervical cancer in which the x's, or independent variables, are: oral contraceptive use—yes or no, actual age, age at first sexual intercourse, and number of cigarettes smoked per day. Suppose that the final diagnosis of the disease occurred in a woman 4 years and 6 months after follow-up began. This woman would be compared only with women who were still under observation at the 4-year 6-month point. Suppose that the next case occurred at the 6-year 2-month point. She would be compared with only those women still under observation and at risk at that time. Any women who had died, who had developed cervical cancer, or who were otherwise lost to follow-up earlier would not be included. These comparisons with the women still under observation and at risk would be repeated every time a new case occurred. Then they would be combined in the overall model. The b's for oral contraceptive use, age, age at first intercourse, and cigarette smoking would be calculated to maximize the likelihood that the women who developed cervical cancer were accurately distinguished from those who did not develop it in all the comparisons.

As with other regression methods, any independent variable, not just oral contraceptive use, can be viewed as the factor of primary interest; each b tells how strongly its independent variable is related to disease with the others controlled or held constant.

Unlike the multiple logistic regression model, the proportional hazards model takes into account the time at which an event occurs, not just whether it occurs. Thus, a group in which a disease develops earlier will show a higher risk in proportional hazards analysis even if the group's cumulative incidence by the end of follow-up is no greater than that in a comparison group. Another valuable feature of proportional hazards analysis is its ability to accommodate independent variables that are measured more than once and are found to change with time (so-called *time-dependent covariates*).

A well-known early application of the proportional hazards model was in a clinical follow-up study of ventricular premature beats (VPBs), a common irregularity of heart rhythm, in relation to mortality after myocardial infarction (Ruberman et al., 1977). A total of 1739 men with prior myocardial infarction who were subscribers of the Health Insurance Plan of Greater New York were followed up for periods ranging from 6 months to 4 years after an examination, which included careful electrocardiographic monitoring. Predictors of sudden cardiac death were evaluated by the proportional hazards model to take into account the variable length of follow-up in the study. In this analysis, VPBs with certain features, termed "complex," proved to be the most powerful predictor among the 17 characteristics studied. The beta coefficient for complex VPBs was 1.204 ($p < 0.001$). Exponentiating, the authors found the relative risk estimate to be 3.33, indicating that men with prior heart attack had more than a threefold increased risk of sudden death if they had complex VPBs, as compared to men with prior heart attack without complex VPBs.

Some Commonly Encountered Concepts

In studies employing multivariate analysis techniques, the following concepts and terms are frequently encountered.

Stepwise Regression Analysis   To determine which independent variables contribute substantially to the prediction of an outcome, investigators sometimes add variables to a model one at a time, or in a stepwise fashion. If predictive ability is substantially improved when a new variable is added—that is, if the model fits the data better—the new variable is retained. If not, it is dropped unless the investigator forces it to be included for other reasons, as will be mentioned below. Developing a model by successively adding and evaluating variables is called a *forward* stepwise approach. A *backward* approach may also be employed. This involves starting with all variables under consideration and noting what happens when they are dropped, one at a time. If excluding one variable has little effect on the fit of the model, it is deemed unimportant and considered no further.

Note that the stepwise approach employs purely statistical criteria to determine whether variables are included in the model. It may be important to incorporate certain variables for clinical or biological reasons. Such reasons are ignored in a pure stepwise approach.

Conditional Regression Analyses   Regression analyses that examine relationships within subgroups that meet specific conditions are called *conditional regression analyses.* An example of this type of analysis is the proportional hazards model, in which the determination of regression coefficients is based on comparisons of only those people still at risk when each case occurs. Regression analyses of relationships in the study group as a whole, not within subgroups, are termed *unconditional.*

Conditional Regression Analysis in Studies of Matched Subjects   Conditional regression analysis is used most often in studies of matched subjects, for example, in case-control studies in which each case is matched with one or more controls. Here the condition to be met in the model is that subjects belong to the same matched pair or matched set. What happens across matched sets is of no concern; only relationships within matched sets are evaluated.

Interaction   Interaction was defined in Chap. 11 and illustrated in cross-classification tables. Interaction can also be studied in regression models, usually by including interaction terms. Each term is the product of the two or more variables whose interaction is to be evaluated. Thus, to give the simplest possible example, consider two dichotomous independent variables, sex (male = 0, female = 1) and current marital status (not married = 0, married = 1), in a study of determinants of emotional depression. One x, call it x_1, would represent sex; another x, call it x_2, would represent current marital status, and a product term, x_1x_2, would represent the interaction between the two. You can easily confirm that $x_1 x_2 = 0$ for unmarried men, married men, and unmarried women and that $x_1 x_2 = 1$ for married women. If the analysis revealed a large and statistically significant b for $x_1 x_2$, this would indicate that the difference between men and women in the occurrence of depression varied according to whether or not they were married, or conversely, the relationship of marital status to depression differed between men and women.

Indicator Variables   Some characteristics are qualitative and have three or more subcategories that are not arranged in any quantitative order. Examples are race (Asian, black, white, etc.) and occupational grouping (white collar, blue collar, retired, student, homemaker, other). Such characteristics can be represented by indicator variables, which are set at either 0 or 1, according to whether the characteristic is absent or present.

The number of indicator variables needed is one fewer than the number of categories. So, for example, in a study of alcohol use and risk of esophageal cancer, alcohol drinkers might be categorized according to whether they prefer beer, wine, or liquor. With beer as the reference category, there would be two indicator variables, one for wine and one for liquor. For those who prefer beer, both would be set at 0. For those who prefer wine, the wine indicator would be set at 1 and the liquor indicator would be set at 0. For those who prefer liquor, the liquor indicator would be set at 1 and the wine indicator at 0. The multiple logistic regression coefficient for the wine indicator can be used to determine the relative odds of developing esophageal cancer among wine drinkers as compared to beer drinkers. The coefficient for the liquor indicator can be used in an analogous fashion.

Indicator variables can be put to other valuable use. For example, if a continuous variable is thought to have a complex relationship to disease, with ups and downs in risk, it would be advisable to break the variable's distribution into segments and to assign an indicator variable to each. The ups and downs could then become apparent, whereas they could not if the variable were entered as a single term. A good example may be found in the multiple regression analysis of alcohol and other beverages in relation to blood pressure shown in Table 12-1. When alcohol consumption was entered into the model as one continuous quantitative variable, its regression coefficient was 1.08, indicating an average increase of 1.08 mmHg in systolic pressure per drink of alcohol per day. However, when alcohol consumption was entered at several levels, each represented by an indicator variable, with abstention as the reference category, a different picture was revealed. The resulting regression coefficients were 1.2 for less than 1 drink per day, 2.8 for 1 to 2 drinks per day, 5.6 for 3 to 5 drinks per day, 9.1 for 6 to 8 drinks per day, and 4.8 for 9 or more drinks per day. Although, as expected, blood pressure rose with increasing alcohol consumption up through 6 to 8 drinks per day, there was a downturn in the 9-or-more drink category that was not apparent when alcohol consumption was represented by one quantitative variable.

Correlated Variables   As we have seen, multivariate analysis is useful in identifying the specific contribution to risk of variables that are correlated with each other, such as alcohol drinking and cigarette smoking. Problems can arise, however, when the model contains highly correlated variables that measure the same or a closely linked attribute. As we saw in the multiple logistic regression analysis of Framingham Study data (Table 12-2), systolic blood pressure is a good predictor of coronary heart disease. However, when both systolic and diastolic levels, two strongly correlated aspects of blood pressure, are put in the model, the relation of systolic blood pressure to coronary heart disease is considerably weakened. The same would be true for diastolic blood pressure. Similarly, in a stepwise analysis, whichever aspect of blood pressure was put in the equation first would be judged to be significantly related to coronary heart disease; the other aspect would be passed over as unimportant.

Multicollinearity is the term often used when a model contains highly correlated independent variables. In such cases it is difficult to estimate their true effects.

Standardized Regression Coefficients   To compare different independent variables with respect to their strength of association with the dependent variable, standardized regression coefficients are sometimes used. This involves expressing the independent variables in standard deviation units rather than in their ordinary units, such as millimeters of mercury (mmHg) for blood pressure or years for age. For example, in a multiple logistic analysis of the relation of systolic blood pressure to coronary heart disease, the standardized regression coefficient, when exponentiated, indicates how much the risk of coronary disease is multiplied when the systolic blood pressure increases by one standard deviation, based on the distribution of blood pressure in the population studied.

As noted by Greenland et al. (1986), when a characteristic is measured in standard deviation units, the apparent strength of its association with an outcome depends on its variability in the particular group studied and can be misleading for between-group comparisons or for judging the relative magnitude of a biological effect. Therefore, this approach should be used with caution, if at all.

Log-linear Models   A form of multivariate analysis, the log-linear model requires that all variables be entered as categorical variables. This model examines both the direct and the interactive relationships of all variables to each other, without requiring that one be specified as the dependent variable. Its results are usually similar to those of multiple logistic regression analysis.

Poisson Regression   An increasingly used method of multivariate analysis of factors affecting incidence or mortality rates in cohort studies is *Poisson regression*. It can be employed when, as usually happens, the number of outcome events, new cases or deaths, is relatively small compared to the size of the cohort, or number of person-time units. Under these conditions it is assumed that the probability of events occurring follows what is known as the *Poisson distribution*. The statistically sophisticated reader can refer to Breslow and Day, 1987, pages 131–136.

R^2   It is sometimes desirable to determine how much of the variability in an outcome variable, such as the occurrence of a disease, can be explained by the independent variables in a model. When one variable is related to another one, as expressed by a correlation coefficient, r (described in Chap. 11), the amount of variation (technically, of the variance) of one that is explainable by variation in the other is r^2. So, for example, if $r = 0.4$, then $r^2 = 0.16$ and we say that 16 percent of the variance in one variable is explained by variation in the other. When more than one independent variable is involved, r^2 becomes R^2, sometimes referred to as *multiple* R^2. The overall multiple linear regression equation for determination of blood pressure level, from which the beverage consumption data in Table 12-1 were extracted, had an R^2 of 0.19, indicating that 19 percent of variation in systolic blood pressure could be explained by the entire model.

The levels for R^2 often appear disappointingly small in epidemiologic studies. However, there is so much measurement error and random variation in epidemiologic data that this is to be expected, even when the model clearly indicates that causal or predictive factors are present, as evidenced by large and statistically significant regression coefficients.

A Final Note

Multivariate methods have proved to be invaluable in analyzing complex epidemiologic data. Although at first they seemed to the uninitiated like "black boxes," which processed data in a totally incomprehensible way, years of experience and comparisons of results with those of simpler methods have indicated their basic validity when used appropriately. It should be clear from the foregoing discussion, however, that each of the main methods rests on assumptions. These assumptions must be understood by the user and the consumer because they might or might not apply to the disease and other variables under investigation. Lack of care in conducting and reporting multivariate analyses is frequent (Concato et al., 1993).

It is regrettable when researchers rely solely on multivariate analysis techniques. Much greater familiarity with, and understanding of, the data are attained when analysis is carried out with straightforward tables, the format used to present most data in this book. Such simple cross-classifications usually allow the investigator to observe most of the important relationships and interactions that are present.

With multivariate methods now so readily accessible, it is tempting to throw data into a computer, together with a "packaged" analysis program, in the hope that the coefficients and other numbers that come out will somehow reveal a new secret of life. It must be stressed, however, that no method of analysis, no matter how mathematically sophisticated, can substitute for a careful evaluation of data based on good scientific judgment and knowledge of the disease process being studied.

PROBLEMS

12-1 Examine Fig. 12-2. Where does the simple linear regression model fit the data better, when body fat was relatively low or when it was relatively high? Do you consider that, overall, the model fits well, or not?

12-2 Assuming that the mean systolic blood pressure in men who drink neither coffee, tea, nor alcohol is 120 mmHg, use the regression coefficients in Table 12-1 to determine the mean systolic blood pressure in men who drink two cups of coffee, one cup of tea, and two alcoholic cocktails per day. Do the same for men who drink six cups of coffee per day but no tea or alcohol.

12-3 Place the data concerning the attack rates of gastroenteritis among eaters and noneaters of the four food items shown in Table 15-1 into separate two-by-two tables as shown in the example below for milk. (Note that the number of milk consumers who became ill was $0.62 \times 55 = 34$; always round all decimals to the nearest whole number.)

Milk	Ill	Not ill	Total
Eaten	34	21	55
Not eaten	48	23	71

Compute the odds ratio for each food; for example, $(34 \times 23)/(48 \times 21) = 0.8$ for milk. Each of the four tables was analyzed using simple logistic regression with the independent variable, x, being eating the item and the dependent variable, y, being illness (for either, no = 0, yes = 1). The logistic equation was:

$$\log \text{ odds } y = \alpha + \beta x$$

For the four food items (in different order than in Table 15-1), the fitted equations were as follows:

I. $\log \text{ odds } y = 0 + 1.195239x$
II. $\log \text{ odds } y = 0.735707 - 0.253869x$
III. $\log \text{ odds } y = -1.722767 + 3.715197x$
IV. $\log \text{ odds } y = 0.064539 + 0.813180x$

Determine which regression equation applies to which food, using either a pocket calculator that can handle logarithms or a printed logarithm table. For readers without either, the necessary conversions from β to e^{β} are given in the following table.

β	e^{β}
1.195239	3.3
−0.253869	0.8
3.715197	41.1
0.813180	2.3

Using the entire equation, determine the odds of illness associated with eating each food (remember, when the food is eaten, $x = 1$) and compare them with the odds in the two-by-two tables. How well does the logistic analysis agree with the traditional analysis of the two-by-two tables? Readers who lack the means of calculating with logarithms may use the table below.

Log odds	Odds
1.195239	3.3
0.481838	1.6
1.992430	7.3
0.877719	2.4

12-4 For each of the studies described below, indicate which method of multivariate analysis would ordinarily be used: multiple linear regression analysis, multiple logistic regression analysis, or the Cox proportional hazards model. Assume that several confounding variables have to be controlled in each study.

a A cohort study of alcohol use and death from automobile crash injury in which all students in several large high schools are given an alcohol questionnaire to be completed sometime during the first month of the school year and each student is followed up for 6 months from the date that the questionnaire is turned in.

b The same study described in the preceding example except for the following: the students may turn in the questionnaire anytime during the school year and the follow-up of all students is ended on December 31 of the following year.

c A study of pregnant women in which a dietary questionnaire is given during the first trimester and the intake of various dietary constituents is related to the total amount of weight gained during the pregnancy.

d The same study described in the preceding example except for the following: the outcome variable is the birth weight of the infant.

e Again the same study, except that the outcome variable is whether the baby has a congenital anomaly.

f A case-control study to determine whether cholecystectomy (surgical removal of the gallbladder) increases the risk of cancer of the large bowel.

BIBLIOGRAPHY

Boyar RM, Ramsey J, Chipman J, Fevre M, Madden J, Marks J: Regulation of gonadotropin secretion in Turner's syndrome. *N Engl J Med* **298:**1328–1331 (1978).

Breslow NE, Day NE: *Statistical Methods in Cancer Research. Volume 1. The Analysis of Case-Control Studies* (Lyon: International Agency for Research on Cancer, 1980).

Breslow NE, Day NE: *Statistical Methods in Cancer Research: Volume II. The Design and Analysis of Cohort Studies* (Lyon: International Agency for Research on Cancer, 1987).

Concato J, Feinstein AR, Holford TR: The risk of determining risk with multivariable models. *Ann Int Med* 118:201–210 (1993).

Cox DR: Regression models and life-tables (with discussion). *J R Stat Soc B* **34:**187–220 (1972).

Greenland S, Schlesselman JJ, Criqui MH: The fallacy of employing standardized regression coefficients and correlations as measures of effect. *Am J Epidemiol* **123:**203–208 (1986).

Kelsey JL, Thompson WD, Evans AS: *Methods in Observational Epidemiology* (New York: Oxford University Press, 1986).

Klatsky AL, Friedman GD, Armstrong MA: The relationships between alcoholic beverage use and other traits to blood pressure: A new Kaiser Permanente study. *Circulation* **73:**628–636 (1986).

Kleinbaum DG, Kupper LL, Morgenstern H: *Epidemiologic Research: Principles and Quantitative Methods* (Belmont, Calif.: Lifetime Learning Publications, 1982).

Rothman KJ: *Modern Epidemiology* (Boston: Little, Brown, 1986).

Ruberman W, Weinblatt E, Goldberg JD, Frank CW, Shapiro S: Ventricular premature beats and mortality after myocardial infarction. *N Engl J Med* **297:**750–757 (1977).

Schlesselman JJ: *Case-Control Studies: Design, Conduct, Analysis* (New York: Oxford University Press, 1982).

Shurtleff D: Section 30. Some characteristics related to the incidence of cardiovascular disease and death: Framingham study, 18-year follow-up, in WB Kannel, T Gordon (eds.), *The Framingham Study: An Epidemiological Investigation of Cardiovascular Disease,* DHEW Publication No. (NIH) 74-599 (Washington: U.S. Government Printing Office, 1974).

Truett J, Cornfield J, Kannel W: A multivariate analysis of the risk of coronary heart disease in Framingham. *J Chron Dis* **20:**511–524 (1967).

Chapter 13

How to Carry Out a Study

Many health care professionals wish to conduct a modest clinical or epidemiologic study. Hoping to answer one or more interesting questions, they find themselves in a good position to collect and analyze some appropriate data. However, to someone without previous research experience, the task often appears awesome, and it is not at all clear how to proceed.

This chapter is written as a general guide for the novice who wishes to carry out such a study. Obviously, each research project and each study setting presents unique problems that cannot be dealt with here. What will be presented is a general approach that emphasizes the practical difficulties that are frequently troublesome to the beginner.

Defining the Problem

The first step—and one of the most difficult ones—is defining the problem and choosing the question or questions to be answered. There is a tendency for the novice at research to ask questions that are diffuse or vague. Instead, the problem must be stated in terms of clear, simple, answerable questions. An example of a vague unachievable goal for a specific study would be *to elucidate the role of psychological factors in coronary heart disease*. It is not clear whether the "role . . . in coronary heart disease" refers to causation of the disease, the outcome of the disease, the patient's attitude toward the disease, or something entirely different. Furthermore, both "coronary heart disease" and "psychological factors" are very broad terms. Better, because they are clear and answerable, are specific aims or questions such as: *Determine the proportion of patients with myocardial infarction who develop severe emotional depression during hospitalization. Do attacks of angina pectoris occur more frequently during periods when patients are anxious?* Or: *Is there an increased risk of sudden cardiac death within a year of the death of a spouse?* It is desirable to express a study question in quantitative terms, such as whether a specified increase in incidence will be observed. This aids both in achieving the needed clarity and specificity and in determining what measurements are needed.

Intimately involved in the asking of vague, overly broad questions is the tendency to be too ambitious. The new researcher wishes to make important discoveries and solve big problems. These unrealistic expectations can lead only to failure and disappointment. For the most part, medical science progresses gradually by very small steps. So much of health care is based on tenuous evidence and incomplete knowledge that a careful study of even a simple question will be a worthwhile contribution, of which any scientist should be proud.

Reviewing the Relevant Literature

Once a problem has been selected, the scientific papers describing previous related work should be read carefully. In addition to learning what is already known about the question, the investigator will become familiar with problems that other researchers have faced, using various study methods. One should be especially alert for potentially confounding variables, which can be measured or controlled in the planned study so that embarrassing spurious correlations can be recognized or avoided. For example, no investigation of a possible etiologic factor in lung cancer would be respectable if smoking habits were not measured or taken into account.

The usual result of a literature review is a realization of how *little* is known about the particular topic one wants to investigate.

Seemingly authoritative statements and accepted medical doctrines, perpetuated through textbooks and lectures, often turn out to be supported by the most meager evidence, if any can be found at all! For example, in my own experience of reviewing the literature for an epidemiologic study of gallbladder disease, I was unable to find any evidence for the "fair" and "forty" parts of the doctrine that persons who are "fair, fat, and forty" are especially prone to gallstones. Indeed, the study did not confirm these traits as predisposing factors.

Many other examples could be mentioned of beliefs that are based on little or no evidence or on the results of poorly conducted studies. In these instances, a literature review will provide encouragement for proceeding with the proposed study. However, if it is evident that the question has already been well answered, a related problem may come to mind—one that can be studied just as well.

Preparing a Protocol

The next essential step is the preparation of a study protocol. Even though the beginning investigator may have a plan clearly in mind, it is extremely important to set it down in writing.

A written protocol serves three major purposes. First of all, when one writes the protocol, ideas and procedures must be clearly defined and spelled out. Usually the plan in one's mind is not as clear and logical as was hoped, and the gaps and flaws are easier to recognize and correct when the plan is seen on paper. Second, a written protocol can be studied by anyone whose advice is desired or whose approval is required. Third, any person involved in carrying out the study, even the investigator, may forget some method or procedure to be followed. The written protocol constitutes a permanent record that can be referred to, so that methods do not change unnecessarily during the conduct of the study.

Some persons have such an abhorrence of writing that the preparation of a protocol is an almost insurmountable obstacle to performing a study. If so, it is probably better just to quit at this point, since even if some data are collected and analyzed, the results will probably never be written up, and no one else can adequately study the findings. Another alternative for a nonwriter with a good idea for a research project is to team up with a co-investigator who is willing and able to write the protocol and the final report.

Contents of the Protocol   Research grant applications may require strict adherence to prescribed contents arranged in a particular order. For example, a recent communication from the U.S. National Institutes of Health listed the following required elements for a grant application (somewhat condensed):

Description (abstract) and personnel
Detailed budget for initial period
Budget for entire proposed project
Biographical sketches for all professional personnel
Other support for professional personnel
Resources and environment
Research plan
    1. Specific aims
    2. Background and significance
    3. Progress report/preliminary studies
    4. Research design and methods
    5. Human subjects
    6. Vertebrate animals
    7. Consultants/collaborators
    8. Consortium/contractual arrangements
    9. Literature cited
Appendix (various supplementary descriptions, papers, etc.)
A protocol prepared for local use may be shorter and simpler but should contain at least the following elements, unless there is good reason for omitting any.

1   A brief statement of the specific question(s) to be answered and/or the specific aim(s) of the study.

2   Background and significance of the study. This should be a pertinent nonrambling discussion of what is known and not known about the problem and why the proposed study would be worthwhile or important.

3   Methods. Included should be a description of the study subjects—how they are to be selected and how many there are likely to be. The data to be collected and the methods for collecting them should be described. Uniform criteria for diagnosis of disease and for decisions as to the presence or absence of a characteristic or outcome should be listed. Data analysis methods should also be presented, preferably with some sample blank tables showing how the data will be organized. Plans for safeguarding the rights and welfare of the subjects and the method of obtaining their informed consent (if needed) should be explained.

4   An approximate time schedule for carrying out the various aspects of the study.

5   A budget, if financial support is being requested, with explanation of any personnel and other costs whose requirement is not obvious.

Consultation

After a draft of the protocol has been written, it is wise to seek some expert consultation before proceeding further. Many potential problems and difficulties will be quickly spotted by knowledgeable persons reviewing the protocol and discussing the proposed research.

It should be no reflection on one's intelligence and skill to ask advice. No one can foresee all the problems that may develop in a study. A consultant will respect the investigator who draws up a protocol as well as possible and then admits to being fallible.

Help can come from persons in a number of disciplines. An experienced investigator who has worked in the area to be studied can perhaps provide the most comprehensive view of the problem. A clinician who specializes in the area of study will often provide some fresh insights into the subject matter derived from the experience with patients and from familiarity with the current literature. Epidemiologists and biostatisticians are professionally concerned with study design and data analysis and can provide guidance on these aspects of the study. The choice of appropriate statistical tests and the determination of whether the proposed sample size is adequate to obtain meaningful information are of particular concern to the biostatistician.

The protocol should now be revised, taking into account the suggestions of the consultants.

Presenting the Study Plan to Other Key Individuals

At this time the investigator should inform all the responsible persons whose approval or cooperation is either required or desirable. Proposed research in medical or academic institutions should be presented to appropriate departmental heads and/or hospital administrators. Often there will be a committee specially designated to review and approve of studies. Epidemiologic studies in the community should be described to local health officials and to the medical society.

In addition to gaining the required approvals, the investigator may receive valuable practical suggestions and other assistance from these individuals, such as introductions to physicians who may permit the study of their own patients. The investigator may also learn of other similar or related research that is under way. Cooperation with other investigators may help avoid duplication of effort and may lead to sharing of resources and, possibly, even of data.

Data-Collection Methods

The data to be collected—whether by observation or interview of subjects, by chart review, laboratory tests, or other means—must be recorded in a systematic and orderly manner. The usual method of bringing order into the data-collection process is by the use of standard forms. Careful attention to preparation of a form, even if only a few items need to be recorded on it, will save the investigator much trouble and grief later on.

One or more forms will be used for each study subject. Each form should provide space for identification of the subject and for recording necessary data.

If computers are to be used for analysis, the format for recording data on the form should meet their requirements. Each unit of information must be recorded in a particular space on each form. Each space is ordinarily assigned a column number that corresponds to a particular space in the computer data file. (The term *column* is used because in the era of punch cards, each digit or letter was represented by a hole in one column of each card.)

For recording quantitative information, specific spaces or boxes should be designated so that the same digit (e.g., the "ones," "tens," or "hundreds" digit) is entered into the same space on each form and the location of the decimal point is uniform. If the value to be recorded is relatively small and does not require all the assigned spaces, zeros should be written in the spaces to the left, which would not otherwise be filled in. Adequate spaces should be provided for all possible values of any particular measurements and for recording that the value is unknown. Special instructions for recording each measurement may be located on the form itself or in an accompanying manual.

For example, suppose that for recording the serum glucose level at admission to the hospital the investigator provides three spaces on the form, to be transferred, say, to cols. 20 to 22 of the data file, as follows:

Serum glucose (mg/100 mL) □□□
Cols. 20–22

At first glance this may seem adequate, but consider what might go wrong if a research assistant tries to use these spaces for three patients, one with a value of 72, one with 1021, and one for whom the test was not done. Without special instructions to use the two boxes on the right for two-digit numbers, the value of 72 might be recorded as 7 2 □, which will be treated by the computer as 720. In recording the value of 1021 the naive research assistant might well write 1 0 2 1, not realizing that what is outside the three boxes will be lost in data processing. The investigator should have anticipated the possibility of the occasional extremely high value for a patient suffering from diabetic acidosis and provided four boxes instead of three. If there is a good reason to limit the spaces to three, an alternative, though less satisfactory, is to make a rule for high values such as "Code 999 for values of 999 or greater.

Write actual value below." The value can then be referred to if needed. However, the computer will not be able to compute an accurate mean if 999 is always substituted for greater values.

For the patient with no glucose determination the research assistant may leave the space blank. But 6 months later when the data are to be analyzed and the research assistant has moved to another city, the investigator will not be sure whether the blank spaces represent an unknown value or whether the assistant forgot to fill in the spaces. It is better to indicate "test not done" with a particular number that could not represent a possible value of the variable. Consideration of these potential problems leads to the improved version of the portion of the form for recording serum glucose as follows:

Serum glucose (mg/100 mL)   ☐☐☐☐
                                             Cols. 20–23

(Record one-, two-, and three-digit numbers
as far to the right as possible, and
fill in the left boxes with zeros.
If test not done, record 9999.)

(Note to reader: If you wish to convert the above glucose values or those that appear later to mmol/L, multiply by 0.05551.)

Qualitative data, such as diagnostic categories, and "yes" or "no" responses usually require the assignment of code numbers to each response if computers are to be used. Consider marital status, for example. Without coding, a data-collection form might show marital status as follows:

Marital status (check appropriate category)

☐ Single   ☐ Widowed
☐ Married   ☐ Divorced
☐ Separated   ☐ Unknown

The responses could be coded into a single digit if a number were assigned to each category. The digit could be recorded in a space or box on the same sheet or onto a separate code sheet. For example, note how marital status can be coded into one digit to be transferred to, say, col. 17.

Marital status (enter appropriate number into box)   ☐
Col. 17

1 Single	**4** Widowed
2 Married	**5** Divorced
3 Separated	**6** Unknown

Precoded forms permit the correct category to be marked and coded automatically. For example:

Marital status (circle number next to appropriate category)

Single	1
Widowed	2
Married	3
Divorced	4
Separated	5
Unknown	6

Col. 17

There are advantages and disadvantages to each type of form. Some general principles to consider are:

The less rewriting or transcribing of data that is needed, the less chance for error.

The less complex the form, the less chance for error.

Most physicians and other professionals neither like to code nor do a good job of coding. If such individuals are to record data, it is often necessary to design a form they are willing to use and pay someone else to do the coding.

In preparing to record qualitative data, a category should be provided for every possibility except the very rare ones. Writing of additional information on the form in longhand should be kept at a minimum because this sort of information is difficult to analyze and relate to other variables. Consider, for example, a study of factors related to adverse reactions to anticoagulant drugs. One item of information that will be desired about each patient is the medical condition for which the anticoagulant was given. The investigator could set up the code sheet as follows:

Condition for which anticoagulant was given: _____

_____

_____

However, it might later become difficult to summarize these data and combine patients into categories. Using clinical experience to anticipate the possibilities, the investigator would find the data easier to analyze and present by providing several mutually exclusive categories, as follows:

Condition for which anticoagulant was given: □□
01 Pulmonary embolism   Cols. 32–33
02 Thrombophlebitis
03 Pulmonary embolism and thrombophlebitis
04 Myocardial infarction
05 Myocardial infarction with mural thrombosis and peripheral embolism
06 Rheumatic heart disease
07 Rheumatic heart disease with peripheral embolism
08 Atrial fibrillation or flutter
09 Atrial fibrillation or flutter with peripheral embolism
10 Atrial fibrillation or flutter with therapeutic conversion
11 Prosthetic heart valve
12 Transient cerebral ischemic attacks
13 Other cerebrovascular disease, specify _____
14 Other disease, specify _____
15 Combinations of above, specify _____

Note the last three categories, which involve some specification in longhand. These permit the recording of unanticipated conditions. But provision of the other common categories will reduce the need for longhand recording to a very small fraction of the cases.

When specifying categories for data-collection forms, it is wise to avoid making these categories too broad. Overly broad categories lead to the loss of valuable information. For example, categories 08, 09, and 10 above might have been combined under a more inclusive category "atrial fibrillation or flutter," but then important clinical distinctions among these cases could not be made without referring to the chart again. Frequently the investigator assumes that broad categories will be adequate for the needs of the study. Later on when the data are analyzed, unanticipated questions arise which could have been answered if narrower categories had been used.

Broad categories may prove especially troublesome when quantitative variables are recorded. In providing for the coding of serum glucose, it might seem reasonable to have only seven categories:

1   Less than 50 mg/100 mL
2   50–99
3   100–199
4   200–499
5   500–999
6   1000 +
7   Test not done

With luck, this might be perfectly adequate. However, if another investigator's study shows an important difference in findings between persons whose glucose level is less than 350 mg/100 mL and those whose glucose is 350 mg/100 mL or greater, the broad categories chosen will not permit data analysis to determine whether the breakpoint at 350 mg/100 mL can be confirmed. Furthermore, it is not possible to compute accurate means and standard deviations with the crude breakdown as shown above.

Thus it is best to record quantitative values exactly as they come from the measuring device. This allows for maximum flexibility and permits the investigator subsequently to use any desired grouping.

Pretesting of Data Collection

No matter how carefully the data collection is planned, problems will come to light after starting. That is why it is important to pretest procedures and forms before the study formally begins.

Suppose, for example, that data for a study of cardiovascular disease are to be collected in a mobile facility in which volunteer subjects are scheduled to pass from station to station every 5 minutes for a series of procedures. It may turn out that the electrocardiogram takes 8 minutes, on the average, instead of the planned 5 minutes. As a result, subjects may pile up at earlier stations if there is no provision for a waiting area in case of delays. It may therefore be necessary to slow down the examination schedule, or provide two electrocardiographic stations, or set up a waiting area. This problem should be uncovered and solved during pretesting. If not, and the subjects have to wait or get the impression that the study is disorganized, cooperation may be seriously impaired.

Similarly, a series of interview questions may seem perfectly clear and appropriate when they are written down. Yet when study subjects are actually asked these questions, they may not understand, or they may be offended, or they may give responses that were not anticipated. In a study of radiation exposure, for example, the investigator may consider it perfectly reasonable to ask, "Have you ever received x-ray or isotope therapy?" It will undoubtedly turn out that some subjects answer "yes" because they misinterpret the question to mean x-ray examinations. The question will have to be reworded and supplemented with additional clarifying questions in case of a "yes" response. Problems such as these quickly become apparent when an interview is tried out on friends and associates first and then on some persons similar to the potential study subjects but not officially part of the study.

Even abstracting data from charts requires pretesting. It seems perfectly reasonable to ask a research assistant reviewing hospital charts to record the patient's blood pressure at the time of admission. When the assistant looks at the first few charts, it will be noted that some, but not all, patients are admitted to a ward from the emergency room, where the blood pressure was recorded by the resident physician. Admission blood pressure is also recorded as the first of a series of blood pressures on the nurse's vital signs chart. In addition, a junior and a senior resident on the ward each performed an initial physical examination in which the blood pressure was recorded. It is apparent that some rule will be required for selecting the blood pressure to be used if any consistency is to be achieved. Review of a few charts will also reveal that one of the physicians has recorded two diastolic pressures, one at the muffling and one at the disappearance of Korotkov's sounds. Thus another decision is required—which one to use.

To mention other examples, the investigator may ask a chart reviewer to indicate whether the patient has a history of hypertension—yes or no. The chart reviewer will find, for a particular patient, that one physician records such a history and another does not. Which physician's history should be used? Or, on a previous hospitalization one blood pressure of 150/105 was recorded. Does this constitute a history of hypertension? Again, decisions and further clarification are needed. Or, the form was constructed so as to provide spaces for three digits for recording systolic pressure and two for diastolic, because it was forgotten that the diastolic is frequently greater than 99 mmHg. Pretesting will reveal the need to change the form.

Data Collection

If the investigator is relying on others to collect and record the data, he or she should supervise this aspect of the study closely, especially during the early stages. The work of persons collecting the data should be observed, and completed data-collection forms should be checked carefully. In this way, the investigator can ensure that the study plan is being followed. Where possible, data collection and recording procedures should be duplicated throughout the study on at least a sample of subjects to measure the error rate.

Not all problems will have been discovered during pretesting. Further changes in the procedures and forms may have to be made after the study officially begins. These modifications should be kept to a minimum to avoid inconsistencies in the data. Any changes or new rules to be followed should be recorded as additions to the protocol.

Data Editing

No matter how carefully data collection is performed, errors and omissions are inevitable and will have to be dealt with before analysis. First, someone should carefully check, and edit as needed, each form before the data on it are entered into computer storage. After entry, individual data items, their distributions, and their selected relations to one another should be checked in computer storage to look for omissions, unbelievable values (e.g., height = 300 cm), and inconsistencies (e.g., pregnant men). Usually, these errors can be corrected by going back to the source data, but if not, decisions are required as to how they should be handled.

Data Analysis

For most epidemiologic or clinical-outcome studies, data analysis mainly involves sorting into categories, counting, and computing proportions, rates, means, odds or rate ratios, and other group characteristics.

To proceed in an orderly fashion and end up with the answers that were desired in the first place, it is often helpful to draw up some blank tables showing the format for displaying the results of data analysis as they would be presented in a final report. These tables are then filled in with the appropriate counts, rates, and so on when these results become available.

For the novice, preparing blank tables is often quite difficult, requiring a good deal of patience and self-discipline. However, the results are well worth the effort and, with experience, subsequent table-making becomes much easier.

Data analysis tables should show the results broken down by age, sex, and other pertinent variables. In addition to showing the key results that one is after, they should show the numbers upon which the results are based. For example, Table 13-1, showing just incidence rates, is inadequate. The counts upon which these rates are based should also be listed, as in Table 13-2. Similarly, when means and standard deviations are shown, the number of persons entering into each of these computations should be given.

The actual work of data processing can be carried out in a variety of ways. The choice of a proper method depends on how many subjects are involved and the complexity of the analysis. If

**Table 13-1   Incomplete Table Showing
Only Incidence Rates by Age and Sex**
(Fictitious Data)

Age	Annual incidence per 1000
Men	
20–29	16.5
30–39	22.8
40–49	23.4
50–59	42.4
60–69	77.1
Total	33.3
Women	
20–29	5.5
30–39	8.6
40–49	10.5
50–59	20.9
60–69	40.6
Total	16.2

only a few counts and proportions are to be determined for a few dozen subjects, manual counting of items on the data-collection forms will be quite adequate. Electronic calculators can be used to perform much or all of the analysis for a small study. Even fairly complex epidemiologic computations can be accomplished with the programmable variety. Rothman and Boice (1982) and Abramson and Peritz (1983) have developed useful sets of calculator programs for epidemiologic analysis.

For small to medium-sized clinical and epidemiologic studies, microcomputers and appropriate data-base and statistical analysis programs can rapidly perform the data handling and calculations required.

However, for large studies, in which voluminous data for many hundreds or thousands of subjects are to be analyzed, the assistance of a mainframe computer is usually necessary. An investigator who cannot program a computer must hire a computer

Table 13-2 Complete Table Showing Incidence Rates by Age and Sex and the Numbers upon Which They Are Based
(Fictitious Data)

Age	Population at risk	Number of new cases during the year	Annual incidence per 1000
	Men		
20–29	1,572	26	16.5
30–39	1,494	34	22.8
40–49	2,012	47	23.4
50–59	1,629	69	42.4
60–69	1,077	83	77.1
Total	7,784	259	33.3
	Women		
20–29	1,827	10	5.5
30–39	2,203	19	8.6
40–49	2,570	27	10.5
50–59	1,912	40	20.9
60–69	1,698	69	40.6
Total	10,210	165	16.2

programmer and describe to him or her in meticulous detail exactly what analyses are wanted. Statistical program packages such as the SAS, BMDP, and SPSS systems can usually be mastered by nonprogrammers. With these systems, investigators themselves can conduct multivariate, survival, and other complex analyses on large computers.

Preparing the Final Report

The difficult job of preparing the scientific paper describing the study becomes a much less imposing task if the investigator writes portions of it during the course of the investigation.

The introductory section of the paper briefly outlines the problem and the purpose of the study. Note that this material has already been set down in preparing the written protocol. All that has to be done is to make any modifications that seem necessary for a final paper or that come to mind once data collection and analysis are completed.

Similarly, the Methods section of the paper can be readily adapted from the protocol. It should describe exactly what was done and, in addition, inform the reader as to how subjects were selected for study, how many subjects were included or excluded, and what the reasons were for exclusion. Criteria for classifying subjects and for decisions as to outcomes should be spelled out. Methods of measurement should be clearly described.

Writing the Results and Discussion sections is simplified if the investigator takes advantage of the fact that the results usually appear in stages. Tables of data are usually completed one at a time. When each table is prepared or received, one should immediately write a paragraph or two describing it for the Results section and a paragraph or two discussing the implications of this result for the Discussion section. Then, by the time the data are completely analyzed, most of the writing will be done. The Results and Discussion sections will still have to be organized and edited, but the task of writing them will not have to be faced all at once.

In the Discussion section the implications of the study and its relation to previous work should be described. In addition, the difficulties, problems, and potential errors and biases of the present investigation should be reviewed. All investigations have some obvious limitations and others that are not so obvious. It is best if the investigator recognizes and points these out, before someone else does.

Importance of Good Communication

Science is a *social* process. Each investigation is related to previous work, either attempting to confirm it or, usually, to build upon it. Investigators need to know and understand what others have done and are doing. It is, therefore, an important responsibility to present a study as fully and clearly as possible.

A paper or an oral presentation at a meeting should be clear and simple (Friedman, 1990). Jargon and unnecessarily complex or obscure terminology should be avoided. Although tables of data in a written paper should be complete, they need not be repetitious. Thus, after the basic numbers have been shown once (as in Table 13-2), they do not need to be repeated over and over again. Some relationships may be communicated most clearly by means of graphs and figures; these visual aids should be used freely.

In preparing slides or charts to accompany an oral presentation, the temptation to crowd a lot of information into one slide should be resisted. Each slide should have only a few lines or numbers displayed with large characters that are easily seen by those in the back of the room.

Importance of Investigator Worry

Many things can go wrong and many errors can occur during a study. Therefore it is essential that, preferably, the investigator, or a conscientious person responsible to the investigator, *worry about details*. The careful investigator might well adopt a questioning or even a suspicious attitude toward each phase of the effort.

In addition to observing the process of data collection, as recommended earlier, the investigator should see to it that every data-recording form is checked carefully by someone other than the person who filled it out to detect and correct omissions and obvious errors. Copies should be made of all completed data-collection forms so that the original information will still be available if any forms are lost. Complete lists and counts of all study subjects should be maintained to provide a check against lost forms. It is surprising how often forms become misplaced or fall behind a desk. Key-entry of data should be verified, which involves independent reentry of the data, preferably by a different person, to reveal discrepancies.

All mathematical calculations should be done twice by two different persons. The investigator's own work should be double-checked by a conscientious individual. Newly written computer programs should be tested on small samples of data and the results compared with hand calculations.

Data tables should be checked to make sure that all the numbers are correct and add up to the totals shown. Surprising or inconsistent results should provoke redoubled efforts to check whether something has gone wrong.

Finally, it would be sad, indeed, if after all this work, the resulting paper were to contain misleading typographical or printing errors. The manuscript and galley proofs should be proofread carefully.

PROBLEMS

13-1 Scientific studies directed at which of the following specific questions have a reasonable chance of being completed successfully? Explain your selection(s).

    a Does taking large doses of vitamin E enhance human sexuality?

    b Does taking 1 g/day of vitamin C decrease the incidence of group A streptococcal pharyngitis?

    c What is the best method of delivering medical care: private fee-for-service, prepaid health maintenance organizations, or a national health service?

    d If coffee drinking were given up by the next 50 coffee-drinking patients attending an insomnia clinic, would their use of sleeping pills over the following year be decreased by as much as 10 percent?

13-2 The following precoded form, shown in its entirety, is to be used to collect data on the age, weight, height, use of microwave ovens, and menopausal status for a study of lens opacities among women in their fifties. A physician's assistant is to weigh and measure each subject and obtain the remaining information by interview. The data will then be key-entered. What problems and deficiencies do you notice?

Age ☐ ☐ years   Weight ☐ ☐ kg   Height ☐ ☐ ☐ ☐ cm
    1 2   3 4   5 6 7 8

Do you have a microwave oven in your kitchen? ☐   0=no
                                                    9 1=yes

How long have you had it?   ☐   0=less than 10 years
                            10   1=10–20 years
                                 2=over 20 years

On the average, how many hours   ☐   0=0–4
per day do you use it?   11   1=5–9
                                     2=10–14
                                     3=15 or more

Have your menstrual periods stopped yet?   ☐   0=no
                                          12   1=yes

At what age did they stop?   ☐   ☐   years
                            13   14

13-3   Design your own clinical or epidemiologic study. Write a proposal following either the outline for grant applications required by the National Institutes of Health or the simpler format given in this chapter. Be sure to include some sample blank tables to show how you would analyze and display the data. Students might aim for a simple research project that could be completed during a summer recess from classes. (Preparing a proposal provides valuable experience. However, this can be a difficult and time-consuming task for the novice and would be most instructive if the proposal were reviewed by a knowledgeable person. If you are using this book as part of a course of study, your instructor may consider this an appropriate activity for small groups of students.)

BIBLIOGRAPHY

Abramson JH, Peritz E: *Calculator Programs for the Health Sciences* (New York: Oxford University Press, 1983).

Friedman GD: Be kind to your reader. *Am J Epidemiol* **132:**591–593 (1990).

Rothman KJ, Boice JD, Jr: *Epidemiological Analysis with a Programmable Calculator,* 2d ed. (Chestnut Hill, Mass.: Epidemiology Resources Inc., 1982).

Chapter 14

Epidemiology and Patient Care

Epidemiology is quite important in patient care. We have already seen (Chap. 10) how clinical studies of disease outcome, based on epidemiologic principles, can determine factors related to prognosis and demonstrate which treatments are best. In addition, clinical decisions are greatly affected by knowledge of the patterns of disease occurrence in populations. Some of the ways that diagnosis and treatment are, or should be, related to epidemiologic knowledge and principles will be discussed in this chapter.

Epidemiology and Diagnosis

In making a diagnosis, the physician must select from the hundreds of known diseases the one that most probably fits the patient's clinical picture. In assessing the probability of a given condition being present, the physician is strongly influenced by an awareness of what diseases are prevalent in the community at the time. During an influenza epidemic, for example, a patient exhibiting fever, headache, weakness, and myalgia would be promptly diagnosed as having influenza; whereas, in the absence of such an epidemic, laboratory tests would probably be ordered to rule out other explanations for the illness. Similarly, at the present time in the United States when a patient presents with congestive heart failure, diphtheritic or Chagas' myocarditis need rarely be considered.

Descriptive epidemiologic findings indicating subgroups of the population in which a disease has a low or high prevalence are also useful for diagnosis. Knowing that a patient is of a particular age or sex or occupation or that he or she comes from a certain part of the country is very helpful in narrowing down the probable diseases that might be present. For example, if a patient has lived in the San Joaquin Valley of California, coccidioidomycosis should be strongly suspected as the disease responsible for a nonspecific lung lesion observed in the chest x-ray.

The use of epidemiologic knowledge in the diagnosis of heart disease was well described by Dry (1943), who quoted a "cardiologist of long experience" as follows:

When I am called to see a patient with heart disease that is not of almost self-evident nature I find out certain things before I enter the room. I know whether the patient is a baby, a child, an adolescent, or an adult. If he is an adult, I find out in what age range he falls. There are certain heart diseases found commonly in certain ages and rarely found in persons of other ages. I have made my first step in probable diagnosis right then.

Then, particularly if the patient is an adult, I must know whether he is male or female, for there is a sex predilection for certain diseases of the heart. That's my second step and I have narrowed the probable diagnosis down further.

Next, I find out from the history what he has been exposed to. What diseases has he had? What kind of life has he lived? Has he suffered important hardships, been a rounder? Is he or she a successful, hard driving person? How much does he eat, smoke and drink? In what condition is his general health? Such questions as these narrow the problem down further. I am pretty well along in logical diagnosis by exclusion before I cross the threshold.

Then I do cross it but I'm in no hurry. I shake hands with the patient, feel his pulse. I get certain impressions that way. I look at him, talk to him and size him up as a man and a doctor rather than as a cardiologist. I ask him questions about his specific complaints and continue to ply him with questions until I have the picture in my own mind of just what he has been experiencing subjectively. It is not enough to know, for instance, that he has pain in his chest or shortness of breath because either may indicate serious heart disease or a condition that is relatively innocent. Thus I have secured further background and some of what already was in my mind when I was standing in the hall has been either reinforced or refuted.

Then I put my hands and my stethoscope on his chest in the course of a complete and thorough examination. Next I review the x-ray and the electrocardiogram. I ought to get every bit of evidence I can, but I honestly doubt if any of it is usually as important as the thinking I did in the hall and at the bedside before I touched the patient or had any apparatus applied to him.

Analytic Studies to Improve Methods of Diagnosis

Population studies, quite analogous to analytic epidemiologic studies, have been used to refine diagnostic methods. Just as epidemiology traditionally studies the associations between a disease and etiologic or predictive factors, the same approach may be used to study the associations between a disease and symptoms, signs, or laboratory tests. These, after all, constitute the information that is used to make a diagnosis.

Because of the current popularity of laboratory tests, one need only glance through a volume of issues of any leading medical journal to find examples of studies showing how a particular test may be used to help distinguish between persons with and without a particular disease or between different categories of patients with the same disease. Ordinarily, the test will be performed on different patient groups, plus some "normal controls." The distributions of the test results in each of these groups are then compared. When any two distributions appear quite different and show little overlap, the test is valuable in discriminating between the two groups, that is, in determining whether a patient belongs to one group or the other.

The value of a symptom in distinguishing between persons with and without a disease may be investigated similarly. Two population studies are examples of great interest because they showed that certain traditional clinical teachings about the relationship between a disease and a symptom are probably incorrect.

One of these studies (Price, 1963) looked closely at the relationship between various types of indigestion, or dyspepsia, and gallbladder disease. It had long been taught by some authorities that chronic epigastric pain, flatulence, heartburn, and intolerance to fatty and other types of foods could often be due to a diseased gallbladder. A total of 204 women aged 50 to 70 were identified in one urban general-practice patient roster in the United Kingdom. Of these women, 142, or 70 percent, agreed to be interviewed concerning these symptoms. Each patient later had an x-ray of the gallbladder, by means of which 24 were shown to have gallstones or a poorly functioning gallbladder.

The relative frequency of fatty-food intolerance and of each of the other "typical" symptoms was quite similar in the groups with normal and abnormal gallbladders. Altogether, dyspepsia was quite a common symptom, afflicting about half of each group. The type of indigestion experienced by the abnormal group did not differ appreciably from that reported by normals. The author concluded that among women aged 50 to 70 the presence of both gallbladder disease and dyspepsia is coincidental and that these symptoms cannot assist in the diagnosis of gallbladder disease and should not influence its treatment.

In another study of this type, Weiss (1972) analyzed data from the 1960–1962 U.S. National Health Survey to explore the relationship between hypertension and certain symptoms long regarded as being due to this condition. Responses to questions about these symptoms on a self-administered questionnaire were studied in relation to blood pressure subsequently measured by a physician. Headache, epistaxis, and tinnitus showed no relationship to either systolic or diastolic pressure. A history of dizziness was more prevalent only in those hypertensives with a very high diastolic pressure. Fainting was inversely related to blood pressure, being reported more frequently by those with lower pressures.

It is not surprising that many physicians have accepted the teaching that gallbladder disease produces fatty-food intolerance and that hypertension produces headache. First of all, these relationships, particularly the former, can be "explained" physiologically. Second, these symptoms are quite common; thus it is not surprising to find patients complaining of them. Nevertheless, by examining these symptom-disease relationships in general population groups, the epidemiologic approach can put them in proper perspective.

"Normal" Values

Returning again to laboratory tests and other quantitative measurements, practicing physicians and laboratory directors are in the habit of dividing the distributions of these findings into two parts, the "normal" and the "abnormal." Having a clear dividing line, or "normal limit," between the two alternatives makes it easier to make decisions. If the patient is normal, he or she can be reassured; if abnormal, some action must be taken. Thus, it is important to understand how normal limits are arrived at.

Unfortunately, much confusion surrounds this area because the term *normal* has more than one meaning. As used above, it means "good" or "desirable" or "healthy." Another important meaning is "usual" or "frequent." In this sense, it is normal for an older person to have gray hair. This says that the occurrence is common but implies nothing either way about desirability. As if these two definitions did not cause sufficient confusion, there is a third meaning having to do with the shape of a distribution curve that is often observed in studies of human characteristics. This symmetrical, bell-shaped curve is referred to as the *gaussian,* or *normal, distribution curve.*

One method that has been used to define the "normal-healthy" is to determine the "normal-usual." That is, the particular test is applied to a large population. A cutoff point is applied to one or both ends of the distribution curve so that an arbitrary, small percentage, say 5 percent or 1 percent of the population, will be called abnormal. Clearly, by this method, the normal range is merely the usual range; but it is easy to drift into the view that normal-usual means normal-healthy.

This method for determining normal-healthy limits can be improved by finding the normal-usual values in a population that is known to be healthy. Unfortunately, the healthy group studied is often small and select—for example, a group of medical or nursing students. Thus it is hard to be sure whether test values associated with health in these groups would also be associated with health in persons of different ages and circumstances.

Even better than studying a healthy group alone is to determine the test values in two groups, one that is healthy and one that has the disease being tested for. The resulting distributions usually overlap, as shown in Fig. 14-1. Outside the area of distribution overlap, a test result clearly identifies the presence or absence of disease. If a patient's value falls into the area of overlap, there is a chance of belonging to either the normal or the abnormal group. Choosing one cutoff point will thus result in errors in classification; that is, there will be some truly normal individuals on the abnormal side of the cutoff point who will be called abnormal, and there will be some truly abnormal individuals who will be considered normal.

These two types of classification errors can be expressed quan-

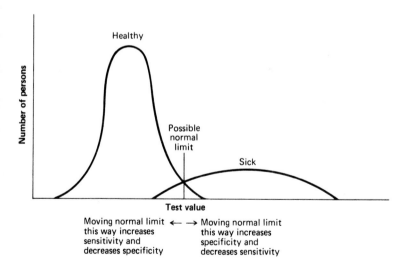

Figure 14-1   Typical example of the overlapping distributions of a test value in the healthy and the sick. Effects of shifting cutoff point on sensitivity and specificity.

titatively in terms of the *sensitivity* and the *specificity* of a test. Sensitivity is the proportion of truly diseased persons who are called diseased by the test. Specificity is the proportion of truly non-diseased persons who are so identified by the test. In the example shown in Fig. 14-1 it is apparent that these two measures are inversely related to one another. Shifting the cutoff point to the left will increase sensitivity at the cost of specificity. That is, a higher percentage of sick persons will be called sick but a smaller percentage of well persons will be called well. Moving the cutoff point to the right will increase specificity while decreasing sensitivity. More of the well will be called well but less sickness will be detected.

In setting the normal cutoff point, then, attention must be paid to the purpose of the test. If it is very important not to miss a particular disease which is both treatable and serious, one usually favors sensitivity over specificity, hoping to correctly identify as many cases as possible. On the other hand, if detecting a disease results in little benefit, while falsely labeling normal persons as sick results in much worry and cost, specificity is to be preferred.

A graphic display of this inverse relation between sensitivity and specificity is useful in indicating how accurate a test is. Originally used in electronics, this diagram is called a receiver operating characteristic (ROC) curve. Sensitivity, or true positive rate, is plotted against $(1 - \text{specificity})$ or false positive rate, as the cutoff point varies from one end of the region of overlap to the other (Fig. 14-2). If the test discriminated perfectly, there would be no overlap between positive and negative results. As a result there would already be 100 percent true positives (sensitivity) when there were no false positives. As shown in Fig. 14-2, it could not be improved by changing the cutoff point to increase the false positive rate (i.e., to decrease specificity); the perfect test would be represented by the Y axis of the graph plus a horizontal line across the top. At the other extreme, a useless test cannot discriminate between true positives and true negatives; the two distributions would coincide and any cutoff point would yield as many true positives as false positives, as shown by the diagonal line in Fig. 14-2. ROC curves for most tests appear like the curved line in Fig. 14-2, and the better the test, the closer the curve approaches the depiction of the perfect test. Like the overlapping distributions in

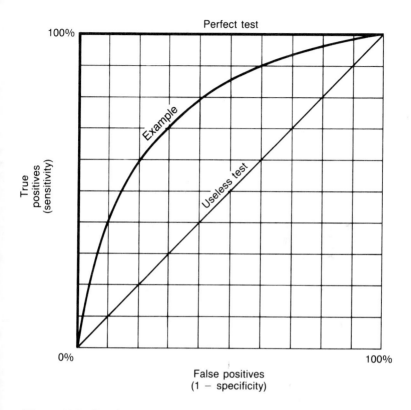

Figure 14-2   Receiver operating characteristic (ROC) curve.

Fig. 14-1, the ROC curve can also be used to determine the cutoff point that yields the desired proportions of false positives and false negatives. The cutoff point at which the curve slopes at 45 degrees is where the total number of errors is lowest (Streiner et al., 1989).

Unfortunately, the physician's desire for a nice cutoff point has been dealt a rather serious blow by recent epidemiologic studies, particularly in cardiovascular disease. For important coronary risk factors such as blood pressure and cholesterol, it appears that within the range usually observed in this country there is no cutoff point between a safe and unsafe level. That is, the lower the level, the lower the coronary disease risk. There is no single level above which treatment should be given. Decisions to treat an elevated coronary risk factor must be based not only on the level of the risk factor itself but on the presence or absence of other indicators of risk. Thus, one is more apt to try to lower a serum cholesterol level of 240 mg/100 mL if it is found in a middle-aged man who also smokes cigarettes and has a blood pressure of 150/95.

Serum cholesterol provides an excellent demonstration of the distinction between normal-usual and normal-healthy. It is not at all unusual to find a middle-aged man with a serum cholesterol level that should hardly be considered as indicative of good health, even if the man feels well. Specifically, there is abundant epidemiologic evidence that *one-fourth* of men, that is, those who happen to belong to the highest quartile of the cholesterol distribution, have 3 to 4 times the risk of developing clinical coronary heart disease as men in the lowest quartile. Knowing that about one in every five middle-aged men in this highest quartile will develop clinical coronary heart disease in the next 10 years hardly leads to confidence that they are normal-healthy, especially since there is mounting evidence that medical attention to their diet and living habits may reduce their high risk.

Epidemiologic studies have shown that many characteristics that have been regarded as normal because they are usual in persons who presently feel well are associated with a high probability of *future* disease. A preventive approach implies that these characteristics can no longer be regarded as consistent with good health.

Practicing Preventive Medicine in the Office or Clinic

Epidemiologic knowledge fosters the practice of preventive medicine in the medical office. Knowledge of the factors and characteristics that *cause* or *predict* the development of a disease permits identifying individuals who are at high risk of developing it. It may then be possible to prescribe measures for these patients that will prevent or at least delay the onset of the disease.

For years, pediatricians have been quite comfortable with the office practice of preventive medicine. Immunizations and well-baby care constitute an important phase of their work. In adult care the trend toward preventive medicine has only recently taken hold. In the hope of hastening this process, the simplicity and ease of preventive care for one of the major threats to adult health, coronary heart disease, will be described.

Based on our current knowledge of coronary risk factors, identification of high-risk individuals entails little cost and effort. Age, sex, family history, and pertinent habits such as cigarette smoking and exercise are simple historical items that can be obtained by paramedical personnel or self-administered questionnaires. Likewise, height and weight or simple observation to detect obesity and a blood pressure measurement can be done by anyone in the office with minimal training. All that remains is an electrocardiogram and the drawing of a blood specimen for measuring cholesterol and glucose. The cholesterol measurement should include a determination of how much of it falls into the beneficial high-density lipoprotein (HDL) and the harmful low-density lipoprotein (LDL) fractions.

Most authorities presently believe that persons with elevated levels of correctable risk factors should receive remedial therapy. As mentioned earlier, there is no safe cutoff point for each measure. The physician must form an overall impression of the patient's risk and act accordingly.

The prophylactic measures for the most part appear to be safe and consistent with good general health. Where appropriate, advice should be given to stop smoking, to eat less rich food, and to get more exercise without going to sudden extremes. These changes in diet and activity may be sufficient to reduce weight, blood lipids, and blood pressure to low-risk levels. Some individuals also experience beneficial effects on blood pressure by reducing their salt or alcohol intake. If these lifestyle changes are insufficient, relatively safe drugs are available to lower blood pressure and blood lipids.

The point that requires emphasis is that the detection and treatment of high coronary risk is simple and should be well within the scope of office medical practice. It would be naive to assume that all high-risk patients will stop smoking, or eat less, or exercise more, if a doctor tells them to. But some will, and it would be a shame if they were not given the opportunity and encouragement to lower their risk for a frequent, often fatal, disease.

CRITICAL READING OF THE MEDICAL LITERATURE

You believe that easily which you hope for earnestly.
    Terence

Most health care professionals do not have enough time for the careful study of the many medical and scientific articles that come to their attention. It is important, however, to be able to evaluate critically reports and papers that can influence clinical decisions or practice.

It is not intended, in this brief discussion, to cover all the errors and pitfalls that can occur in medical papers. Evaluating methods, observations, and interpretations in specialized fields such as surgery or biochemistry often requires knowledge and experience in the particular discipline.

An understanding of epidemiology does foster a critical approach to certain aspects of papers involving the study of populations or patient groups. The following discussion will focus primarily on some common problems and fallacies of an epidemiologic or statistical nature. The basic principles involved have been presented in previous chapters.

Need for an Adequate Control Group or Basis of Comparison

Many papers report findings showing the apparent benefits of a preventive or treatment measure, based on what appear to be good results when the measure has been used on a study group. In viewing these "good results," the reader should always ask: *Compared to what?* This initial question will usually imply others such as: *Was there a control or comparison group? Who constituted the control group? Were they similar to the treated group in all important aspects other than the treatment?* The author should have provided clear and satisfying answers to these questions in the paper. If not, there is good reason to doubt the claimed benefits.

It might be found, for example, that 95 percent of those given a certain hypnotic drug reported the next day that they slept soundly. Although, at first glance, this in itself seems like impressive evidence for the efficacy of the drug, we must know what percentage of similar but untreated persons would report sleeping soundly on the previous night. Furthermore, to rule out a placebo effect, we also need to know what percentage, given an inactive "sleeping pill," would report sound sleep.

The demonstration of harmful effects also requires a basis of comparison. It may be recalled (Chap. 7) that it was not sufficient to show that a large proportion of fatally injured pedestrians have high blood-alcohol levels to incriminate alcohol as a contributor to being struck and killed by a motor vehicle. It was also necessary to demonstrate that noninjured pedestrians, otherwise similar to those killed, had, on the average, less alcohol in their blood.

Requirement of Denominators for Statements Comparing Risks

Statements implying that a factor involves greater or less risk of a certain outcome are often made using only "numerator" data. The reader should "think epidemiologically" and remember that statements concerning risk should be based on *rates,* which require *denominators* as well as numerators. An example, again regarding motor vehicle injuries, comes from a radio advertisement promoting the use of auto seat belts. A statement was made to the effect that 75 percent of all motor vehicle fatalities occurred within 25 miles of home. The implication seemed to be that it was especially risky to drive on short trips close to home. However, note that motor vehicle fatalities constitute only the numerator of a mortality rate, which needs also an appropriate denominator, such as passenger-miles. If, say, 95 percent of all passenger-miles were driven within 25 miles of home, it could easily be shown that the *risk* of getting killed per passenger-mile is *less* within 25 miles of home than it is farther away.

Failure to choose the appropriate denominator in drawing conclusions about risk is an easy error to fall into. In noting the age distribution of a large series of 500 myocardial infarction cases (Table 14-1), it would be tempting but erroneous to conclude that the risk of myocardial infarction rises with age into the sixties and then falls sharply. Statements about risk at various ages must be related to the underlying population from which the cases are drawn. Incidence rates should be constructed by using the number

Table 14-1 Hypothetical Age Distribution of Myocardial Infarction Cases

Age	Number of cases	Percent
20–29	10	2
30–39	40	8
40–49	75	15
50–59	125	25
60–69	175	35
70–79	50	10
80+	25	5
Total	500	100

of cases at each age as the numerator and person-time, or the number of persons at risk per unit of time as the denominator. These will permit an appropriate comparison of risk at different ages. Fallacious inferences about risk, of the type illustrated here, are frequent and should be watched for.

Other Problems

Among the special problems involving particular concepts, measurements, or study designs discussed in previous chapters are: selection and information bias, the possibility for spurious correlations due to uncontrolled confounding variables, the need to distinguish statistical from biological significance (Chap. 11), and the likelihood of biased comparisons of survival when the starting point for follow-up is different in two groups (Chap. 10). Perhaps the reader's attention should again be called to the discussions in Chap. 3 on the limitations of medical observations, to the sections in Chaps. 4 to 10 concerning the conduct and interpretation of various types of studies, and to the interpretation of statistical associations as described in Chap. 11. In addition, much of the advice on conducting a study in Chap. 13 is also pertinent to the evaluation of the studies of others. Further discussion of problems and fallacies can be found in Huff (1954), Schor and Karten (1966), Hill and Hill (1991), Ludwig and Collette (1971), Colton (1974), Riegelman (1981), and Gehlbach

(1982). In addition to concerns regarding epidemiologic factors, critical readers should also consider the following general points in evaluating reported studies.

Need for Adequate Information

It is important to determine whether the methods of selecting subjects and of collecting and analyzing data have been described by the author in sufficient detail to allow their evaluation and replication. Others who try to repeat the study need to understand why their findings might differ. By close attention to these methods, the critical reader may also be able to determine whether the study was done with care or in a haphazard fashion.

Evidence of Objectivity

Some attempt should be made to determine whether the author is objective or is an advocate of a particular point of view. Is the presentation slanted toward a particular viewpoint? Would the author have published the paper if the opposite findings had been observed? Some knowledge of the author's previous work may be helpful in answering these questions.

One way a lack of objectivity may be expressed is through a selection process. Without intending to mislead, an investigator may emphasize those observations that support his or her point of view and discard those that do not. Referring again to Fig. 11-1, which shows a moderate correlation between coronary heart disease mortality and per capita cigarette consumption in 44 states, note that the points for Utah, Arkansas, Kentucky, Indiana, and Connecticut fall along a straight line. If one wanted to show that the two variables had a nearly perfect correlation, one could prepare a graph showing these five states only. These five points would indeed present an impressive picture if it were not mentioned that they were selected out of all the available data.

Selection for Publication

Viewing the medical literature as a whole, it is clear that positive findings are more apt to appear than are negative findings (Dickersin, 1990). It must be remembered that positive findings may occur by chance where there is no relationship. Even when the authors are objective, chance positive findings are more apt to find their way into the literature than are truly negative findings, at least until controversy makes negative findings just as important and interesting as positive findings.

PROBLEMS

14-1 Reread the quotation by Dry starting on page 269, substituting for heart disease a pulmonary problem, such as chronic cough and dyspnea, or a gastrointestinal complaint, such as abdominal pain or jaundice. Note how epidemiologic knowledge is applicable to a variety of diagnostic problems.

14-2 Easy fatigue is said to be a frequent result of anemia. How would you determine whether anemia is indeed associated with this symptom?

14-3 A urologist in a teaching hospital has developed a new blood test for detecting occult prostatic cancer. The cancerous cells produce a substance which can get into the bloodstream, and the test measures the concentration of this substance in the patient's serum. To establish normal values, the urologist performs the test on all healthy male interns and residents at his institution who are 25 to 29 years old. He finds that 99 percent of them have test values ranging from 32 to 66 units. He therefore concludes that values of 67 or greater are positive test results that warrant an extensive diagnostic evaluation of the patient. What major deficiencies do you see in his approach to establishing normal values?

14-4 The currently accepted risk factors for breast cancer include nulliparity or late age at first pregnancy, early age at menarche, late age at menopause, higher socioeconomic status, large doses of radiation to the chest, a history of breast cancer in close relatives, obesity, and certain benign breast tumors. Design a simple procedure to be used in a family practitioner's office to detect high-risk women. What prophylactic measures should be recommended for them?

14-5 What possible fallacies or problems can you detect in the following statements?

    a Of the patients with disease X in our hospital, 92 percent are of Mediterranean extraction. Therefore, Mediterranean people are clearly predisposed to disease X.

    b Our toothpaste is very effective. Three-quarters of the employees of a large firm who use it received personal appearance ratings of "above average" or better by their supervisors.

    c A large-scale study of 10,000 schoolchildren indicates that the drinking of soft drinks instead of milk significantly stunts their growth. The mean height of 7000 ninth graders who regularly drank milk was 162.6 cm, whereas the 3000 who regularly drank soft drinks was 162.5 cm. The difference was highly significant ($p < 0.0001$).

    d The modified total gastrectomy operation developed by surgeons in our institution is much safer than the traditional operation. After 1 year, 96 percent of patients who were followed up from the time of hospital discharge were still alive. Recent 1-year survival figures reported from other institutions average only 82 percent.

14-6 Dr. X noted that several of his patients with appendicitis had been frequent eaters of barley soup. He developed the hypothesis that barley irritates the opening of the appendix, which leads to spasm and the resultant trapping of foreign matter in the appendiceal lumen. After feeding barley to hamsters, Dr. X observed that histologic examination of their cecums revealed some inflammatory cells. He presented his findings at medical and surgical meetings, published several journal articles on the subject, and went on to write a book on the dangers of eating barley. Two years later, because of the resulting controversy, a governmental agency decided to fund a large-scale study to determine definitively whether eating barley could cause appendicitis. Someone suggested that Dr. X would be the ideal person to direct such a study since he was an expert on the subject and "obviously not on the payroll of the barley-growers association." Do you agree that he would carry out an objective evaluation?

14-7 If you were trying to prove that cigarette smoking helped prevent coronary heart disease, what data points would you select from all those shown in Fig. 11-1?

BIBLIOGRAPHY

Colton T: *Statistics in Medicine* (Boston: Little, Brown, 1974), chaps. 12, 13.

Dickersin K: The existence of publication bias and risk factors for its occurrence. *JAMA* **263:**1385–1389 (1990).

Dry TJ: *Manual of Cardiology* (Philadelphia: Saunders, 1943), pp. 1, 2.

Gehlbach SH: *Interpretinng the Medical Literature: A Clinician's Guide* (Lexington, Mass.: Collamore Press, 1982).

Hill AB, Hill ID: *Bradford Hill's Principles of Medical Statistics,* 12th ed. (London: Edward Arnold, 1991).

Huff D: *How to Lie with Statistics* (New York: Norton, 1954).

Ludwig EG, Collette JC: Some misuses of health statistics. *JAMA* **216:**493–499 (1971).

Price WH: Gall-bladder dyspepsia. *Br Med J* **2:**138–141 (1963).

Riegelman RK: *Studying a Study and Testing a Test* (Boston: Little, Brown, 1981).

Schor S, Karten I: Statistical evaluation of medical journal manuscripts. *JAMA* **195:**1123–1128 (1966).

Streiner DL, Norman GR, Blum HM: *PDQ Epidemiology* (Toronto: Decker, 1989).

Weiss NS: Relation of high blood pressure to headache, epistaxis, and selected other symptoms: The United States health examination survey of adults. *N Engl J Med* **287:**631–633 (1972).

Epidemiology, Medical Care, and the Health of the Community

Health and disease in the community are important concerns not only of medical and public health professionals but of the general public as well. To illustrate the important role of epidemiology in community health, three types of epidemiologic investigations will be described briefly: the time-honored investigation of infectious-disease epidemics, some recent efforts to detect unsuspected environmental hazards, and follow-up studies of occupational exposures. Then, the limited effects of medical care on community health will be discussed. Finally, screening for disease and other ways of increasing the benefits of health care for the community will be described.

Investigation of Epidemics of Infectious Disease

Until a few decades ago, epidemiology had focused primarily on infectious diseases, which have been the major scourges of humankind. Recently, in the more affluent nations, most infectious diseases have been brought under reasonably good control, and the leading causes of death and disability have become the noninfectious conditions. Thus, in these areas, the attention of many epidemiologists has been directed toward chronic degenerative and neoplastic diseases. Other diseases or conditions of great interest and importance include physical trauma or "accidents," mental illness, and congenital defects. Additional concerns that have recently engaged the epidemiologist are studies of medical care and health services, and studies that focus on general health status irrespective of the particular diseases responsible for departures from good health.

Despite this shifting emphasis in the more affluent nations, infectious diseases remain extremely important problems in the "less developed" parts of the world. Furthermore, dangerous infectious-disease outbreaks continue to occur in industrialized nations. This is well illustrated by the epidemic of the acquired immune deficiency syndrome, or AIDS, an infectious disease that became a major public health problem in the 1980s, particularly in certain large cities in the United States. Even though the principal causes of many of these diseases are fairly well understood, epidemiologists, health officers, and other physicians and public health nurses are still called upon to investigate specific disease outbreaks to determine the particular conditions or factors that are responsible.

Investigation of the variety of epidemics that might occur cannot be described by a single step-by-step "cookbook" approach. However, certain principles are followed sufficiently often to deserve at least a brief summary here. The interested reader should consult Anderson et al. (1962) or Mausner and Kramer (1984) for more details.

The typical field investigation of an epidemic involves, first, a study of the cases. Clinical examination and appropriate laboratory tests are needed to determine or verify the diagnosis. Once the disease is identified, knowledge of the usual sources of infection and common modes of spread for that disease will help point the investigation toward the most likely explanations of the epidemic. A convenient reference book that summarizes the important information for most infectious diseases is *Control of Communicable Diseases in Man* (Benenson, 1990).

In addition to verifying the diagnosis, the patients are studied further, usually by interview. Their basic characteristics such as age, sex, and occupation should be determined, as should the onset and time course of the disease. Personal contacts at home, work, school, and other places, special events such as parties and trips, foods eaten, and exposures to other common vehicles are items that will frequently be inquired about, depending, of course, on the disease believed responsible for the outbreak. Particular emphasis should be placed on the time period when the patient was most probably infected. This period precedes the disease onset time by an interval equal to the usual incubation period for that disease.

The subsequent investigation will be guided by information gained from the known cases. For example, plotting the dates of disease onset graphically, as seen earlier in Figs. 5-7, 5-8, and 5-9, will help determine if the epidemic had a point source or involved person-to-person spread. Or, if the disease involves a gastrointestinal infection and several cases mention going to the same restaurant or party, further investigation of possible food contamination at the restaurant or party would be in order. Pursuing the party further, apparently well persons who also attended might be given appropriate laboratory tests to detect subclinical infection. Comparisons of what the infected and uninfected persons at the party will help determine which foods were contaminated.

Data analysis concerning possible causative factors in an epidemic will usually take the form of either a case-control study or a cohort study. In the case-control approach, persons who developed the disease are compared with those who did not, with regard to various exposures. The suspect sources or vehicles are those to which a much higher proportion of cases than controls were exposed. In the cohort study approach, the *attack rates* of persons exposed to possible sources or vehicles are compared with those of persons not exposed. (Attack rates are cumulative incidence rates without specification of time in the denominator.) If the rates are much higher in the exposed, the source is highly suspect. For example, Table 15-1 shows the findings in connection with an epidemic of gastroenteritis among persons who ate lunch in a cafeteria in Chattanooga, Tennessee, on March 2, 1973 (Jensen et al., 1973). The foods under investigation as possible sources were potato salad, hamburger, baked beans, and milk. The only food with a large and statistically significant difference in attack rate between

Table 15-1 Food-specific Attack Rates of Gastroenteritis—Chattanooga, Tennessee, March 2, 1973

Food item	Persons eating it		Persons not eating it	
	Total no.	Attack rate, %	Total no.	Attack rate, %
Potato salad	100	88	33	15
Hamburger	126	71	31	51
Baked beans	99	77	10	50
Milk	55	62	71	68

Source: Data from Jensen et al. (1973).

eaters and noneaters was the potato salad (88 percent versus 15 percent ill), and this proved to be the main vehicle for the infectious agent.

It is hoped that investigation of the epidemic will reveal correctable problems. A major accomplishment would be the identification of infected persons who can continue to spread disease if not attended to, such as typhoid carriers working in restaurants or hospital employees with staphylococcal skin infections. The recognition of other factors leading to the spread of disease, such as improper food-handling practices, contaminated water supplies, or segments of the population who have not received the usual vaccinations, can also lead to effective control measures.

The Detection and Evaluation of Environmental Hazards

In recent years there has been considerable concern that we are poisoning ourselves with our technology. It is well known that our land, water, and air are being polluted by such substances as industrial wastes, exhaust products from burning fuels, trace metals, chemicals, pesticides, and radioactive materials. Furthermore, the population now ingests a variety of chemicals in such forms as preservatives and medicinal drugs.

What is less clear is the extent to which these substances affect human health. Epidemiologic studies can play an important role in the quantitative determination of the risks involved.

The usual investigations have employed standard epidemiologic methods to assess the relationship between specific substances, drugs, energy sources, or occupational exposures and particular disease outcomes of interest. Examples are the Berlin, New Hampshire, cross-sectional study of chronic respiratory disease in relation to air pollution and smoking, described in Chap. 6; the case-control study of thromboembolic disease in relation to oral contraceptives, described in Chap. 7; and the cohort study of occupational exposure to x-ray, described in Chap. 8. (For further examples, see Goldsmith, 1972, and Whittenberger, 1981.)

These studies involve an assessment of environmental hazards that are *already under suspicion*. The proliferation of new chemicals and energy sources to which we are exposed has led to serious concern that there are many hazards that we are not aware of. Sometimes, unsuspected hazards come to light only after considerable damage has been done. A dramatic example involved the drug thalidomide, which, when given as a tranquilizer to pregnant women, resulted in the birth of thousands of seriously deformed babies. Other classic instances were the occurrence of retrolental fibroplasia in premature infants who received oxygen therapy and the development of bone cancers in radium-dial painters.

As a result of concern about the unsuspected, epidemiologists have developed a new area of research, sometimes called *monitoring*. The purpose of monitoring is to detect unsuspected adverse or undesired effects of components of the environment as soon as possible after these effects appear, and thus provide an "early warning system." Because broad areas are to be covered, this type of investigation usually involves initially a search for hypotheses. Suspicious relationships can then be subjected to more intensive study.

Some of the experience to date in monitoring environmental hazards has been gained from monitoring adverse reactions to medicinal drugs (*Report of the International Conference on Adverse Reactions Reporting Systems,* 1971; Gross and Inman, 1977; Venning, 1983). Despite careful testing of drugs before they are marketed, many drug reactions do not become recognized until the drug has been extensively used by large numbers of patients. Monitoring of drug reactions will be used to illustrate some of the methods to be described.

A number of methods or systems of monitoring are available.

These have been tried with varying degrees of success. They involve the assembly and analysis of data on morbid events, usually, but not always, in relation to various exposures.

Spontaneous Reporting Systems   Many hypotheses come from the observation by individual physicians of patients who develop what seems to be an adverse reaction to a drug. Ordinarily, if sufficiently concerned, the physician might report this to the drug manufacturer or publish a letter or brief case report in a medical journal.

Programs known as spontaneous reporting systems have been established to encourage physicians to send such reports to a central agency or clearinghouse where they can be assembled and evaluated. Examples are the reporting programs that have been set up by the Food and Drug Administration in the United States and the Committee on Safety of Drugs in the United Kingdom.

While some useful information has been obtained at low cost from spontaneous reports, certain deficiencies are apparent. Despite promotional efforts to get physicians to respond, the number of reports submitted and the amount of information contained in each report have often been disappointing. Furthermore, it is very difficult for the physician to determine the cause of a serious untoward event in a single patient. While it could be an adverse effect of a drug, it could also be a worsening or complication of the disease being treated or even the result of a different disease that has developed independently. Physicians tend to recognize and interpret as drug reactions events known to be drug-related, such as skin rash following penicillin therapy or aplastic anemia following chloramphenicol; they tend not to report unsuspected relationships. Finally, the lack of any denominator, or population-at-risk, information makes it difficult to determine whether the reaction might be rare or relatively common.

Changes in Disease Frequency   If a population is being exposed to a new environmental hazard or to increased levels of an old hazard, suspicion can be aroused by monitoring disease frequency. Populations or special subgroups may be kept under systematic surveillance to determine time trends in incidence, prevalence, or mortality from any or all diseases. A good example is the monitoring of congenital malformations in newborn infants. The prevalence of various malformations among newborn infants in several cooperating hospitals can be recorded on a monthly basis. If the occurrence of one or more malformations shows a distinct increase beyond the fluctuations usually noted due to chance or seasonal variations, then an inquiry into prenatal exposures might be initiated, much as one would investigate an epidemic of infectious disease (Hook, 1972).

Although probably less accurate than special programs to monitor disease frequency, the surveillance of vital statistics can also provide useful information about changes in disease occurrence. Increases in mortality rates in communities or increases in congenital malformations reported on birth certificates can provide useful clues that something is happening in the environment.

Intensive Surveillance of Both Exposures and Disease   Procedures can be established to collect extensive information concerning both exposures and disease frequency. In this way a variety of exposure-disease relationships can be explored to look for unsuspected relationships and to develop quantitative information about known relationships. This form of investigation has been applied extensively in the study of adverse drug reactions. Examples of drug-reaction monitoring programs are the Boston Collaborative Drug Surveillance Program (Jick et al., 1970) and the Drug Epidemiology Unit of the Boston University Medical Center (Shapiro and Slone, 1977), which collect and analyze data about drug administration and untoward events from several hospitals, and the Kaiser Permanente Drug-Reaction Monitoring System, which emphasizes drug use and drug reactions in outpatients (Friedman et al., 1971). The latter system is now being employed in the long-term follow-up of users of prescription drugs to check for possible carcinogenic effects (Selby et al., 1989). The application of epidemiologic principles to drug-reaction monitoring has been discussed by Finney (1965), Jick (1977), Shapiro and Slone (1977), Jick and Vessey (1978), and Strom (1989).

Evaluation of Occupational Exposures

A growing concern about occupational hazards has recently led to increased efforts to investigate and ensure the safety of the workplace. Spurred by government, unions, lawsuits, and their own sense of responsibility, industrial organizations are developing data-collection systems to assess both the health status of employees and the physical and chemical hazards to which employees are exposed. All the analytic study methods described in Chaps. 6 to 8 can be applied to these data in the epidemiologic evaluation of suspected occupational hazards.

Since much of the recent concern is with long-term health effects manifested years after the onset of exposure, there is considerable reluctance to wait for evaluation by cohort studies carried out prospectively. Clues or initial impressions can be gained from proportional mortality studies (Thun, 1991). Since occupations are ordinarily recorded on death certificates, one can determine whether a particular cause of death is seen disproportionately among persons in a given occupation. For example, brain cancer was found to occur more frequently than expected among the causes of death of employees who had worked at least 10 years at a facility that manufactured missile and aircraft guidance systems. The standardized proportional mortality ratio (PMR) was 4.4 based on 12 observed and 2.7 expected brain cancer deaths. This led to suspicion of fluids involved in the assembly of gyroscopes (Park et al., 1990).

Studies that are more rigorous but still retrospective, and thus accomplished fairly quickly, usually take the form of case-control or cohort investigations. The retrospective cohort study is used especially frequently in occupational health. One example is the study of mortality of radiologists described in Chap. 8. Another is the study of coke-plant workers by Lloyd (1971). In this classic investigation of mortality of steelworkers it was originally noted that the death rate from respiratory (chiefly lung) cancer for those who worked in coke plants (where bituminous coal is heated in ovens and transformed into coke for use in blast furnaces) was about twice the rate of steelworkers in general. By progressively narrowing the focus of attention to specific categories of coke-plant employees, Lloyd identified subgroups with increasingly higher risk. First, within the coke plant some men worked at the coke ovens, and some did not. All the excess risk of respiratory cancer in coke-plant workers was limited to the coke-oven workers, who showed about a 2.5-fold increase. Coke-oven workers could further be subdivided into those who worked on top of the ovens and had a large exposure to coal-tar fumes and those who worked at the side of the ovens with considerably less exposure. The topside workers experienced about a sevenfold increase in lung cancer mortality and accounted for almost all the excess risk of lung cancer among coke-oven workers. Still further subdivision by duration of employment revealed a tenfold increase in risk for men who worked topside for 5 or more years. This study is one of a series of epidemiologic investigations beginning two centuries ago that has linked occupational exposure to coal tar to the development of cancer. The first was the observation by Percivall Pott (1775) of the occurrence of scrotal cancers among London chimney sweeps.

The coke-oven-worker study points up some potential problems in occupational epidemiology. Available data may permit classification of workers only by broad occupational grouping. This can mask or markedly dilute an association between an occupational hazard and a disease among a subgroup of workers who experience an intense or specific exposure. Note how the sevenfold increase in lung cancer among topside coke-oven workers was seen as only a twofold increase among all coke-plant employees. Then, too, job titles may be uninformative, obsolete, misleading, or varying across different plants or over time within a plant, making it difficult to distinguish those workers who experienced the exposure of concern. Lloyd found that the great majority of coke-plant workers could be classified according to their discrete work areas by investigation of their work histories. Other investigators may not be so fortunate.

A common problem in occupational epidemiology is an inability to account for pertinent variables other than the occupational exposure itself. Retrospective occupational data often do not include measurements of confounding factors. It would be helpful, for example, to know whether coke-oven workers included relatively more cigarette smokers than other steelworkers before concluding that topside coke-oven exposure itself led to a tenfold increase in lung cancer mortality. Differences in smoking habits would probably not account for a tenfold excess, but they could explain part of it, or all of a smaller excess in lung cancer risk, such as that in the 1.5-fold range found in certain aluminum workers who were exposed to coal-tar fumes. Also, occupational exposures may operate synergistically with other factors, as was found for workers exposed to both asbestos and cigarette smoking. The combination of both exposures led to enormous increases in the incidence of lung cancer—92 times higher than that among nonexposed nonsmokers (Selikoff and Hammond, 1975).

Another problem with retrospective cohort studies of the occupationally exposed is the difficulty in finding appropriate comparison groups. Death rates in the general population are often used as a standard of comparison, but because the severely ill and disabled are ordinarily excluded from employment, workers usually exhibit lower overall death rates than the general population. This "healthy-worker effect" may amount to a 10 to 40 percent decrease below general population death rates.

It is hoped, then, that the ongoing collection and computerization of occupational health data will lead to an improvement in follow-up studies by capturing relevant nonoccupational characteristics and exposures and by including data on nonexposed but otherwise comparable workers.

Limited Effects of Medical Care—Historical Perspective

With the impressive technical advances in medical care that have become available in recent decades, it is easy to forget that the quality and quantity of medical care have only a limited influence on community health. That medical care is not the only determinant of health is well illustrated by the observed long-term trends in mortality from certain diseases. As will be shown, these trends appear to bear little relationship to changes in medical care.

One example is the marked decline in mortality from tuberculosis in the United States during the twentieth century (Fig. 15-1). As pointed out by Winkelstein (1972), the only treatment available

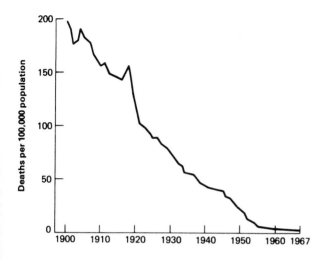

Figure 15-1   Annual age-adjusted tuberculosis death rates per 100,000 population, death registration states of the United States, 1900–1967. (Adjusted to the age distribution of the U.S. population in 1940.) *(Reproduced, by permission, from Winkelstein, 1972.)*

at the beginning of the century was rest therapy in sanatoriums, accessible only to the wealthy. This was made available to all economic classes in the 1930s, and during the same decade, collapse therapy was introduced. Chemotherapy became widely available in the 1950s. Figure 15-1 shows that the downward trend in mortality was clearly evident before these new therapies were widely applied. Winkelstein also cited data from a study by Terris (1948) showing that the isolation of cases in treatment facilities was probably not a major determinant of tuberculosis mortality. Thus, even though therapy and isolation of cases may have accentuated the decline shown in Fig. 15-1, other important factors also must have been operating.

Other diseases have also shown major secular changes that are difficult to attribute to the benefits of medical care. For example, McKeown and Lowe (1966) presented a graphic picture of the decline in mortality from pertussis (whooping cough) among English children, which is similar to that shown for tuberculosis in Fig. 15-1. Mortality declined rather steadily from about 1400 deaths per million per year in 1870 to a negligible number in the 1960s. Relevant medical landmarks during this decline were the identification of the causative organism in 1906, sulfonamide and antibiotic therapy beginning in 1939, and the general availability of immunization beginning in 1952. By the time drug therapy and immunization became available, the whooping cough mortality rate was only a small fraction of what it had been in the late nineteenth century, when it was a very important cause of death.

The rather striking time trends over the last few decades in lung cancer and stomach cancer mortality rates (see Fig. 5-10) are also largely independent of the effects of medical care. To date, medical, surgical, and radiation therapy cannot save the lives of the vast majority of victims of these two malignancies.

It is obvious from these examples and from the usual incurability of the degenerative and neoplastic diseases, which cause most death and disability, that if we are to bring these conditions under control and improve the health and longevity of the population, we cannot rely solely on increasing the availability of medical care as we know it today. More important will be an increase in our understanding of the environmental and social factors that foster these diseases and, using this knowledge, to apply effective preventive measures.

Two Aspects of Disease Prevention

One approach to disease prevention is through medical care of individual patients. As an example of this approach, a simple method for preventing coronary heart disease, to be used in the clinic or the physician's office, was described in Chap. 14. It involved, first, detecting individuals who are at high risk of developing the disease, and second, attempting to reduce their risk by changing their dietary and other habits and by judiciously prescribing drugs, when indicated.

The second avenue of disease prevention does not focus on the individual. Rather, it involves large-scale social and environmental changes, such as improving housing conditions, requiring pasteurization of all milk sold commercially, adding fluoride to community water supplies, or conducting educational programs through the mass media. For coronary heart disease, possible preventive approaches on this scale might include changing food processing to decrease the amount of saturated fat and cholesterol in animal food products, discouraging cigarette smoking by increased taxes or by other forms of persuasion well known to the advertising industry, or discovering the harmful agents in tobacco smoke and removing them, or banning automobiles from certain areas so as to force many people to walk or ride bicycles. Recently, some successes in lowering coronary risk factor levels has been achieved by innovative community education programs (Farquhar et al., 1990; Perry et al., 1992; Salonen et al., 1989).

Because many people do not go to doctors routinely and because many others who do go either do not follow medical advice or find it extremely difficult to break pleasurable habits, one is forced into a rather pessimistic view about the impact that office preventive medicine can have on the health of the general population. Even special intensive programs to change patient behavior have not had as much long-term effect as had been hoped. For example, a variety of methods have been tried to help people stop smoking cigarettes. However, despite high initial success rates, follow-up 1 year later usually reveals that only about one-fifth of those originally treated still refrain from smoking.

The health care professional must do everything possible to help individual patients. Certainly a success rate of one out of five is better than nothing. Nevertheless, since medical care often has so little impact on major health problems of the community, many believe that large-scale social and environmental changes are required.

The Physician's Limited View of Disease in the Community

One reason that medical care has less influence than one might expect is that much disease never comes to the attention of medical personnel. Using prevalence survey data obtained in Great Britain and the United States, White, Williams, and Greenberg (1961) showed how illness in the community gets filtered to various physicians and institutions in the medical care system. As shown in Fig. 15-2, of 1000 adults in the community, 750 reported one or more illnesses each month. Of those with illnesses, one-third, or 250, consulted a physician. Only 9, or 1.2 percent, of the ill were admitted to a hospital, and only 5, or 0.7 percent, were referred to another physician. Particularly striking from the viewpoint of medical education is the fact that only 1 of these patients was seen at a university medical center. Although these proportions may have changed somewhat, this marked selection process undoubtedly still operates.

Not only do just a portion of the sick get seen medically, but each medical specialty and medical setting attracts a selected group of patients out of all those seen. For example, in the outpatient clinic one is especially apt to encounter patients with mild acute

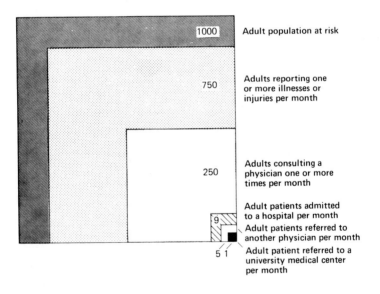

Figure 15-2   Monthly prevalence estimates of illness in the community and the roles of physicians, hospitals, and university medical centers in the provision of medical care (adults 16 years of age and over). *(Reproduced, by permission, from White, Williams, and Greenberg, 1961.)*

and chronic illness and patients with symptoms for which no organic basis can be found. In the hospital, patients are, on the average, much more seriously ill with diseases that are farther advanced. As pointed out by White et al.: "Each practitioner or administrator sees a biased sample of medical care problems presented to him; rarely has any individual, specialty or institution a broad appreciation of the ecology of medical care that enables unique and frequently isolated contributions to be seen in relation to those of others and to the over-all needs of the community."

Efforts to Bring More Disease to Medical Attention: Screening

In the hope of increasing the impact of current medical knowledge and technology on disease in the community, medical and public health facilities have established *screening* programs to detect persons with early, mild, and asymptomatic disease.

As stated by Thorner and Remein (1961): "The basic purpose of screening for disease detection is to separate from a large group of apparently well persons those who have a high probability of having the disease under study, so that they may be given a diagnostic workup and, if diseased, brought to treatment." Since screening tests are designed to be applicable to large population groups, they must be simple, rapid, and inexpensive. As a result, they are generally less accurate and definitive than the examinations and tests used by physicians to arrive at a final diagnosis.

Screening is carried out in the belief that the detection of disease in an early or asymptomatic stage will lead to appropriate treatment which, in turn, will lead to less disability and/or mortality from the disease. After an initial period of enthusiasm in some quarters, considerable skepticism developed concerning the benefits of screening, based on doubts as to whether it would really lead to favorable modifications in the course of disease.

Critics pointed out that many persons with diseases discovered by screening did not receive adequate or appropriate treatment afterward. Or, even if the accepted treatment were to be given for some diseases detected by screening, such as mild maturity-onset diabetes mellitus, it has not been shown that persons so treated live happier, healthier, or longer lives. Also, persons correctly or incorrectly labeled as having a disease would be caused considerable worry and anxiety, often to no good purpose. Furthermore, careful analysis showed that the apparently good results of screening could be misleading, due to self-selection for screening of those persons who take better care of themselves or due to fallacies such as lead-time bias (Chap. 10), wherein persons would *seem* to survive longer merely because the diagnosis was made earlier.

Another pitfall in evaluation, *length bias,* has to do with the fact that a screening program, like a prevalence survey, initially picks up a disproportionate number of long-duration cases—cases who would survive longest even without screening (Chap. 6 and Prob. 6-2). Screening programs can also look better than they really are due to overdiagnosis; if some of the small breast tumors picked up by screening are called malignant when they really are not, the patients with screen-detected cancer will appear to have an especially favorable outcome. Ethical questions have also been raised (McKeown, 1968), since in contrast to traditional medical care which is sought by the patient, disease detection by screening is initiated by medical or public health professionals, who, therefore, are under special obligation to make sure that screening does more good than harm.

Thus, whenever possible, screening programs should be evaluated by carefully controlled experimental studies in which relevant disease outcomes in a group receiving screening and in a comparable unscreened group are measured and compared. Any benefits found for screening programs should be compared to costs involved (McKeown and Knox, 1968; Wilson, 1968; Cochrane and Holland, 1971; Morrison, 1992). Although it is more an evaluation of periodic comprehensive health checkups than of screening per se, the Kaiser Permanente Multiphasic Health Checkup Evaluation Study, described in Chap. 9, illustrates the approach that is needed if screening programs are to prove their merits. Other examples of well-controlled experimental evaluations of screening or disease detection methods are the study of breast cancer screening by the Health Insurance Plan of New York (Shapiro et al., 1988) and the Canadian National Breast Screening Study (Miller et al., 1992). When applied carefully, the more efficient case-control evaluations of screening tests can also be quite informative, as illustrated by investigations of screening for cervical cancer by Pap smear (Clarke and Anderson, 1979) and of screening for colorectal cancer by sigmoidoscopy (Selby et al., 1992).

A generally accepted principle is that screening should be done only if it can be integrated with the medical care program where it is carried out. In practice this means not only that adequate treatment and follow-up be available for those who screen positive, but that the screening test results must be acceptable to the practicing physicians in the area. The characteristics of screening tests that relate to accuracy and acceptability will be discussed briefly.

Sensitivity and specificity, two measures of the accuracy of diagnostic tests, were defined in Chap. 14. These measures are also important features of screening tests. The relationship of a screening test to the final accurate diagnosis is conveniently shown in a fourfold table (see Table 15-2). In the table, a represents persons with the disease who are correctly labeled by the screening test. Persons denoted by b are *false positives,* that is, the test is positive, but they do not have the disease. The letter d denotes persons free of disease who are correctly labeled by the test. The letter c represents *false negatives,* that is, persons with the disease for whom the test is negative.

Sensitivity, the proportion of true positives that are labeled as positive, is thus $a/(a + c)$. Specificity, the proportion of true negatives that are labeled as negative, is $d/(b + d)$. Both of these measures are important, since the test should detect as much disease as possible while avoiding false labeling. False negatives, persons incorrectly labeled as disease-free, may be deprived of valuable therapy.

Table 15-2   Relationship of Screening-Test Results to the Final Accurate Diagnosis

Screening test	Final diagnosis		Total
	Disease present	Disease absent	
Positive	a	b	$a + b$
Negative	c	d	$c + d$
Total	$a + c$	$b + d$	$a + b + c + d$

False positives, persons incorrectly labeled as diseased, are subjected to needless worry and expensive diagnostic evaluations until their freedom from the disease is established. With all quantitative screening tests, the level above or below which a person is called positive will affect the sensitivity and specificity. Modifying this cutoff level to improve one of these characteristics will adversely affect the other, as shown in Fig. 14-1.

Physicians evaluating patients who have been screened are especially sensitive to another measure, $a/(a + b)$, the proportion of positive tests that are true positives. This is sometimes called the *predictive value* of a positive test or, more simply, the *positive predictive value*. (Correspondingly, the *negative predictive value*, $d/(c + d)$, is the proportion of persons with negative tests who are truly negative.) Since physicians are usually asked to evaluate only the positive screenees, they understandably become irritated and critical of the screening program when most of their follow-up diagnostic evaluations turn out to be negative.

If the disease is infrequent in the population—and most chronic diseases are—even a screening test with a high degree of specificity will yield positives of which a large percentage turn out to be false. Thorner and Remein (1961) showed an example of a population of 10,000 with an assumed prevalence of diabetes mellitus of 1.5 percent, screened with a random blood glucose (not drawn at any particular time in relation to eating). Using a cutoff point of 130 mg/100 mL (7.2 mmol/L), the test had been shown previously to have a sensitivity of 44.3 percent and a high specificity of 99.0 percent. The results are shown in Table 15-3. Note, that of the 164 positives, 98, or 60 percent, turned out to be false positives.

If, in order to decrease the number of false positives, the screening level is raised to 180 mg/100 mL (10.0 mmol/L), the specificity will be improved to 99.8 percent. The test will now yield only 54 positives, of whom only 20, or 37 percent, are false positives. However, there is a marked decrease in sensitivity. Only 34 of the 150 diabetics will be detected. This illustrates the trade-off between sensitivity and specificity when the cutoff point is changed.

For a test with a given sensitivity and specificity, the higher the disease prevalence, the higher the positive predictive value. One

Table 15-3   Results of Screening for Diabetes Mellitus in a Population of 10,000*

Screening test	Final diagnosis		Total
	Diabetic	**Not diabetic**	**Total**
Positive	66	98	164
Negative	84	9752	9,836
Total	150	9850	10,000

*In this population the disease prevalence is 1.5%, and the sensitivity and specificity of the test are 44.3% and 99.0%, respectively.

Source: Data from Thorner and Remein (1961).

strategy for increasing the prevalence of disease in the population screened is to restrict screening to high-risk individuals. For example, screening for diabetes by measuring blood sugar may be carried out only among persons who are obese or who have a family history of the disease.

Screening for High Risk   As more emphasis is being placed on disease prevention, community programs for disease control may well include screening programs to detect persons at high risk of developing disease. In this way, preventive measures can be applied before the disease occurs. For example, programs are now under way in industry and communities to identify persons with coronary risk factors such as high serum cholesterol and blood pressure levels, so that myocardial infarction and other manifestations of coronary heart disease can be prevented. The long-term effects of these programs need to be evaluated.

Before setting up such a program it is necessary, as with screening for early disease, to make sure that suitable care and follow-up will be available for positive screenees. That is, the screening must fit in with the local medical care program so that more will result than anxiety due to labeling.

Evaluating a Changing Health Care System

We are living in a period of great change in health care, marked by great advances in technology, unacceptably high and rapidly increasing costs, and growing empowerment of patients in medical decision making. As a result, many old methods are being questioned or discarded and new approaches are being introduced.

Innovations can and should be evaluated by well-controlled experiments whenever possible. Where particular circumstances or meager resources prohibit rigorous experiments, less formal evaluations such as before/after comparisons can be conducted. However, careful attention should then be paid to extraneous influences and biasing factors that may affect the apparent outcomes of the innovation.

A few of the health care issues of current interest are modes of payment for services, selection of treatments that produce the best outcomes—with careful attention to their costs, use of nurses and other paramedical personnel for tasks traditionally performed by physicians, content and frequency of health checkups and preventive services; control of drug overuse and abuse, and provision of optimal care for persons living in inner cities and remote rural areas. Defining and describing these problems and identifying and evaluating possible solutions, all involve studies of health-related characteristics, events, and outcomes in groups of people.

Whether these studies are labeled as *epidemiology,* or *medical care research,* or *health services research* makes little difference. What is important is that we are guided by careful observations and wise judgment to make necessary improvements while preserving the many good methods and approaches that we now have.

PROBLEMS

15-1 a An epidemic of gastroenteritis due to staphylococcal enterotoxin occurred after breakfast on an airliner, as previously described in Prob. 5-4 and Fig. 5-13. The occurrence of illness among the eaters and noneaters of each food served for breakfast is described in Table 15-4. Complete the table and determine which food was contaminated.

b The source of the food contamination was probably an irritated lesion on a finger of one of the cooks who

Table 15-4 Illness Experience of Eaters and Noneaters of Individual Breakfast Foods Aboard an Airliner

Food	Persons eating food				Persons not eating food			
	No. ill	No. not ill	Total no.	Attack rate, %	No. ill	No. not ill	Total no.	Attack rate, %
Omelette	169	133			23	14		
Ham	190	139			2	8		
Yogurt	147	98			45	49		
Roll	166	135			26	12		
Butter	137	130			55	17		
Cheese	103	94			89	53		

prepared the breakfast for the airline-owned catering company. The bacteria could multiply and produce toxin because the food was stored for several hours without adequate refrigeration. Fortunately, none of the pilots became ill, since they received a different meal. Besides following standard sanitary procedures for handling and storing anyone's food, what additional safety precautions would you suggest for pilots' food on future flights?

15-2 Would you regard Prohibition, under which the manufacture and sale of alcoholic beverages was forbidden by law, as an approach to prevention of disease on the individual or societal level? What do you suppose its effects were on the mortality rates from cirrhosis of the liver?

15-3 The free thyroxin index (FTI) is said to be an excellent screening test for thyroid dysfunction (both hypothyroidism and hyperthyroidism), with sensitivity and specificity each over 99 percent. Assume that both are exactly 99 percent and that the prevalence of thyroid dysfunction in a population of 1000 persons is 1 percent. Set up a fourfold table, like Table 15-3, to show the results of the screening test in this population. How many false negatives are there? How many false positives? What is the predictive value of a positive test?

15-4 Describe four types of bias that can occur in evaluations of screening that are not randomized controlled trials.

BIBLIOGRAPHY

Anderson GW, Arnstein MG, Lester MR: *Communicable Disease Control: A Volume for the Public Health Worker,* 4th ed. (New York: Macmillan, 1962), chap. 10.

Benenson AS (ed.): *Control of Communicable Diseases in Man,* 15th ed. (Washington: American Public Health Association, 1990).

Clarke EA, Anderson TW: Does screening by "Pap" smears help prevent cervical cancer? A case-control study. *Lancet* 2:1–4 (1979).

Cochrane AL, Holland WW: Validation of screening procedures. *Br Med Bull* **27**:3–8 (1971).

Farquhar JW, Fortmann SP, Flora JA, Taylor CB, Haskell WL, Williams

PT, Maccoby N, Wood PD: Effects of communitywide education on cardiovascular disease risk factors: The Stanford Five-City Project. *JAMA* **264**:359–365 (1990).

Finney DJ: The design and logic of a monitor of drug use. *J Chron Dis* **18**:77–98 (1965).

Friedman GD, Collen MF, Harris LE, Van Brunt EE, Davis LS: Experience in monitoring drug reactions in outpatients: The Kaiser-Permanente Drug Monitoring System. *JAMA* **217**:567–572 (1971).

Goldsmith JR: Statistical problems and strategies in environmental epidemiology, *Proceedings of the Sixth Berkeley Symposium on Mathematical Statistics and Probability,* vol. VI, *Effects of Pollution on Health* (Berkeley: University of California Press, 1972), pp. 1–28.

Gross FH, Inman WHW (eds.): *Drug Monitoring* (New York: Academic Press, 1977).

Hook EB: Monitoring human defects, methods and strategies, *Proceedings of the Sixth Berkeley Symposium on Mathematical Statistics and Probability,* vol. VI, *Effects of Pollution on Health* (Berkeley: University of California Press, 1972), pp. 355–366.

Jensen RL, Lewis HG, Yinger HV, Jr, Failing FW, Foley JM, Young MM, Smith L, Hutcheson RH, Jr: Staphylococcal foodborne disease— Tennessee. Centers for Disease Control. *Morb Mortal Wkly Rep* **22**:141 (1973).

Jick H: The discovery of drug-induced illness. *N Engl J Med* **296**:481–485 (1977).

Jick H, Vessey MP: Case-control studies in the evaluation of drug-induced illness. *Am J Epidemiol* **107**:1–7 (1978).

Jick H, Miettinen OS, Shapiro S, Lewis GP, Siskind V, Slone D: Comprehensive drug surveillance. *JAMA* **213**:1455–1460 (1970).

Lloyd JW: Long-term mortality study of steelworkers: V. Respiratory cancer in coke plant workers. *J Occup Med* **13**:53–68 (1971).

Mausner JS, Kramer S: *Mausner & Bahn Epidemiology: An Introductory Text,* 2d ed. (Philadelphia: Saunders, 1984), pp. 287–299.

McKeown T: Validation of screening procedures, in *Screening in Medicine: Reviewing the Evidence: A Collection of Essays* (London: Oxford University Press, 1968), pp. 1–13.

McKeown T, Knox EG: The framework required for validation of prescriptive screening, in *Screening in Medicine: Reviewing the Evidence: A Collection of Essays* (London: Oxford University Press, 1968), pp. 159–173.

McKeown T, Lowe CR: *An Introduction to Social Medicine* (Philadelphia: Davis, 1966), pp. 86–87.

Miller AB, Baines CJ, To T, Wall C: Canadian National Breast Screening Study, parts I–II. *Can Med Assoc J* **147:**1459–1488 (1992).

Morrison AS: *Screening in Chronic Disease,* 2d ed. (New York: Oxford University Press, 1992).

Park RM, Silverstein MA, Green MA, Mirer FE: Brain cancer mortality at a manufacturer of aerospace electromechanical systems. *Am J Ind Med* **17:**537–552 (1990).

Perry CL, Kelder SH, Murray DM, Klepp K-I: Community-wide smoking prevention: Long-term outcomes of the Minnesota Heart Health Program and the Class of 1989 study. *Am J Public Health* **82:**1210–1216 (1992).

Pott P: Cancer scroti, *Chirurgical Observations* (London: Hawes, Clark and Collings, 1775). Reproduced in W Winkelstein, Jr, FE French, JM Lane (eds.), *Basic Readings in Epidemiology,* 2d and 3d eds. (New York: MSS Educational Publishing, 1970 and 1972).

Report of the International Conference on Adverse Reactions Reporting Systems, National Academy of Sciences, Washington, 1971.

Salonen JT, Tuomilehto J, Nissinen A, Kaplan GA, Puska P: Contribution of risk factor changes to the decline in coronary incidence during the North Karelia project; A with-in community analysis. *Int J Epidemiol* **18:**595–601 (1989).

Selby JV, Friedman GD, Quesenberry CP, Jr, Weiss NS: A case-control study of screening sigmoidoscopy and mortality from colorectal cancer. *N Engl J Med* **326:**653–657 (1992).

Selikoff IJ, Hammond EC: Multiple risk factors in environmental cancer, in JF Fraumeni, Jr (ed.), *Persons at High Risk of Cancer: An Approach to Cancer Etiology and Control* (New York: Academic Press, 1975), pp. 467–483.

Shapiro S, Slone D: Case-control surveillance, in FH Gross, WHW Inman (eds.), *Drug Monitoring* (New York: Academic Press, 1977), pp. 33–48.

Shapiro S, Venet W, Strax P, Venet L: *Periodic Screening for Breast Cancer. The Health Insurance Plan Project, 1963–1986, and Its Sequelae* (Baltimore: Johns Hopkins University Press, 1988).

Strom BL (ed.): *Pharmacoepidemiology* (New York: Churchill Livingstone, 1989).

Terris M: Relation of economic status to tuberculosis mortality by age and sex. *Am J Public Health,* **38:**1061–1070 (1948).

Thorner RM, Remein QR: *Principles and Procedures in the Evaluation of Screening for Disease.* U.S. Department of Health, Education, and Welfare, Public Health Monograph 67, 1961.

Thun MJ: Measuring occupational effects: How could we do it better? *Epidemiology* **2:**5–7 (1991).

Venning CR: Identification of adverse reactions to new drugs, parts I–IV. *Br Med J* **268:**199–202, 289–292, 458–460, 544–547 (1983).

White KL, Williams TF, Greenberg BG: The ecology of medical care. *N Engl J Med* **265:**885–892 (1961).

Whittenberger JL: The physical and chemical environment, in DW Clark, B MacMahon (eds.), *Preventive and Community Medicine,* 2d ed. (Boston: Little, Brown, 1981), pp. 481–494.

Wilson JMG: The evaluation of the worth of early disease detection. *J R Coll Gen Pract* (Suppl.), **2:**48–57 (November 1968).

Winkelstein W, Jr: Epidemiological considerations underlying the allocation of health and disease care resources. *Int J Epidemiol* **1:**69–74 (1972).

Chapter 16

Quick Review

This chapter offers a brief listing of the main points and principles found in the main text. Its purpose is to aid the reader in reviewing the contents of this book and in preparing for examinations.

Chapter 1   Introduction to Epidemiology

Epidemiology is the study of disease occurrence in human populations.

Epidemiology focuses on groups rather than individuals.

Traditional epidemiology is concerned with the causes of disease development in populations. Clinical epidemiology, at least in part, is concerned with factors affecting the outcome of illness in groups of patients.

Epidemiology, which approaches disease at the population level, is at least equal to other medical sciences in its ability to determine the causation of disease.

Each disease has multiple interrelated causes, usually viewed as a web of causation, but sometimes conveniently placed into the categories: agent, environment, and host.

Disease names reflect arbitrary and transitory ways of classifying ill people. Some are descriptive and some relate to causal factors.

Chapter 2   Basic Measurements in Epidemiology

Measures of the occurrence of disease in groups are frequently proportions, and many of these proportions, particularly but not exclusively those with time in the denominator, are called rates.

The most important of these measures to remember are:

(Point) Prevalence: Proportion of group with a disease at one point in time

Instantaneous incidence: New cases of a disease per number of persons per unit of time, idealized to an instantaneous rate of change

Person-time incidence: New cases of a disease per person-time. This is equivalent to instantaneous incidence

Cumulative incidence: Proportion of group at risk who develop a disease in a specified period of time

Mortality rate: May consist of either form of incidence with death rather than disease onset as the event of interest

Other rates with special features include period prevalence, case fatality, proportional mortality, and maternal mortality rates.

One important way to compare rates is in terms of their difference, often called attributable risk. When this difference is specified in relation to an exposed group or to a total population, it is called attributable fraction.

Another important way to compare rates is in terms of their ratio, often called rate ratio, risk ratio, relative risk, morbidity ratio, or mortality ratio. When standardized for another characteristic, they are so labeled, e.g., standardized morbidity ratio (SMR).

Measures that lie on a quantitative scale are also used frequently. These can be described by their distribution, mean, standard deviation, and range. Quantiles, such as quartiles or percentiles, divide groups into equal parts along a quantitative scale. The median separates the upper half from the lower half of the group.

Chapter 3   Observations Used in Epidemiology

Data inevitably contain some errors.

Validity, one measure of data quality, indicates how closely the observations correspond to reality.

Reliability, another measure of data quality, indicates how closely observations of exactly the same thing match one another.

Reliable data may be invalid. The mean of several unreliable measurements may have high validity.

Commonly used measures of reliability include the coefficient of variation for quantitative measurements and Cohen's kappa for qualitative measurements.

In addition to lack of validity or reliability due to measurement errors, data vary because of differences among subgroups, differences among individuals, and differences within individuals.

Another source of variability in data is sampling variation due to chance. This can be assessed by confidence intervals, or p values. The larger the number of people studied, the less the sampling variation.

Clinical observations, including those of trained specialists such as radiologists and pathologists, are quite prone to error.

Clinical diagnoses can also be quite unreliable and invalid. Specific criteria should be used in determining the presence or absence of a disease for a study.

Organized recording of diagnoses, as by abstraction of medical records or legally required reporting of diseases and deaths, is affected by inaccuracies in diagnosis as well as by inherent problems.

Other important sources of epidemiologic data—questionnaires and laboratory tests—also suffer from error to varying degrees.

Studying large groups of people can help overcome some of these errors. Relationships can be discerned in data that contain errors that clinicians find intolerable in individual patient care.

Nondifferential misclassification generally results in the reduction in the apparent strength of an association.

Differential misclassification, i.e., affecting one subgroup more than another, can change the apparent strength of associations in either direction.

Chapter 4   Basic Methods of Study

Much of science involves the study of relationships between one or more independent variables and a dependent variable.

In observational studies these relationships are observed as they occur naturally. In experiments the investigator actively introduces or changes an independent variable, keeps the others constant, and observes the effect on the dependent variable.

Because of the difficulties in conducting experimental studies on humans, most epidemiologic studies are observational, and control of extraneous variables is usually accomplished through data analysis.

Observational studies consist of descriptive and analytic studies. Although the distinction is not always clear, descriptive studies try to describe the occurrence of a disease, while analytic studies try to determine its causes.

There are three types of observational epidemiologic study designs: cross-sectional, case-control, and cohort studies.

Cross-sectional, or prevalence, studies examine the relationships between diseases and other characteristics or variables of interest as they exist in a population at one point in time.

Case-control studies compare persons with a disease (cases) with a sample of persons without the disease (controls) with respect to the proportion with, or level of, the other characteristic(s) of interest.

Cohort or incidence studies measure attributes in a population free of the disease and relate them to the subsequent development of the disease in the population as it is followed up over time.

Prospective and retrospective are terms that are sometimes used incorrectly as synonyms for cohort and case-control, respectively. Actually, they refer to the timing of the recording of data in relation to when a study begins. In a prospective study, be it cohort or case-control, the planned collection of data occurs after the study is started. A retrospective study uses data that were recorded beforehand.

Chapter 5   Descriptive Studies

Descriptive epidemiologic studies show patterns of disease occurrence in populations as related, generally, to personal characteristics (person), place, and time.

Descriptive data assist in making diagnoses, planning health care resources, and suggesting hypotheses regarding causal factors.

Personal characteristics commonly related to disease occurrence include age, sex, race, marital status, and socioeconomic status.

Tabulations of the relationship of age to disease occurrence can be current or cross-sectional, i.e., at one point in time, or cohort, i.e., following a population as it ages through time. Changes in cohort age trends may reveal past changes in exposure to etiologic factors. Calculations of life expectancy are usually cross-sectional, that is, based on the assumption that current mortality rates at each age will apply to persons born now, as they age.

Differences between females and males in disease occurrence often reflect environmental factors as well as hormonal and other physiologic differences between the sexes. Similarly, racial differences may be caused by constitutional or environmental factors.

Many diseases show a socioeconomic gradient. Generally the higher classes do better, but for some diseases the opposite is true.

Disease occurrence can vary widely from place to place. When a group that migrates from a lower-incidence to a higher-incidence area, or vice versa, shows a disease incidence that is closer to that of long-term inhabitants in the new location, this suggests that one or more environmental factors that changed as a result of the move plays a role in causing the disease.

Climate, sun exposure, and living conditions may play a role in the north-south gradient in the occurrence of some diseases. Place-to-place variations may involve much smaller areas such as parts of a city or of a building.

Short-term changes in disease occurrence are usually measured in hours, days, weeks, or months. Long-term changes taking many years are called secular changes.

An epidemic is the occurrence of a disease clearly in excess of the prevalence or incidence usually seen in the population of concern. The magnitude and time course of an epidemic are related to the means of introduction and spread of the disease in the afflicted population and the proportion of the population that is susceptible.

When most of a population are immune to a particular infection, the remaining susceptible individuals may be sufficiently protected from exposure to benefit from so-called herd immunity.

Examples of recurrent or periodic time trends include seasonal variation and weekly patterns.

Chapter 6   Cross-sectional Studies

Sampling for cross-sectional and other types of studies involves selection of a representative fraction of a study population. Commonly used samples include simple random and stratified random samples, cluster samples, and systematic samples. Multistage sampling may combine different types of samples.

The usual way to tabulate the data in a cross-sectional study is to subdivide the population according to the suspected predisposing factors being studied and compare the disease prevalence rates in each subgroup.

Factors related to existing or prevalent disease may not correspond to factors causing disease to develop. Prevalent cases tend to overrepresent cases of longer duration; correlates of prevalence may be correlates of disease duration rather than disease development. Prevalent cases may differ from incident cases in other ways, too.

Care is required in judging whether a factor associated with disease prevalence truly preceded the disease, as is required for a factor to be causal.

Under stable conditions a disease's prevalence usually equals its incidence times its mean duration.

Repeated cross-sectional surveys can be used to assess time trends.

A cross-sectional study can be used to begin a cohort study. The population at risk, i.e., free of the disease under study, is determined, and the baseline characteristics to be related to subsequent disease development are measured.

Chapter 7   Case-Control Studies

Cases may be identified from a variety of sources. Diagnostic criteria should be specified and described. If possible, in a study to identify factors leading to disease development, incident cases should be used to avoid the possible unrepresentative nature of prevalent cases.

Control selection is often difficult. When possible, controls should be selected from the population from which the cases emerged. They should be persons who would have been cases had they developed the disease of interest. When population-based controls are not available, other controls may be used, but ways in which they might differ from the source population should be considered.

Controls should be similar to cases with respect to the availability and quality of information they can supply about the causal and other factors being studied.

Controls may be selected to be matched to the cases for some characteristics that improve comparability. Overmatching, which may make studies less efficient or may tend to conceal real case-control differences, should be avoided.

Matching may be performed as individual or frequency matching. When the number of cases is limited, more than one control can be selected per case to increase statistical reliability, but little is gained by having more than five or six controls per case.

Every effort should be made not to let the subjects' status as cases or controls influence the collection of information about them.

Incidence or absolute risk cannot be determined directly from a case-control study. The usual objective is to measure relative risk. Attributable fraction in either the exposed or the total population can also be determined.

In case-control studies relative risk is usually estimated by the odds ratio, although when a study is suitably designed, the instantaneous rate ratio or cumulative incidence ratio may be directly measured.

The odds is the number of subjects exposed to a factor divided by the number not exposed. The odds ratio is the odds in cases divided by the odds in controls, which simplifies to exposed cases times unexposed controls, all divided by unexposed cases times exposed controls. In studies of matched case-control pairs, the odds ratio is simply the number of pairs in which *only* the case is exposed divided by the number of pairs in which *only* the control is exposed.

When controls are selected to be matched to cases, a matched-pair or matched-group data analysis should be performed.

The case-control study is usually the least expensive and most readily performed type of investigation. It may be the only feasible approach to the study of a rare disease.

Case-control studies may be nested within cohort studies. These usually require the collection of additional data not available for the entire cohort.

Chapter 8   Cohort Studies

Initially a study population or cohort to be followed up is defined. In a prospective cohort study, this cohort is characterized at the start of the study and followed up into the future. In a retrospective or historical cohort study, a cohort characterized in the past is followed up toward the present.

No one may be added to a closed cohort once the cohort is defined at the start of follow-up. In contrast, new members may join an open cohort.

A cohort study focuses on factors related to the development of disease. Incidence rates are readily determined among all or among subgroups of the cohort. These rates may be compared between, say, those exposed and those not exposed to a suspected causal factor. Or, if the entire cohort has been exposed, as in an occupational group, it may be contrasted to the general population or other suitable comparison group.

An initial examination of a cohort may be used to assess exposures and other relevant characteristics and to identify and exclude individuals who already have the disease(s) being studied.

The length of follow-up required depends on the number of new cases of the disease needed to yield statistically significant results. It also depends on the duration of the induction period between exposure to a causal factor and the onset of manifest disease.

Comparisons may be made either of cumulative or of person-year incidence rates. Study subjects may contribute person-years of observation to more than one subgroup as their age or other characteristics change.

Follow-up of each subject continues until the end of the study or until he or she is lost to observation. The investigator should consider whether losses of subjects to follow-up occur in a way that could bias the study. When the disease of interest develops in a subject, he or she stops contributing person-years of follow-up to the population at risk.

Decisions about the development of the disease under study should not be influenced by knowledge about possible causative factors.

Prospective cohort studies may entail considerable time and expense, especially if the study population must be brought in for repeated examinations. Retrospective cohort studies can often be conducted quickly and inexpensively if the necessary data have already been collected and are readily accessible.

In contrast to case-control studies, cohort studies permit the study of several disease outcomes in relation to the exposures or characteristics of interest.

Chapter 9   Experimental Studies

Experiments, in which the investigator intervenes rather than merely observes, are thought to be the best test of a cause-and-effect relationship.

Experimental epidemiology is concerned primarily with testing the efficacy of measures to prevent disease.

A properly conducted experiment requires that, when the intervention or treatment is applied to one group, there be a control group or some other suitable standard against which the results of the treatment can be compared.

Ethics require that experiments be conducted only when there is considerable uncertainty about which of the alternatives is superior. Failure to carry out controlled experiments when they are necessary and feasible may also be unethical. Subjects of experiments or their guardians must give informed consent.

It is usually preferable to conduct randomized experiments in which only chance determines to which of one or more interventions (often including nonintervention) a subject is assigned. Randomization helps to equalize the treated and control groups with respect to both known and unknown factors that might affect the results. It also permits the application of standard statistical tests to determine whether chance could have produced the observed outcome.

If randomization is not feasible, possible nonrandom standards of comparison include persons selected to be similar to the treated group, a community similar to a whole treated community, similar persons treated differently in the past (historical controls), and before-after comparisons of the treated group.

The definitive comparison in an experiment is between the complete groups as assigned—either randomly or otherwise—an *intention-to-treat* analysis. Because of the special characteristics of cooperators, comparisons involving only those actually treated can be misleading and should be done with caution.

To the extent possible, the subjects, the therapists, and those who evaluate the results should be kept blind as to the assignment of each subject.

The number of subjects in an experiment should be large enough to yield statistically reliable results, but not larger than necessary so that both the number of persons receiving the inferior intervention and costs will be kept to a minimum. One way to strike this balance is by sequential analysis. With this method, the findings for each pair of subjects, one treated and one control, are added to the results until a conclusion with the desired precision can be drawn.

Chapter 10   Clinical Studies of Disease Outcome

Epidemiologic methods and measurements can be applied to groups of patients as well as to populations. The purpose is to improve outcomes of disease by learning what treatments or other factors cause or predict various outcomes. These studies are sometimes referred to as clinical epidemiology.

Studies of the natural history of disease are analogous to descriptive studies in epidemiology.

Analytic studies aimed at identifying factors affecting prognosis or outcome of disease can employ cross-sectional, case-control, or cohort designs.

Cohort studies are often more feasible in the clinical setting than in the population because the outcomes of interest are apt to occur with greater incidence, that is, more rapidly and in a greater proportion of the subjects studied.

The clinical or therapeutic trial is an experiment carried out on patients in the clinical setting. Random and blind assignment to alternative treatments and blind assessment of the results are greatly preferable whenever feasible.

In clinical studies, rates of development of unwanted outcomes including death are often measured in terms of survival, that is, the proportion of the study group remaining free of the outcome as time passes. This can be depicted graphically as a survival curve.

Appropriate methods such as life tables should be used to analyze survival. These make use of data on all subjects including those who are observed for only a portion of the entire duration examined.

When comparing groups with respect to survival, it is necessary that the same starting point is used for each group.

As the preferences of patients have come to play a greater role in decisions about therapy, survival measurements can be adjusted for quality of life. In forming quality-adjusted life years (QALYs) a year of life with illness or disability is valued at some fraction of a year of healthy life.

Chapter 11   Making Sense Out of Statistical Associations

The fact that there is an association between two variables or between a characteristic and a disease may be expressed in a number of ways. Most commonly one finds contrasts between rates or proportions; for example, the incidence of a disease may be higher in a group with, than without, a certain environmental exposure. Or two variables may be correlated to the degree expressed by their correlation coefficient.

In contrast to the ordinary, or Pearsonian, correlation, which measures how much linear relationship one quantitative variable has to another, the intraclass correlation reflects the degree of agreement between two quantitative variables within specified categories.

Ecological correlations between variables that are properties of groups may not accurately reflect the corresponding correlation,

if any, that exists at the individual level. F
to demonstrate the association of a causa
comparing populations when there is co
the factor within individuals.

When a statistical association is found
main questions that arise are:

> Could this be due to chance?
> Could this be due to bias?
> Could this be due to confounding?
> To whom does this apply?
> Does the association represent a cause-and-effect relationship?

The possible role of chance in producing the observed association (or lack thereof) is evaluated by statistical significance tests or
confidence intervals. In general, the more subjects a study has, the
smaller the role that chance can play.

Bias is of two main types. Selection bias occurs when study
subjects are selected in a way that can misleadingly increase or
decrease the magnitude of an association. Information bias results
when the method of data collection makes the information obtained from two or more groups differ in some misleading way.
The possibilities for either type of bias must receive careful attention in designing a study.

Confounding, which some regard as a form of bias, implies that
the apparent relationship between two variables is increased or
decreased because of their relationship to some other variable(s).

Confounding can be combatted by prevention, as by selecting
study groups to match for the confounding variable, and in data
analysis. Analytic methods include specification—looking at the
association in specific subgroups or strata of the confounding
variable—and adjustment of the findings to account or control for
differences between groups.

Adjustment of rates can be either direct or indirect. Although
either method usually proves satisfactory, direct adjustment is less
likely to distort comparisons while indirect adjustment is less subject
to variability resulting from very small numbers in certain strata.

Adjusted relative risks include (directly) standardized rate ra-

directly) standardized morbidity or mortality ratios, and tel-Haenszel relative risk estimates. Adjustment by multi-ariate analysis is discussed in the next chapter.

Some variables, related to both of the variables whose association is of primary concern, are not confounding and should not be controlled. An example is a variable that lies along the causal pathway between the independent and the dependent variable or is otherwise a consequence of the independent variable.

Two variables may show interaction in their association with a third variable. This means that the association of one of them with the third variable differs according to the level of the other.

The applicability or generalizability of an association is an important issue. If it exists in one group because the study that showed it has internal validity, does it apply to other groups of concern or to the general population? That is, does it have external validity? Deciding this is often a matter of judgment.

Judging whether a statistical association found in an observational study involves cause-and-effect can be difficult. Criteria that are often used include the strength of the association, the proper time sequence between cause and effect, consistency with other knowledge, and failure to find other explanations. Other criteria that are useful, with limitations, include a gradient of risk or dose-response relationship, consistency in several studies, and specificity.

Associations between diseases, if not due to Berkson's (selection) bias may be helpful in determining etiology or in forming a clinician's diagnostic suspicion.

Chance, bias, and confounding can conceal associations as well as produce or exaggerate them. For evidence that there is no association to be convincing, a study must have adequate statistical power to detect the degree of association that is of interest. Otherwise the association's apparent absence may be due to chance. Another way to add assurance that an association is absent is to show that the confidence interval around its measure (e.g., relative risk = 1.0) is narrow.

Chapter 12   Introduction to Multivariate Analysis

The simplest approach to controlling for more than one confounding variable is to subdivide the study group into strata according to the categories or levels of each of the confounders and then apply standard adjustment methods. If one were controlling for age, sex, and race, for example, one such stratum might be black women, age 50 to 54 years.

Multiple subdivisions often result in strata that have zero or very few subjects, which, respectively, are uninformative or yield very imprecise information.

Multivariate analytic methods can provide an accurate view of the relationships between possible causal factors and disease, while adjusting simultaneously for several confounding variables and smoothing out the irregularities and uncertainties that small or nonexistent strata introduce into stratified analysis or ordinary adjustment procedures.

Most multivariate analyses involve regression, i.e., a relationship expressed as the dependent variable, y, being equal to some function of the independent variables, the x's.

Multiple linear regression is usually used to describe a linear relationship between the x's and a continuous dependent variable, y, expressed as $y = a + b_1x_1 + b_2x_2 + b_3x_3 +$ and so on. The b (or beta) coefficients indicate how strongly their respective x's relate to y—how much y changes for each unit change in x.

For dichotomous outcomes such as presence or absence of a disease, multiple logistic regression analysis is often used. It expresses the odds of disease versus no disease as a function of the independent x variables such that log odds $= a + b_1x_1 + b_2x_2 + b_3x_3 +$ and so on. Exponentiating each b (that is, taking e^b) yields an odds ratio, which indicates how much the odds of having or developing the disease increases with each unit change in the corresponding x.

In addition to estimating the strength of the association of each independent variable with the outcome variable, while controlling for all the others, multivariate equations allow one to estimate the overall risk of a particular individual by substituting his or her values for the x's.

To take into account different lengths of follow-up for the subjects of a cohort study or experiment, the Cox proportional hazards model may be used. The outcome variable is the instantaneous incidence rate which is a function of time, t, as well as the independent, x, variables. The equation is log rate $= a(t) + b_1x_1 +$

$b_2x_2 + b_3x_3 +$ and so on. As each new case occurs during follow-up, that person is compared to all others still free of the disease at that time.

Other aspects of multivariate analysis that are briefly introduced include stepwise regression analysis, conditional regression analyses including those of matched subjects, assessment of interaction, indicator variables, correlated variables, standardized regression coefficients, log-linear models, Poisson regression, and R^2.

Multivariate analysis should supplement, and not replace, the inspection and analysis of a study's basic data in simple tables.

Chapter 13 How to Carry Out a Study

A study's objectives or questions to be answered should be specific, and, if possible, stated in quantitative terms.

An early step is to review the relevant literature. Often it is surprising how little is known about the study questions.

A written protocol is essential. It serves to clearly spell out ideas and procedures, to obtain consultation and approval, and to document methods so that they can be applied consistently.

Although funding agencies often require more elaborate write-ups, essential components of any protocol are objectives, background and significance, methods for selecting subjects and for collecting and analyzing data, plans for safeguarding human subjects, time schedule, and budget with justification if financial support is sought.

Inexperienced investigators should seek consultation with experts including investigators and clinicians familiar with the areas of study and with epidemiologists or biostatisticians who can help with study design, data analysis methods, and sample size.

The study plan should then be presented to others whose approval or cooperation is needed.

Data must be collected in a consistent, organized manner, usually on prepared standard forms. For recording qualitative variables, it is helpful to specify in advance as many categories within them as possible, still allowing for the unexpected and unknown. Quantitative variables should be recorded in original form to allow maximum flexibility in creating categories during analysis.

Pretesting of data collection is essential since unanticipated problems almost always occur.

Data collection requires close supervision. Duplication of collection on at least a sample aids in quality control. If changes in procedures are required, they should be added to the protocol.

Collected data need to be checked and edited, before and/or after entry, to correct or allow for the inevitable errors. Data entry into computer storage should be verified by reentry.

Data analysis is accomplished by sorting, counting, and calculating, and may be accomplished by hand, supplemented by electronic calculator as needed, or by micro- or mainframe computer, depending on the volume of data and the complexity of the analysis.

It is easier to write portions of the final scientific report or paper as soon as the necessary information becomes available. The investigator should strive to communicate the study effectively, whether writing a paper for publication or making an oral presentation; this requires clarity, simplicity, and brevity of expression.

The lead investigator, or some other conscientious member of the team, must check all details carefully throughout the investigative process.

Chapter 14   Epidemiology and Patient Care

Knowledge of the prevalence of diseases in one's community and of other descriptive epidemiologic findings assists in diagnosing a patient's illness.

Just as epidemiologic methods may be used to associate a disease with causal or predictive factors, they may also be used to study associations between a disease and the symptoms, signs, or laboratory test findings. Sometimes the findings of these studies contradict long-held beliefs about the symptoms a disease may cause.

The concept of *normal* values of tests or measurements can be confusing because normal can be interpreted as healthy or desirable on one hand, or frequent or usual on the other. These two meanings do not always coincide.

The best way to determine normal values for a test is to examine the distribution of results in persons who do and do not have the condition being tested for. Select a cutoff point in the area where the distributions overlap which results in the sensitivity and specificity that best serve the purposes of the test.

Sensitivity of a test is the proportion of true positives that it labels as positive. Specificity is the proportion of true negatives that it labels as negative. Changing a cutoff point to increase sensitivity reduces specificity and vice versa.

The ability of a test to distinguish true positives from true negatives and how the cutoff point affects the test results is conveniently depicted by a receiver operating characteristic (ROC) curve.

The physician's desire to have a clear cutoff point between abnormal and normal (indicating intervention versus no intervention) can be frustrated by measures that reveal graded abnormality or graded risk of future disease with increasing (or decreasing) levels of the test result.

Factors that elevate one's risk of developing common serious diseases in the future can often be readily detected in the clinical setting, and preventive intervention there can be effective.

In reading the medical literature critically, some important considerations are the need for an adequate control group or basis of comparison in asserting benefit or harm; the requirement of denominators in statements comparing risks; selection and information bias; spurious correlations (or lack thereof) due to uncontrolled confounding; the need to distinguish statistical from biological or clinical significance; the need for comparable starting times in follow-up studies of survival or other outcomes; the need for description of a study sufficient to permit evaluation and replication; evidence of the investigator's objectivity; and the likelihood that publication bias will favor the dissemination of positive, as compared to negative, findings.

Chapter 15   Epidemiology, Medical Care, and the Health of the Community

Although epidemiologists in industrialized countries are tending to focus more on the causes of chronic noninfectious diseases, infectious diseases continue to be major public health problems in all nations.

An investigation of the causes of an epidemic of an infectious disease typically starts with studying the cases to verify the diagnosis and determine other relevant characteristics such as disease onset times and common experiences and exposures. Cases and noncases are then compared with respect to suspicious factors, or attack rates can be determined for both the exposed and non-exposed. Strong and plausible associations with the disease suggest that factors are causal.

Suspicions about environmental factors causing illness have led not only to *ad hoc* studies but to ongoing monitoring programs to detect and evaluate environmental hazards. Monitoring includes systems for spontaneous reporting of suspicious events, noting changes in disease frequency, and linking information about exposures and disease occurrence.

Occupational epidemiology makes frequent use of proportional mortality studies and retrospective cohort studies, each of which may present problems in interpretation. Increased proportional mortality due to a particular cause of death may be caused by a relative deficiency of other causes. Difficulties frequently encountered in retrospective occupational cohort studies include poor measurements of the workers' specific exposures of concern, lack of data on important confounding variables, and less-than-ideal comparison groups.

Medical care is only one among many factors that determines the health of a population, and for many diseases its importance is less than is commonly believed.

Prevention of disease may be approached either through care of individual patients or by large-scale social or environmental changes.

Much disease in the community never comes to the attention of health care providers, and that which does is often unrepresentative of the full spectrum in the population.

Screening involves the application of relatively simple and inexpensive tests to distinguish those who probably have a disease from those who probably do not have it. It is generally applied to asymptomatic people in an effort to detect disease early when treatment should be more effective. Problems frequently encountered include lack of adequate follow-up, failure of the recommended treatment to improve health or longevity, and unnecessary anxiety provoked by labeling.

Pitfalls in the evaluation of screening include self-selection of those with either a better or worse prognosis to be screened; lead-time bias, whereby making an earlier diagnosis seems to, but actually does not, prolong life; length bias, whereby screening preferentially detects cases with more slowly progressive disease; and overdiagnosis or inclusion in the screen-detected cases of some who do not really have the disease. The best way to overcome these problems is to evaluate screening procedures by randomized controlled trials. Observational studies of screening, whether cohort or case-control, may also be informative, but they must take these biases into account.

Supplementing the measures, sensitivity and specificity, of screening or other tests, is the positive predictive value, which is the proportion of those who test positive who prove to be truly positive. If the positive predictive value is low, positive tests will lead to many negative workups, which can be costly and discouraging to patients and physicians alike. The lower the disease prevalence, the lower the positive predictive value. Negative predictive value is the proportion of true negatives among those who test negative.

Screening can be directed at high risk of a disease as well as at the disease itself.

Health services research or medical care research is related to epidemiology and requires the same careful application of measurement and judgment.

Chapter 17

Answers to Problems

CHAPTER 1

Problem 1-1

a B   **b** C   **c** A   *d* C   **e** B   **f** A

Problem 1-2

Environmental factors: social pressures, industrial society, cigarette smoking.
Host factors: hereditary factors, obesity, personality, lack of exercise.

Some of these factors are difficult to assign to either the environment or the
host category. For example, obesity and personality seem to be host characteristics, but both are affected by environmental factors and, in the case of obesity, by
the agent, too.

If this web of causation is reasonably accurate, regular exercise would help
prevent myocardial infarction by improving myocardial collateral circulation,
decreasing catecholamine levels, and decreasing obesity. Obesity is in turn associated with diabetes, hyperlipidemia, and hypertension. This can be seen by following the arrows leading from "lack of exercise."

Problem 1-3

a Manifestation—appearance
b Manifestation—gross and microscopic pathological findings
c Manifestation—symptoms (wheezing and difficulty breathing)
d Cause—the organism, leptospira
e Cause and manifestation (pathologic)

329

CHAPTER 2

Problem 2-1

  a In January 1976, the prevalence was 8/1000, or 0.008. In January 1978, the prevalence was 13/999, or 0.013. Note that the person who died of myxedema heart disease was no longer in either the numerator or the denominator in 1978.

  b The annual incidence was 6 new cases per 992 persons at risk in a 2-year period = 0.003, or 3 cases per 1000 per year.

  c The 2-year-period prevalence was 14/1000, or 0.014.

  d For the cases detected in 1976, the case fatality rate was 1/8, or 0.125. No follow-up information is given concerning mortality of the cases detected in 1978.

  e The proportion of newly detected cases was 7/14, or 0.5.

  f For part *a*, the prevalence in January 1978 would now be 13/900, or 0.014. For part *b*, the denominator population at risk dropped from 992 to 900 over the 2 years and would be approximated by the midpoint between the two values, or 946. The annual incidence would now be 6 per 946 cases in a 2-year period, or 0.003 (changed from the previous answer in the fourth decimal place—from 0.0030 to 0.0032). For part *c*, the denominator population would be 950, a midpoint estimate between 1000 and 900. The 2-year-period prevalence would now be 14/950, or 0.015. The other answers would be unaffected.

Problem 2-2

  a The incidence of hearing loss was 40 cases per 100 in a 4-year period in the nonwearers and 16 cases per 400 in the wearers or, on an annual basis, 0.1 in the nonwearers and 0.01 in the wearers. The attributable risk was 0.1 − 0.01 = 0.09, or 9 cases per 100 per year.

  b The attributable fraction in the nonwearers was 0.09/0.1 = 0.9. That is, nine-tenths of the cases of hearing loss were attributable to the nonwearing of earplugs.

  c The attributable fraction in all the workers was (0.028 − 0.01)/0.028 = 0.64. (The annual incidence in all workers was calculated thus: 56 cases/500 workers/4 years = 0.028.)

  d The relative risk was 0.1/0.01 = 10.

Problem 2-3

The answers are provided in Table 17-1 and Fig. 17-1. Note that in drawing the histogram, the extreme left bar is twice as wide and the extreme right bar is 3 times as wide as the other bars. The respective bar heights are therefore scaled

Table 17-1

Serum uric acid, mg/100 mL	Distribution		Cumulative distribution	
	Number	**Percent**	**Number**	**Percent**
1.0–2.9	29	0.8	29	0.8
3.0–3.9	214	6.2	243	7.0
4.0–4.9	720	20.8	963	27.8
5.0–5.9	1107	31.9	2070	59.7
6.0–6.9	842	24.3	2912	84.0
7.0–7.9	368	10.6	3280	94.6
8.0–8.9	133	3.8	3413	98.4
9.0–11.9	56	1.6	3469	100.0
Total	3469	100.0		

down to one-half and one-third of the percent as shown on the ordinate to make the areas of the wide bars proportional to the areas of the other bars.

Problem 2-4

Mean: 12.0 patients
Standard deviation: 4.3 patients
Median: 13 patients (halfway between the sixth and seventh highest numbers)
Range: from 3 to 18, or 15 patients
Interquartile range: from 9 to 15, or 6 patients

CHAPTER 3

Problem 3-1

a Device B.
b Device A.
c Device A, since you are more interested in the *trend* than the absolute level.
d Device B. Device A will consistently miss many persons with counts in the high 3000s.
e Device B, being more valid, will give the more accurate mean.
f Device A, being more reliable, will more often be correct in ranking individuals.

Problem 3-2

Merely flipping a coin 20 times on two occasions would lead to assigning 50 percent to each category about 3 times in 100. In order to evaluate the validity and reliability of their murmur assessment, we need to know the students' find-

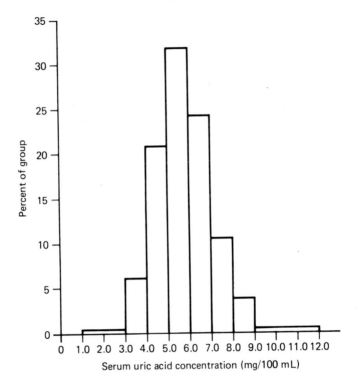

Figure 17-1　Histogram showing percent distribution of uric acid levels among a group of cigarette smokers (answer to Problem 2-3).

ings for *each* patient. A student's readings would be invalid if the wrong 50 percent were chosen as systolic or diastolic, and they would be unreliable if a different 50 percent were chosen each time.

Problem 3-3

The probability is less than 1 in 100 that the difference could have been due merely to chance sampling variation.

Problem 3-4

The major potential sources of error in the study data included errors and inconsistencies in diagnosis by individual physicians, differences among the physicians in the clinic as to diagnostic criteria for each condition, difficulties in reading and interpreting physicians' notes in charts, and intra- and inter-abstractor differences in information derived and recorded from a chart. If these errors and differences were not equally frequent in the data for the two groups being compared (persons with and without stroke), the study could have been biased. Bias could also be introduced if the abstractors were aware of the hypotheses under study and could distinguish the patients with stroke from those without. Fortunately, there were some additional, more objective, sources of information about cardiac status, such as the chest x-ray to determine heart size and the electrocardiogram. However, even these are subject to errors and inconsistencies in measurement and interpretation.

Problem 3-5

The underlying cause of death would be recorded accurately for a larger proportion of 45-year-olds. In elderly persons there are more often multiple diseases present at the time of death, making it difficult to select the primary cause accurately. Also, if an elderly patient is quite senile, there is often less effort made to arrive at an accurate diagnosis.

Problem 3-6

a Some persons consuming moderate or large amounts of alcohol are apt to underreport their intake.
b This bias by itself could not produce the reported association. Suppose that those with higher and lower alcohol consumption (referred to now as the high-alcohol and low-alcohol group) actually had the same average blood pressure. The underreporting of alcohol consumption would misclassify some who belong in the high-alcohol group into the low-alcohol group, but the average blood pressure of the two groups would be unchanged and, therefore, still equal. If the reported association between alcohol consumption and blood pressure did exist, then misclassification of some high-alcohol consumers into the low-alcohol group would raise the average blood pressure of the low group, making it closer to that of the high group. Thus, given the misclassification that probably occurred, the results of the study were conservative; the difference in average blood pressure between the groups was actually greater than was apparent in the data. The study results could have been produced by the underreporting of alcohol consumption only if the underreporting occurred more often in persons with lower blood pressures, and there is no reason to believe that this was the case.

Problem 3-7

Actual agreement was—*positive:* $10\% \times 50\% = 5\%$; *negative:* $90\% \times 95\% = 85.5\%$; total $= 90.5\%$. The corresponding assortment of the children is shown in

Table 17-2

	Crime		
	+	−	**Total**
Test positive	10(5%)	10(5%)	20(10%)
Test negative	9(4.5%)	171(85.5%)	180(90%)
Total	19(9.5%)	181(90.5%)	200(100%)

Table 17-2. Calculation of chance agreement—*positive:* 10% (test positive) × 9.5% (commit crimes) = 0.95%; *negative:* 90% (test negative) × 90.5% (do not commit crimes) = 81.45%; total = 82.4%.

$$\text{Kappa} = \frac{.905 - .824}{1 - .824} = \frac{.081}{.176} = .46$$

Notice how much lower kappa is than the actual agreement of 90.5 percent. Since such a large proportion of the children tested negative and such a large percentage did not go on to commit crimes, agreement had to be reasonably good just by chance, as noted above.

CHAPTER 4

Problem 4-1

a Prospective, cross-sectional
b Retrospective, cohort
c Retrospective, case-control (either the manic-depressives or the schizophrenics could be considered the control group)
d Prospective, cohort

Problem 4-2

An experiment

Problem 4-3

1a Independent variable: employment status; dependent variable: prevalence of peptic ulcer
1b Independent variable: branch of Armed Forces; dependent variable: mortality rate
1c Independent variable: type of mental illness; dependent variable: proportion with previous behavior problems in school
1d Independent variable: presence or absence of parental permission; dependent variable: incidence of teenage pregnancy

2   Independent variable: movie or lecture; dependent variable: incidence of teenage pregnancy

Problem 4-4

a Descriptive
b The hypothesis that unemployment leads to peptic ulcer

CHAPTER 5

Problem 5-1

a B. The increase in the incidence of lung cancer suggests some hypotheses for further study and may lead to revisions of plans for prevention and treatment programs and facilities, but it is not likely that a physician would be helped in making a diagnosis by knowledge of this long-term time trend.

b C. The shigella epidemic would alert practicing physicians to consider this disease in diagnosing patients with severe diarrheal illnesses; and, if the epidemic is severe, awareness of it may lead to the setting aside of hospital wards for complicated cases. However, the etiology of the disease is already well understood (although the source and means of spread of the epidemic may require investigation).

c B. The black-white difference in hypertension has spurred programs of education and screening directed especially to blacks and has led to several hypotheses for further study, as described on p. 70–71. However, since the condition is frequent and easily diagnosed in either racial group, the black-white difference is of little value in diagnosis.

Problem 5-2

a The mortality rate increases with age. Note that the mortality rate was plotted on a logarithmic scale, so the age trend is much greater than it appears at first glance.

b A cohort.

c Despite some irregularity, there was a general rise in the mortality rate in all age groups as birth year progressed from 1846–1850 to 1896–1900. For succeeding birth-year groups after 1900 there was a general downtrend.

d The cohort born in 1896–1900.

e Since the death rate has continued to increase in persons aged 70 and over and since they account for the majority of cases of prostatic cancer, the overall death rate is still rising.

f No. During or after the 1980s the preponderance of cases will come from cohorts born after 1900, and the overall mortality rate should start to fall.

g Although difficult, a search for experiences or environmental exposures that were most common in the 1896–1900 birth cohort might prove fruitful. For example, the authors have considered exploring the patterns of migration of blacks from the rural Southeast United States to large cities in the North and West, where they found employment in industry.

h In Fig. 5-3 each birth cohort is represented by a different line, and age is shown on the abscissa. In Fig. 5-11 each age is represented by a different line, and each cohort's 5-year time of birth is shown on the abscissa.

Problem 5-3

There is a North-South gradient with higher death rates in the South. This is consistent with the belief that sun exposure is an etiologic factor for melanoma of the skin. Obviously, there must be other factors involved as well, since the geographic gradient is not uniform throughout the United States.

Problem 5-4

a Staphylococcal enterotoxin—most cases occurred about 1½ to 3 hours after breakfast.

b This is probably a point-source epidemic since it started and ended so abruptly. If additional contaminated food had been served later to the unaffected persons, the epidemic would probably have lasted longer. The short duration and probable cause (staphylococcal enterotoxin) of the epidemic also argue against person-to-person spread.

c They may have saved some contaminated food for later consumption or may have had a different illness.

CHAPTER 6

Problem 6-1

a Stratified random sample, in which the classrooms are the strata
b Cluster sample, in which each page contains a cluster of names
c Systematic sample, even though the digits used for selection are randomly chosen
d Simple random sample

Problem 6-2

a The prevalence was 4/100, or 0.04. (Note that the prevalence would be the same at any time during the period if the cases starting before 1983 and after 1986 were also shown.)
b The incidence was 2 cases per 100 over a 1-year period, or 0.02 per year.
c If $P = I\bar{d}$, then $\bar{d} = P/I = 0.04/0.02/\text{year} = 2$ years. This is the same as the mean duration computed directly.

d Four, or 50 percent, of all eight cases were of long duration. In the cross-sectional study three of four, or 75 percent, were long-duration cases. This illustrates the overrepresentation of long-duration cases in cross-sectional studies.

Problem 6-3

Increased survival time is accompanied by an increase in the prevalence of a disease unless there is a compensating decrease in incidence. Prevalence is a poor index of risk, since it is influenced by disease duration. The two nations might have different average durations of the disease due to differences in quality of medical care; patients in the nation with better care would survive longer and, as a result, the disease would be more prevalent. Incidence is the correct measure of risk of disease development.

Problem 6-4

A cross-sectional study can identify a population at risk, free of the disease under study. It can also supply the measurements of charactistics to be related to subsequent incidence of the disease in this population at risk.

CHAPTER 7

Problem 7-1

The estimated relative risk is $(202 \times 110)/(136 \times 238) = 0.7$ for the "two or less" drink group, $(42 \times 110)/(136 \times 46) = 0.7$ for the "three to five" drink group, and $(11 \times 110)/(136 \times 24) = 0.4$ for the "six plus" drink group. Since the risk declined with increasing alcohol consumption, this is a negative association. Note that even if there are several categories (in this case four), instead of just two (as in the "yes-no," or dichotomous, variable), the odds radio method can be used to estimate relative risk. Simply select one category as the standard and construct separate fourfold tables for each of the other categories using the standard, or reference, category for comparison. The relative risk in the standard category itself is, of course, 1.0.

Problem 7-2

Relative odds method: relative risk = $(67 \times 152)/(23 \times 108) = 4.1$.
Matched = pair method: relative risk = $57/13 = 4.4$.

Problem 7-3

Advantages: quick, inexpensive, easy to conduct, only practical approach for rare diseases.
Disadvantages: cases and/or controls often not representative of all persons

with and without the disease; no direct measure of disease prevalence or incidence rate; change in characteristics after disease has developed (e.g., change in diet, loss of weight) or bias in recall (e.g., occupational exposure is remembered more readily by cases than by controls).

Problem 7-4

a Variables that could usefully be matched are age and sex, as these are related to both risk of bladder cancer and amount of coffee consumed. Another characteristic that could be matched is cigarette smoking, since coffee drinking and cigarette smoking are often correlated, and the latter may play a causal role in bladder cancer. It would be impractical and useless to match for coffee strength and added sugar or saccharin, since these could be determined only after presence or absence of coffee drinking, the dependent variable of primary interest, is established; this occurs during data collection *after* the controls are selected. It may be important to study these as additional related factors; if so, they should be included in the inquiry about coffee drinking. In Chaps. 11 and 12 you will learn of ways, other than matching, to "control" for the effects of extraneous variables.

b Since cancer is believed to require years to develop after exposure to carcinogens, you could ask about usual coffee consumption 10 to 20 years before the disease developed or over the subject's lifetime. Also, recent consumption may have been reduced in the cases due to their illness.

c Examination of the pathology report would be well worth the effort since it would confirm the presence of the disease. Also, you should record the histologic type, since each type (for example, transitional cell, squamous cell) may have a different etiology and can be studied separately.

d Some patients should probably be excluded, for example, those admitted for treatment of peptic ulcer disease. Ulcer patients are often advised to avoid coffee. Including them might therefore artificially lower coffee consumption in the control group. If you would like to read about some completed case-control studies of coffee and bladder cancer, see Cole (1971); Fraumeni et al. (1971); Bross and Tidings (1973); and Morgan and Jain (1974).

Problem 7-5

a The letter a in Table 7-1 = $a + b$ in Table 7-2. Similarly, b (Table 7-1) = $c + d$ (Table 7-2); c (Table 7-1) = $a + c$ (Table 7-2); d (Table 7-1) = $b + d$ (Table 7-2).

b One new set of paired data would be : $a = 5$, $b = 15$, $c = 5$, $d = 75$. There are still $15 + 5 = 20$ of 100 cases with the attribute and $5 + 5 = 10$ of 100 controls with the attribute. The relative risk estimate is $15/5 = 3$. Now try starting with $a = 0$, $a = 1$, $a = 3$, and $a = 10$ in the paired data. Note that $a + b$ must always equal 20, $a + c$ must equal 10, and d must be such that the total number of pairs is 100.

CHAPTER 8

Problem 8-1

a Retrospective cohort study

b The general population, which usually includes a greater proportion of disabled and seriously ill persons than does an employed group. Thus, the general population is often an unsatisfactory comparison group for an employed population, since its mortality rate would be expected to be higher. Unfortunately, there are often no available data from more suitable comparison groups.

c Identify smokers and nonsmokers among the tobacco company employees and compare their mortality rates. Unfortunately, employee health records often lack information on smoking and other health-related habits.

d No. Virtually no environmental causal factor for disease is *invariably* associated with the occurrence of the disease, either in exposed individuals or when groups are compared. For example, not every person or group exposed to the herpes simplex virus will develop the characteristic rash on the skin or mucous membranes, yet there is little doubt that the virus is a causal factor.

Problem 8-2

a 60,000 diabetics. Multiply this population size by the annual incidence rate (0.0002, or twice the general population rate of 0.0001) and then by 5 (years of follow-up) to verify that 60 cases of pancreatic cancer will develop. Solving the problem, of course, requires division of 60 by 0.0002 and 5 rather than multiplication.

b 3 million persons, assuming that about 2 percent of this population are diabetic.

c No. A case-control study would be the most practical approach, unless one can obtain information about a very large number of diabetics followed up for a long period of time. (Restricting the study to older persons would reduce the population size required since both the prevalence of diabetes and the incidence of pancreatic cancer would be higher.)

Problem 8-3

a Prospective cohort
b Cross-sectional
c Case-control
d Retrospective cohort
e Cross-sectional, case-control
f Cross-sectional, case-control
g Prospective cohort
h Prospective cohort

    i Cross-sectional, retrospective cohort, prospective cohort
    j None of these types of observational studies (this is discussed further in Chaps. 9 and 11).

Problem 8-4

The main problem is the strong possibility of bias. The investigator has already formed an opinion about the effects of sugar. This may unintentionally influence her findings when she interviews the patients about symptoms since she knows about their previous sugar consumption. Ideally, information about the symptoms should be obtained in a structured interview by another person who is unaware of their sugar consumption or, if this is not possible, by a self-administered questionnaire which can be scored objectively by the investigator. Also worrisome is the fact that the two groups are evaluated in different months. There may be seasonal variations in the symptoms under investigation; for example, increased fatigue may occur around the Christmas–New Year holiday period. The interviews of the two groups should be intermingled during the same time period.

Finally, to reduce misclassification of sugar consumption, it would be advisable to gather additional information at the follow-up examination to learn whether any of the men's sugar intake changed after the initial interview.

Problem 8-5

Members of the three specialty groups were identified for the study by having joined their respective societies. Joining took place after residency training. Thus, the radiologists in the study were not at risk of dying during residency. The study design guaranteed their survival through training, and it is meaningless to consider this period as part of their follow-up time.

CHAPTER 9

Problem 9-1

    a A group receiving the standard dose of penicillin. Use of less than the standard dose or a placebo would be unethical since some patients might not be cured and might develop serious complications, such as rheumatic fever. The addition of a placebo control group to the penicillin control group would be justified only if the efficacy of penicillin were in doubt.

Problem 9-2

    a Randomization should have been performed *after* the subjects had proved to be cooperative by expressing willingness to inject themselves or, better yet, after a trial period in which they actually performed daily injections on themselves.

b Keep the patients blind by having each one receive both injections and tablets. One group would receive an active injection and inert tablet and the other would receive an inert injection and active tablet. The physicians could be kept blind by having another person randomly assign the treatments, which would be identified only by a code number. The code would not be revealed until the evaluations were complete. If the side effects of the two medications were so different that the treating physician might easily guess which one was being used, a different person should measure the blood pressure used for evaluation.

Problem 9-3

a No. There is no way to have some of the town's inhabitants exposed to the effects of the device and others not.
b A before-after comparison seems the best approach to use here. Base-line monitoring of emergency room visits could be done during the year required for installation.
c Other factors affecting the occurrence of hospital visits for asthma attacks may change during the course of the study. For example, many asthmatics may move from the town. Weather conditions may change. A new therapy for asthma might become available and thus diminish the need for emergency room visits. A new doctor, willing to make house calls, may move into the town.
d Comparable towns with similar factories and similar pollution problems should be sought. The occurrence of asthma in the town with the pollution-control device could then be compared to the occurrence of asthma in the towns without the device.

CHAPTER 10

Problem 10-1

a The 5-year survival rate is the proportion of patients in a given population still alive 5 years after follow-up is started.
b It is often measured since, for many cancers, it is believed that survival for 5 years after treatment means that the disease is cured.
c Yes
d About 45 percent
e 0 percent

Problem 10-2

Were the patients at the two hospitals comparable in all factors pertinent to survival, or did the surgeons at hospital B operate on healthier, better-risk patients?

Did both groups start their 1-year follow-up at the same time in the course of treatment or did the surgeons at hospital B start later—for example, after the operation or after discharge?

Were there differences in medical care other than the surgery, such as better postoperative care for patients at hospital B?

Was follow-up for mortality equally thorough for the two groups, or could some deaths among the patients in hospital B have escaped notice?

Problem 10-3

Articles on the natural history of disease are often written by specialists at academic or referral centers. The patients who are sickest or who develop the most complications are most likely to be referred to these specialists for care. This bias in the medical literature has been well described by Motulsky (1978).

CHAPTER 11

Problem 11-1

There was no apparent association. The fracture incidence rate was the same in the two groups. (Three percent in 6 years is the same as an average annual rate of 0.5 percent per year.)

Problem 11-2

No. A correlation coefficient that is close to -1 shows that there is an almost perfect *inverse* relation between the two measurements; that is, when one is higher, the other is lower. For there to be almost no association, the correlation coefficient would have to be close to zero.

Problem 11-3

An ecological correlation is based on groups of groups rather than on groups of individuals. Statements *a*, *b*, and *d* express such correlations (although the term *ecological* is not commonly applied to correlations in time trends, as in *d*;) *c* does not. To avoid the potentially fallacious conclusions that might be inferred from these ecological correlations, the following study questions would make suitable replacements for *a*, *b*, and *d*.

    a Do individuals eating large amounts of beef have a higher incidence of colon cancer than those who do not?

    b Do patients receiving care from interns and residents experience a higher mortality rate than those who do not receive such care?

    d Do black men exposed to microwave ovens have a higher suicide rate than those who are not similarly exposed?

Problem 11-4

a Yes

b The threefold difference was based on very small numbers—three cases versus one case. This would suggest that chance sampling variation might well have played a role here. To check out this possibility, perform the appropriate statistical significance test, for example, the chi-square test with Yates correction. (Some medical-statistics texts are listed in Chap. 11, Bibliography.) It turns out that the observed difference in proportions, 3/10,000 versus 1/10,000, could occur just by chance about 60 percent of the time. A finding so easily attributed to chance should not generally be taken very seriously.

Problem 11-5

a To prevent selection bias. Controls selected elsewhere might differ systematically from the cases.

b To prevent information bias. Anonymity would help ensure more accurate responses.

c Primarily to prevent selection bias. Since some cases were non-English-speaking, such persons should not be systematically excluded from the control group. Being able to communicate with the controls in their own language should also have helped prevent information bias for variables that were obtained by interview, but not for others such as blood alcohol level.

d To control confounding. In data analysis the investigators determined that age was a confounding variable that explained the other case-control differences mentioned.

e To prevent information bias. Note the importance of doing this even though it required the sacrifice of some information about one of the groups.

f To prevent selection bias. This method was equivalent to random selection and should have prevented systematic differences between the groups.

g To prevent confounding. That was the primary purpose of matching the cases to the controls for these potentially confounding characteristics.

h To prevent information bias, which might have occurred if one group was interviewed in the hospital and the other at home.

Problem 11-6

a No, nothing would be gained. You have already prevented age from being a confounding variable by matching the cases and controls for age (year of birth).

b Even though age is not a confounding variable, it may still be valuable to break down your study group into age-specific subgroups. Sometimes an etiologic factor may have more of an effect at one age than at another.

c Since you have not matched for race, it would be best to look first at the data for specific races, that is, Asians, blacks, whites, etc. If there were sufficient numbers of case-control pairs with both members of the same race, you could restrict your analyses to these pairs. Chances are, though, that for a racial group that is infrequent in the community, you will not have enough matched pairs; you will have to compare all cases of that race to all controls of that race. As a result, you may lose the age and sex matching that you had in the entire group. In studying this infrequent racial group, you will then have to look at specific age-sex subgroups or adjust your data for age and sex.

Problem 11-7

a Urban: 0.0500. Calculations: [(0.05 × 100,000) + (0.06 × 150,000) + (0.04 × 150,000)]/400,000. Rural: 0.0538. Calculations: [(0.02 × 100,000) + (0.05 × 150,000) + (0.08 × 150,000)]/400,000. Note that the rates are still similar, but after adjustment for educational level the rural rate is higher than the urban rate, whereas the crude rate was lower in the rural area.

b Applying the state rates to the totals in corresponding urban subgroups, we get the expected numbers of alcoholics: 1280 for the elementary school level, 3829 for high or trade, and 5577 for college. The sum of these expected numbers divided by the total number of men in urban areas is 10,686/ 220,000, or 0.0486. The standard population's overall rate is 0.0475/0.0486, or 0.9774 times this expected rate for urban areas. Therefore, the crude prevalence of 0.0482 in the urban areas is multiplied by 0.9774, yielding 0.0471 for its adjusted rate.

The corresponding calculations for rural areas yield 1920, 4376, and 2028 expected cases, whose sum divided by 180,000 yields an expected rate of 0.0462. The standard population's overall rate is 0.0475/0.0462, or 1.0281 times this expected rate for rural areas. The crude prevalence for rural areas of 0.0467 multiplied by 1.0281 equals 0.0480, the adjusted rate. Note that indirect adjustment, like direct, makes the rural rate (0.0480) slightly higher than the urban rate (0.0471), whereas the opposite was true for the crude rates.

Problem 11-8

a X. A biological link to stomach cancer is more likely for a food eaten than for a car driven.
b Y. Y is more strongly associated with stomach cancer.
c Y. Y more clearly preceded the cancer. A preference for X may be the result of having stomach cancer.
d X. Although Y shows a somewhat stronger relation to stomach cancer in Helsinki, it is not consistently related to it in diverse populations, as is X.

CHAPTER 12

Problem 12-1

The data points tend to be closer to the regression line, and therefore the model fits better for higher body fat levels. This linear regression model appears to fit the data quite well.

Problem 12-2

For men who drink two cups of coffee, one cup of tea, and two alcoholic drinks per day, mean systolic blood pressure would be: $120 + 2(-0.38) + 1(-0.29) + 2(1.08) = 121.11$ mmHg. For men who drink six cups of coffee per day but no tea or alcohol, mean systolic blood pressure would be: $120 + 6(-0.38) + 0(-0.29) + 0(1.08) = 117.72$ mmHg.

Problem 12-3

The odds ratios are as follows:

potato salad: $(88 \times 28)/(12 \times 5) = 41.1$
hamburger: $(89 \times 15)/(37 \times 16) = 2.3$
baked beans: $(76 \times 5)/(23 \times 5) = 3.3$
milk: 0.8 (calculation shown in Problem)

Since e^β equals the odds ratio, the fitted logistic equations correspond to foods as follows:

I. baked beans
II. milk
III. potato salad
IV. hamburger

The odds from the logistic analyses agree beautifully with those seen in the two-by-two tables. Consider III. potato salad, for example:

log odds $y = -1.722767 + 3.715197 \times 1 = 1.992430$

Exponentiating,

odds $y = 7.3$

From the two-by-two table, we can see that the odds of being ill if potato salad was eaten were 88/12, which equals 7.3. Similarly, the odds of being ill if each of the other foods was consumed were: 3.3 by either method for I. baked beans, 1.6 by either method for II. milk, and 2.4 by either method for IV. hamburger.

Problem 12-4

    a Multiple logistic regression analysis. The outcome, death from auto injury, is dichotomous, and follow-up durations are all equal.
    b Cox proportional hazards model, since the follow-up durations now vary.
    c Multiple linear regression analysis, since the dependent variable, weight gain, is continuous.
    d Multiple linear regression analysis, since this independent variable, infant birth weight, is also continuous.
    e Multiple logistic regression analysis, because the outcome, presence or absence of an anomaly, is now dichotomous. The length of follow-up would ordinarily be considered a completed pregnancy, regardless of its duration.
    f Multiple logistic regression analysis. When multivariate analysis is used in a case-control study, the outcome is viewed as the dichotomous variable, presence or absence of disease—here, large-bowel cancer.

CHAPTER 13

Problem 13-1

Only *b*. In *a*, the dependent variable, enhancing human sexuality, is vague and would probably be impossible to define to most scientists' satisfaction. In *c*, the best method of delivering medical care is not a specific concept. There are many possible criteria for evaluating medical care—mortality rates, recovery rates, costs, patient satisfaction, provider satisfaction, etc. Also, even if the criteria for evaluation are spelled out, what proves to be best for one population may not be best for another. Problem 13-1*d* is a specific question, but it is unrealistic to expect that 50 successive patients could be persuaded to give up coffee for a year.

Problem 13-2

The form has at least the following deficiencies. In the first place, no provision is made for identifying each subject. If there is to be more than one interviewer, he or she should also be identified on the form. Next, three digits should be provided for recording weight for the occasional woman who weighs 100 kg or more. Three digits should also be provided for recording height, since the fourth would never be needed; the unneeded space might lead to the erroneous place-ment of a three-digit number, that is, one space to the left of where it should be.

In the microwave entries, the categories of duration of ownership and hours of use per day are too broad. For example, it would be impossible to distinguish a few minutes' daily use or occasional use from 4 hours' daily use. Probably, use by almost all subjects would fall within the 0- to 4-hour category.

A definition of cessation of menses should be provided, either on the form or in an accompanying set of instructions, for example, menstrual periods that have stopped for at least 6 months or 1 year. Similarly, codes should be indicated for the category "don't know" or "information missing."

Some additional deficiencies, more related to subject matter and not necessar-ily familiar to all readers, are as follows: Some women (for example, flight attendants, hospital dietary personnel) use microwave ovens outside their homes; thus the subjects should be asked about occupational and other exposures to microwaves. A question about natural versus surgical menopause should also be included, especially if information is desired about the women's hormonal status. If the menopause was surgical, one would want to ascertain whether just the uterus or both the ovaries and the uterus were removed.

CHAPTER 14

Problem 14-2

One way would be to question all patients coming to a clinic for a routine checkup about the symptom of easy fatigue. (Be sure to do this before the results of their blood tests are known.) Then measure the hemoglobin level of these patients, and determine whether a greater fraction of those who are anemic complained about fatigue. It may well be that fatigue is associated only with severe anemia. Therefore, the patients should be divided into several subgroups according to their hemoglobin levels.

Problem 14-3

One major deficiency is his failure to perform the test on a series of patients with prostatic cancer, particularly of the occult variety. It may be that patients with prostatic cancer generally have values much higher than 67, which would make 67 too low to use as a cutoff point. On the other hand, patients with occult disease, which is the chief target of the test, may not produce enough of the substance to appreciably elevate serum levels, making the test of little value.

Another major problem is his use of young men as the reference group free of disease. Prostatic cancer occurs mainly in men in their sixties and older. This is the age group that would receive the test in practice. Normal values should be determined by testing men in this age group, both those with the disease and those who are evidently free of it.

Problem 14-4

Most of the risk factors can be detected by inquiry about personal and family history. In addition, height and weight should be measured and the breasts examined. To foster early detection of cancer, high-risk women should have frequent regular breast examinations, by both palpation and mammography. Breast self-examination should be taught and encouraged. Low-risk women should also receive these diagnostic procedures but, given limited time and resources, less frequently. (Age-specific recommendations as to frequency of mammography are evolving, and current guidelines should be consulted. Also, because of lack of demonstrated benefit and because of the false-positive findings and anxiety that frequently occur, routine breast self-examination by all women has been questioned.)

Problem 14-5

a The conclusion about susceptibility to disease X is based only on numerator data on hospitalized patients. It may be that the hospital serves a population that is largely of Mediterranean extraction. One would need to compare the rate of disease in Mediterranean and non-Mediterranean groups.

b There is no basis for comparison. It may be that employees who use other toothpastes, or even no toothpaste at all, receive appearance ratings that are just as good.

c The distinction between statistical significance and biological significance needs more emphasis here. The *p* value indicates only statistical significance, that is, that the difference is not due to chance. A difference in mean height of only 1 mm does not seem biologically or clinically significant or, by itself, a matter of concern. There is also a question of cause-and-effect. Perhaps shorter children prefer soft drinks, and this preference is the reason for the difference rather than an effect of the beverages on growth.

d Survival figures from other institutions may be based on follow-up that starts earlier. Those from our institution start from the time of discharge and therefore do not include operative and early postoperative mortality. Other important possibilities for lack of comparability are given in the answer to Problem 10-2.

Problem 14-6

He might very well be objective if he were an honest individual, interested in determining the truth and willing to admit if it turned out that he was wrong. However, there is good reason to have doubts about this investigator. Monetary gain is not the only factor that can affect a person's objectivity. Often someone identifies with an idea or theory he or she has proposed or believes in strongly and, as a result, becomes its advocate and finds it very difficult to accept contrary evidence.

Problem 14-7

Try South Carolina, Washington, Kentucky, Montana, and Wyoming. Equally convincing might be Pennsylvania, Massachusetts, Maine, Connecticut, Delaware, and the District of Columbia. Note that these sets of data points appear to show a negative correlation, in which greater per capita cigarette consumption is associated with lower coronary heart disease mortality.

CHAPTER 15

Problem 15-1

a The attack rates among eaters and noneaters of the foods were, respectively: omelette—56 and 62 percent, ham—58 and 20 percent, yogurt—60 and 48 percent, roll—55 and 68 percent, butter—51 and 76 percent, cheese—52 and 63 percent. Thus, the only large excess rate among eaters as compared to noneaters was for ham, and this difference proved to be statistically significant ($p = 0.023$).
b The pilot and copilot should each be served different foods, cooked by different cooks.

Problem 15-2

Prohibition was clearly a societal approach. In the United States, Prohibition was associated with a markedly reduced death rate from liver cirrhosis, which began a slow rise back to pre-Prohibition levels after repeal in 1933. Terris (1967) correlated the time trends in cirrhosis mortality with alcohol consumption and other population characteristics in the United States and other countries and concluded that governmental fiscal and regulatory measures that reduce alcohol consumption can markedly lower cirrhosis mortality rates. Thus, despite Prohibition's apparent fostering of social problems, such as bootlegging, organized crime, and disrespect for law, this limitation of personal freedom did have the desired effect of reducing alcohol abuse.

Problem 15-3

See the following table. First you should have entered the totals in the bottom row, based on the fact that the disease prevalence is 1 percent; in the population of 1000 there would be 10 with disease. Since the sensitivity is 99 percent, all 10 would likely test positive, and there would be no false negatives. Since the specificity is 99 percent, 99 percent × 990, or 980, would test negative, and 10 would be false positives. There would be a total of 20 positive tests. Since 10 of the 20 are true positives, the predictive value of a positive test is 50 percent.

Screening test	Final diagnosis		Total
	Positive	Negative	
Positive	10	10	20
Negative	0	980	980
Total	10	990	1000

Problem 15-4

Self-selection bias, in which persons who are healthier or who take better care of themselves are more apt to undergo the screening test.

Lead-time bias, in which survival appears to be, but is not actually, lengthened because the screening leads to earlier diagnosis of the disease.

Length bias, in which more slowly progressive disease is preferentially detected in a cross-sectional screening survey.

Overdiagnosis, in which more benign conditions are mistaken for the targeted disease.

BIBLIOGRAPHY

Bross IDJ, Tidings J: Another look at coffee drinking and cancer of the urinary bladder. *Prev Med* **2:**445–451 (1973).

Cole P: Coffee-drinking and cancer of the lower urinary tract. *Lancet* **1:**1335–1337 (1971).

Fraumeni JF, Jr, Scotto J, Dunham L: Coffee drinking and bladder cancer. *Lancet* **2:**1204 (1971).

Morgan RW, Jain MG: Bladder cancer: Smoking, beverages and artificial sweeteners. *Can Med Assoc J* **11:**1067–1070 (1974).

Motulsky AG: Biased ascertainment and the natural history of disease. *N Engl J Med* **298:**1196–1197 (1978).

Terris M: Epidemiology of cirrhosis of the liver: National mortality data. *Am J Public Health* **57:**2076–2088 (1967).

INDEX

Index